The Medical Mycology Handbook

The Medical Mycology Handbook

MARY C. CAMPBELL, B.A.
Microbiologist in Charge, Mycology Section
Division of Clinical Microbiology, Department of Clinical Pathology
University of Oregon Health Sciences Center
Portland, Oregon

JOYCE L. STEWART, B.S.
Medical Technologist
Regional Microbiology Laboratory
Kaiser Permanente Clinic
Portland, Oregon

Foreword by **HOWARD W. LARSH, Ph.D.**
Research Professor of Microbiology
University of Oklahoma

A WILEY MEDICAL PUBLICATION
JOHN WILEY & SONS
New York · Chichester · Brisbane · Toronto

Cover and interior design: Wanda Lubelska
Production editor: Eileen Tommaso
Editorial supervisor: Marilyn Zirke

Library of Congress Cataloging in Publication Data:

Main entry under title:

The Medical mycology handbook.

  (A Wiley medical publication)
  Bibliography: p.
  Includes index.
  1. Fungi, Pathogenic – Identification – Handbooks,
manuals, etc. 2. Mycoses – Diagnosis – Handbooks, manuals,
etc. 3. Medical mycology – Handbooks, manuals, etc.
I. Campbell, Mary C. II. Stewart, Joyce L. [DNLM:
1. Fungi – Handbooks. 2. Mycoses – Handbooks.
3. Mycology – Methods – Handbooks. QY110 M489]
QR245.M42   616'.015   80–11935
ISBN 0–471–04728–7

Printed in the United States of America

10 9 8 7 6 5 4 3 2 1

This book is respectfully dedicated to those who need it the most, **the medical technologists.**

Foreword

Medical mycology is a fascinating aspect of biological study that has been handicapped because of the lack of well-trained laboratory personnel. Nevertheless, fungi were observed and described long before other types of microorganisms. Unfortunately, bacteria proved more exciting to investigators following the monumental works of earlier bacteriologists and virologists. In the early nineteenth century mycology was progressing very well until the Pasteur-Koch era, at which time it was pushed back into the "dark ages." Then, with the publishing of *Les Teignes* by Sabouraud in 1910, the emphasis on mycology was increased. However, the rapid development of virology again led to less activity in mycology. During World War II, with the increased mobility of individuals, infections caused by mycotic organisms began to be recognized more frequently, and many more people were attracted to the specialization of medical mycology. The rapid expansion of laboratory mycology throughout the world resulted in the use of personnel with little or no training in medical mycology.

Because of mycology's history and because the discipline is still expanding but sorely neglected, there is a place for a manual that has evolved from many years of practical experience. The authors have assembled basic concepts necessary to understanding clinical mycology as well as current information. Morphologic, physiologic, and taxonomic principles are presented in a concise and understandable manner. It is apparent that the authors' many years at the bench have been invaluable in their efforts to develop a practical approach to the isolation and identification of mycological agents.

Throughout the handbook the authors have drawn heavily on their personal experiences, providing accurate, to-scale drawings and individual descriptions of pathogenic and contaminating fungi. There are many refreshing innovations that make this handbook an excellent tool for a person new to the field of medical mycology; the book will also be appreciated as a superior review for the established laboratory worker. The *Handbook* has been prepared in a practical and sincere manner, with the objective of making laboratory mycology a precise and informative branch of science as well as that of recruiting motivated and dedicated people to the authors' field of specialization. There is little doubt that, by mastering the procedures, beginning or experienced laboratory workers will find many opportunities to use their training and qualifications. There remains a dire need for highly qualified medical mycology laboratory workers if mycology is to reach the position it so richly deserves within the medical sciences.

Howard W. Larsh, Ph.D.
Research Professor of Microbiology
University of Oklahoma
Norman, Oklahoma

Preface

We face an ever-increasing threat from fungal disease. Normal defenses against fungi have been lowered by long-term therapies such as antibiotic administration, steroid treatment, immunosuppressive drugs used with organ transplants, and cytotoxic drugs used in cancer treatment. Common yeasts and molds that have always seemed harmless are now becoming opportunistic pathogens. This means that workers in clinical microbiology laboratories are asked to identify a bewildering new assortment of fungal isolates, in addition to the few well-known major pathogens.

Those of us who have developed expertise in this field are largely self-trained. Our bible has consisted of medical mycology texts and laboratory manuals. From these books we have developed a good working knowledge of the major pathogenic fungi and several common molds. Now, with so many unusual isolates coming into our laboratories, we are being led to discover other sources. We are learning exciting new ways of looking at the fungi, a new terminology and new nomenclature, and we are beginning to come to grips with fungal taxonomy.

We are expected to train other technologists to do this work, usually in a very few days. These workers cannot be asked to read so much material in a short time. Neither can the work be shortchanged by oversimplifying the field. In response to the needs of the many technologists and other students who come through our laboratories, we have developed a system of training that follows the rhythm of a clinical laboratory while providing basic background information. This handbook has been written as an aid in this training and as a resource for all workers in this field.

Part 1 sets the stage for the working part of the book. Besides the general characteristics of fungi, new systems of taxonomy are described and compared with earlier systems still used in many texts. With the work of Barron as a background, it has been exciting to follow the proceedings of the first Kananaskis conference (The First International Specialists's Workshop Conference on Criteria and Terminology used in the Classification of Fungi Imperfecti). We hope we have made these systems easily available to our readers. A general description of individual fungal diseases is given, with references to the more thorough clinical descriptions (written specifically for physicians) in the basic mycology texts. A quick look at Table 3, which lists medically significant fungi by disease classification, gives some idea of the range of significant organisms that might be isolated in a mycology laboratory.

Part 2 starts by addressing the question "Where do I begin?" Chapter 4 follows the accepted mycologic techniques now in use, from specimen collection to final identification of fungal isolates. It is written for workers new to mycology who are trained in routine bacteriologic techniques. Setting up of media, microscopic preparations of specimens, what to do when something grows, and systems for identification of yeasts, dermatophytes, systemic and opportunistic fungi are described. Many flow charts and tables (with drawings) are included. While the morphologic recognition of a yeast or mold is always a critical factor in making a fungal identification, several differential tests have been developed, particularly for yeast identification. Procedures for all these tests are precisely written for use in a clinical laboratory. Our system contains elaborate safeguards to protect inexperienced workers from possible inhalation of infectious fungal spores and from accidentally discarding a major pathogenic fungus that "doesn't look very important." While only a handful of fungi are normally pathogenic, they are similar in many ways to those that may be routinely isolated as common molds. A mycology technologist needs to be familiar with all of these, and our system takes this into account. Besides the few primary pathogens, the clinical mycologist is aware that we live in a world of opportunistic fungal disease. Any fungal isolate in a clinical laboratory is potentially significant.

Chapter 5 begins with two guides. A general guide (Table 20) to gross characteristics is arranged primarily by color. The guide to microscopic characteristics, with small key drawings (Table 21), is arranged by kinds of spore or conidium production. Individual descriptions of over 100 fungi are easily located by alphabetical arrangement. Most of these descriptions are illustrated with clear line drawings, done to scale by Joyce Stewart, exactly as seen from clinical isolates. Written gross and microscopic descriptions are given and measurements of critical structures are stated in micrometers or millimeters. Several references are given with each description. Brief statements of known pathogenicity and any known serologic tests are given. While the time-honored system of "matching the isolate with the picture in the book" is still the easiest way to begin to make an identification, we are increasingly aware of similarities between major pathogens and many common molds. We are now better able to differentiate these and we are feeling more confident as we learn to use new skills and better tools for observing these fascinating organisms.

In the appendix, which includes formulae for stains, reagents, and media, emphasis is placed on measures for quality control. We find that even in this highly interpretive field, it is possible to develop a program that leads to quality assurance. This program includes the use of clinical material in testing staining reagents and the use of clinical and stock strains of fungi and bacteria for testing media. We believe that our final and most important quality-control measure is a series of review questions for technologists who are assigned to do this work. This kind of review gives confidence to workers on the bench and reassurance to supervisors.

It is our hope that this manual will help to bring the isolation and identification of medically significant fungi within the easy reach of all clinical laboratories. If we have made it possible for mycotic disease to be more easily recognized and diagnosed, we will feel that our time has been well spent.

Mary C. Campbell
Joyce L. Stewart

Acknowledgments

Grateful acknowledgments of those who have encouraged and supported us in this project are in order. We feel privileged that the distinguished medical mycologist, Dr. Howard Larsh, has agreed to write the Foreword. We thank him for his endorsement of our book and for sharing with our readers his own perspective of this field. We also want to mention specifically Dr. Carlyn Halde, who opened many doors; Dr. Michael McGinnis, who responded quickly and generously to questions; and Dr. Richard Thompson who outlined the material that led to the development of Part 1. Dr. Bryce Kendrick has given a helpful criticism of our drawings of conidium ontogeny.

We are fortunate that several experts in medical mycology and related fields have been willing to take time to review some of our material. While we have gratefully accepted most of their suggestions, they are not responsible for any inaccuracies or oversights. Betty Russell has read drafts of all the chapters. In addition, various parts of the material have been reviewed by Mary Bauman, Sharon DeLong, Nancy Gerhardt, Leanor Haley, Abdel Rashad, Greg Raugi, Michael Saubolle, and Annette Youngberg.

We are grateful to the many dermatologists who have studied with us over the years, beginning with Dr. Jacob Swartz at the Massachusetts General Hospital. We particularly want to mention Dr. Leon Ray, who led in the development of a mycology teaching program at the University of Oregon Medical School and who is the senior author of our first published teaching manual, the *Fungus Syllabus*. We are also grateful to our fellow laboratory workers, whose patience, good ideas, and many questions have led to the writing and organization of much of this material.

We also gratefully acknowledge the release given by the Oregon Department of Higher Education for permission to use the laboratory procedures developed by

Mary C. Campbell at the University of Oregon, Health Sciences Center, Department of Clinical Pathology. Thanks go to Dr. Kirtikant Sheth for the use of his photomicrographic camera and to Phoebe Rich and Jim Phillips for photographic help. Jonathon Newman's wise counsel has been invaluable. We have had the excellent help of several typists, including Fran Hawkins, Amy Nutter, Rob Bellin, and Margaret Campbell.

It has been a pleasure to work with Cathy Somer and Andrea Stingelin, our editors, and the production staff at John Wiley & Sons, Inc.

Last, we would like to thank our friends and families for understanding support throughout this project. It will be nice to see more of them again.

M.C.C.
J.L.S.

Contents

The Medical Mycology Handbook

PART I
UNDERSTANDING IT

1. Introduction

BRIEF HISTORY

Fungal invasion of human tissue was recognized in the early 1800s, well before the science of bacteriology was developed. The fascinating and often complex fungal structures could be studied under the microscope with simple magnification, either in human tissue or in laboratory cultures. Even today, with all of the histologic, biochemical, nutritional, and serologic tests available to us, the identification of a pathogenic fungus is often made by recognition of characteristic structures seen in culture using a low-power objective of the microscope.

As pathogenic fungi were recognized by early physicians, they were described in the literature and given names, many of which were based on the clinical, not the cultural, characteristics. Often the same fungus would be given a new name each time it was isolated in a new clinical setting. This led to a tremendously complicated nomenclature, which is now, happily, becoming unraveled. We owe a great debt of gratitude to the dedicated workers who have been studying and redescribing these organisms and classifying them in agreement with the classification of fungi in general. The laboratory identification of pathogenic fungi is much simpler today than it was 50 years ago.

GENERAL CHARACTERISTICS

Morphologic Features (Yeasts and Molds)

The fungi seen in a medical laboratory are referred to either as *yeasts* or *molds.* These are descriptive, not formal, taxonomic terms. Characteristically, the yeasts have moist-to-waxy colonies in culture, with a predominance of budding cells (3 to 5 μm in diameter). The molds have leathery-to-velvety, powdery, granular, or cottony colonies. These mold colonies are made up of hyphae (tubular cells 2 to 20 μm in diameter), which grow by elongation at the tips or by lateral branching, forming a tangled mass of mycelium. Many kinds of spores and spore production are seen in the molds.

The word *dimorphic* means *two forms.* Five of the major systemic pathogenic fungi are described as dimorphic. Four of the major systemic pathogenic fungi grow as molds in culture at room temperature, as yeasts in culture at 37°C, and also as yeasts in tissue. These are *Blastomyces dermatitidis, Histoplasma capsulatum, Paracoccidioides brasiliensis,* and *Sporothrix schenckii.* A fifth major pathogen, *Coccidioides immitis,* grows as a mold in culture both at room temperature and at 37°C. It grows in a spherule form in tissue and, under special conditions, in culture, at 37° to 40°C. A *spherule* is a structure, bounded by a membrane, in which spores are produced. At maturity, when spores are completely formed, it is called a *sporangium.* Many other fungi are found to have different forms under different conditions. A good example of this is the yeast *Candida albicans,* which can produce either a yeast or a hyphal form, depending on available nutrients and other factors, whether in culture or in tissue. Other fungi have a yeast form in early culture growth and develop a hyphal form as they mature. We want to emphasize that, while it is necessary to demonstrate dimorphism in order to identify some of the major pathogens, dimorphism is not limited to these organisms.

A vexing feature of many of the fungi seen in a medical laboratory is their ability to mutate. On repeated subcultures, characteristic spores will be lost, and only sterile hyphae will remain. The word *pleomorphic* has been used to describe such cultures. They would be more accurately described simply as sterile mutants.

Growth Requirements

Generally speaking, all fungi need a protein source and a carbohydrate source. Sabouraud's dextrose agar, the standard medium for support of yeast and mold growth, contains only dextrose and peptone as nutritional sources. Many common molds and yeasts grow well on fruits, vegetables, grains, breads, and meats. The formation of enzymes that break down complex organic substances causes changes recognized as decay. Some fungi are able to grow better in soil composed of decaying vegetable debris. This kind of material is the source of most pathogenic fungi, many of which prefer specific kinds of organic debris. *Histoplasma capsulatum,* for example, is found most often in association with the excreta of chickens, bats, or starlings. Some fungi may, under special conditions, colonize areas of human tissue, but their growth requirements are better met in the soil where animal excreta or animal or vegetable debris are found. On the other hand, *Candida albicans* is isolated primarily as a parasite on a human host. Different fungi have different nutritional requirements, some of which may be used as an aid in their identification. The ability of yeasts to use combinations of carbohydrates unique to each species provides major criteria for yeast identification.

The fungi are able to tolerate a wide range of pH; many of them can grow in media that have a pH of anywhere from 2.0 to 10.0. Although they prefer a neutral pH, the ability of some fungi to grow under such conditions is useful in developing selective media that inhibit the growth of bacteria and allow the growth of the fungi.

Moisture is necessary for the growth of molds and yeasts. Moist cellars and damp camping gear are two examples of places where molds may be expected to grow. When the cellar or the camping gear dries out, the spores will survive, but the mold will not grow unless moisture is supplied again.

The yeasts and molds prefer moderate temperatures, but the ability of molds to grow on leftover food in the refrigerator demonstrates the fact that they can also grow at lower temperatures. All the fungi isolated routinely in a medical laboratory grow well at room temperature. Some grow well or better at 37°C. *Aspergillus fumigatus* can tolerate temperatures as high as 56°C. Some, as already described, will produce a mold form at room temperature and a yeast form at 35° to 37°C. Some will not grow at all at 35° to 37°C. Generally speaking, a fungus that is able to grow at body temperatures (35° to 37°C) has a greater chance of invading deep human tissue than one that is inhibited at these temperatures.

Reproduction

ASEXUAL (VEGETATIVE) REPRODUCTION

Fungi will grow and reproduce indefinitely so long as a proper food supply is available. The *thallus,* the name given to the main body of the fungus, extends either by repeated budding of yeast cells, by elongated budding of pseudohyphae, or by continued elongation and branching of the true hyphae. Pseudohyphae are distinguished by constrictions between each cell, resulting from the budding process. The appearance has been likened to a chain of sausages. (The pseudohyphae and budding cells of *Saccharomyces cerevisiae* are shown in Fig. 1). True hyphae are recognized by the lack of constrictions. In septate hyphae (which are 2 to 8 μm across) straight cross walls are laid down and branching occurs (Fig. 2). In the much wider aseptate hyphae (which are 5 to 15 μm across), branching and "cleavage lines" may occur, but true cross walls are absent (Fig. 3). As the culture ma-

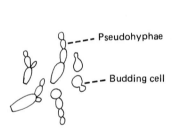

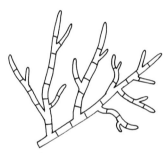

Figure 1. Pseudohyphae and
budding cells.

Figure 2. Septate hyphae.

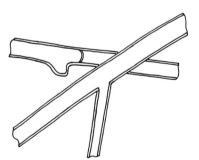

Figure 3. Aseptate hyphae.

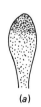
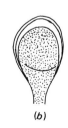
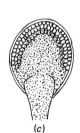
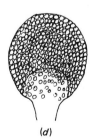
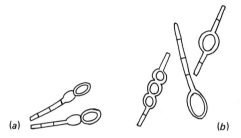

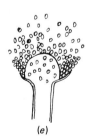

Figure 4. Chlamydospores: (*a*) terminal;   **Figure 5.** Germ
(*b*) intercalary and terminal.   tubes.

tures, large double-walled resting spores (chlamydospores) may be formed (Fig. 4). These spores may appear within the hypha (intercalary, Fig. 4*b*) or in chains, or they may develop at the tip of a hypha (terminal, Fig. 4*a*). The spores may survive for a long time in unfavorable conditions or they may develop into a new organism when the conditions are again more favorable. Fungi will also produce a large variety of vegetative spores, unique to each species. These spores may disseminate widely, being easily blown about in the wind or tossed into refuse piles. When good growth conditions exist, the spores will produce germ tubes (Fig. 5), and a new organism may be formed. These vegetative spores and the way in which they are produced are the basis of the classification of most of the fungi isolated in a medical laboratory.

Endospores (sporangiospores) are spores produced within a sporangium. Figure 6 is a diagrammatic drawing of the development of a sporangium (*d*) in *Rhizopus* sp. The endospores are produced by a separation or cleavage (*c* and *d*) of the cytoplasm (*b*) within the sporangium which develops from the swollen tip (*a*) of the spore-bearing (sporogenous) hypha (sporangiophore). Often the central part of the cytoplasm remains as an entity (*e*) and this is called a *columella*.

Figure 6. Endospore production.

Figure 7. Exogenous spores.

Exogenous spores (conidia) are born on specialized spore-bearing (conidiogenous) hyphae (conidiophores) or directly on undifferentiated hyphae or hyphal projections. Figure 7 is a diagrammatic drawing of the conidia of *Petriellidium boydii.*

SEXUAL REPRODUCTION

Sexual reproduction may occur in the fungi with fertilization taking place after the union of two fungal elements. The nuclei fuse, and meiosis and reassortment of chromosomes occurs. Walls are then laid down and spores are formed. Four basic types of sexual spores are recognized: oospores, zygospores, ascospores, and basidiospores. The four major taxonomic subdivisions of the fungi are based on these types of spores (Table 2, Chap. 2).

Oospores are produced in organisms of the taxonomic subdivision Mastigomycotina. A large, smooth-walled cell called an oogonium is fertilized by a thin tubular cell called an antheridium. The antheridium may be formed on the same branch as the oogonium or it may originate from an entirely separate hypha. After fertilization, oospores develop within the oogonium. Figure 8 illustrates oospore production in *Pythium debaryanum.*

Zygospores are produced in the subdivision Zygomycotina. Fertilization takes place following the union of two specialized hyphal tips (gametangia), often born on the same structure. Figure 9 illustrates zygospore development in *R. stolonifer.*

The production of asci and ascospores, shown in Figure 10, occurs in the Ascomycotina. An antheridium (*a*) fertilizes the ascogonium (*b*). The fertilized ascogonium (*c*) develops short septate hyphae, each septation containing two nuclei, one male and one female. These septated cells crook over, forming "crozier hooks" (*d*) and (*e*). Each hook divides into three cells, the base one containing one nucleus, the central one containing two nuclei, and the terminal one containing one nucleus (*f*). The two nuclei in the central cell form a union and the cell begins to enlarge (*g*). These nuclei divide to form eight nuclei (*h*). Walls are laid down around each

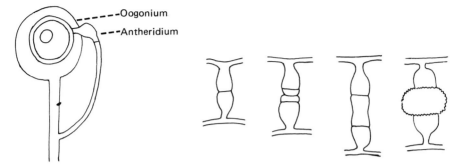

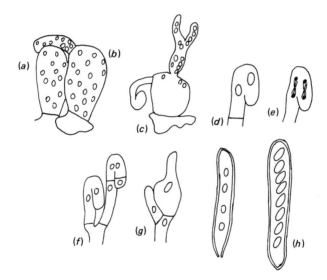

Figure 8. Oospore production (from Alexopoulus, p. 156).

Figure 9. Zygospore production (from Alexopoulus, p. 196).

Figure 10. Ascospore production.

nucleus, separating each into one of eight spores contained in a central cell that is now called an ascus.

Basidiospores are produced in fungi of the subdivision Basidiomycotina, as shown in Figure 11. The basidiospores (*a*) are formed by the uniting of as many as four mating strains. Often, in the fertilized hyphae and at the region of nuclear division, a clamp connection (*b*) will be seen. Very few medically significant fungi

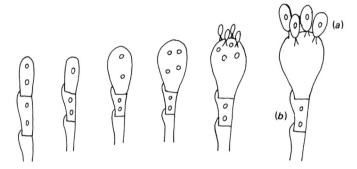

Figure 11. Basidiospore production (from Alexopoulus, p. 433).

are known to produce basidiospores. The major pathogenic yeast, *Cryptococcus neoformans,* has recently been demonstrated to belong in its sexual state to the Basidiomycotina and in this form is known as *Filobasidiella neoformans* (Kwon-Chung, 1975).

BIBLIOGRAPHY

Alexopoulos CJ: *Introductory Mycology,* ed 2. New York: John Wiley & Sons Inc, 1962.

Emmons CW, Binford CH, Utz JP, Kwon-Chung KJ: *Medical Mycology,* ed 3. Philadelphia: Lea and Febiger, 1977.

Kwon-Chung KJ: Description of a new genus, *Filobasidiella,* the perfect state of *Cryptococcus neoformans. Mycologia* 67:1197, 1975.

Rippon JW: *Medical Mycology.* Philadelphia: WB Saunders Co, 1974.

Wilson JW, Plunkett OA: *The Fungous Diseases of Man.* Berkeley: University of California Press, 1974.

2. Taxonomy

PLACE OF FUNGI IN THE BIOLOGICAL WORLD

The relationship of fungi to bacteria, to plants, and to animals has been studied and understood in new ways in recent years. Because the structures seen in fungi correspond to stems, branches, roots, and seeds of plants, it was natural for early workers to classify them as primitive plants. Now that the cell structure and physiology of these organisms are better understood, modern taxonomists are placing the fungi, along with the bacteria and the algae, in a separate group, the protists. The protists are subdivided into the prokaryotes and the eukaryotes, mainly on the basis of the degree of development of their cellular organization. The bacteria and the blue-green algae are classified as prokaryotic protists. The more advanced protozoa, slime molds, fungi, and algae are eukaryotic protists.

The fungi are eukaryotic protists without chlorophyll. As shown in Table 1, they are placed quite separately from the plants and are more closely related to animals. They have true nuclei, which contain several chromosomes confined in a nuclear membrane. This is one of several properties that separate the fungi from the prokaryotic protists, which do not have nuclear membranes or other membrane-bound organelles.

Table 1
RELATIONSHIPS OF BIOLOGICAL GROUPS

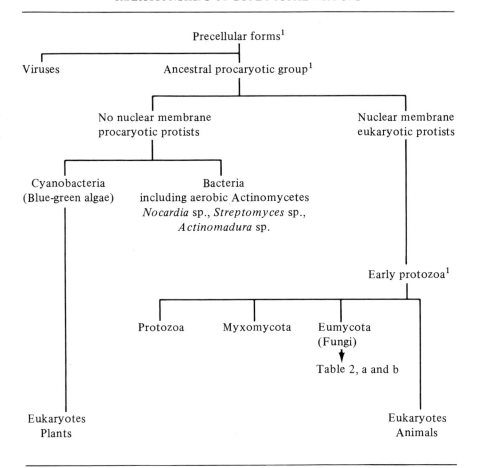

Precellular forms[1]

Viruses   Ancestral procaryotic group[1]

No nuclear membrane   Nuclear membrane
procaryotic protists   eukaryotic protists

Cyanobacteria   Bacteria
(Blue-green algae)   including aerobic Actinomycetes
Nocardia sp., *Streptomyces* sp.,
Actinomadura sp.

Early protozoa[1]

Protozoa   Myxomycota   Eumycota
(Fungi)
↓
Table 2, a and b

Eukaryotes   Eukaryotes
Plants   Animals

[1] Postulated, now extinct.
References:
Joklik and Willett (eds), p. 12.
Davis, Dulbecco, Eisen, et al., p. 14

PLACE OF THE ACTINOMYCETALES
IN THE BIOLOGICAL WORLD

The Actinomycetales (which include *Nocardia, Streptomyces, Actinomadura,* and *Actinomyces* species) were originally thought to be fungi, but are now classified with the bacteria, as Schizomycetes. They are superficially similar to fungi in many ways, producing filamentous branching cells, sometimes forming spores on aerial branches, and producing lesions in human tissue similar to lesions caused by true fungi.

The inclusion of the Actinomycetales in the prokaryotes with the bacteria, rather than in the eukaryotes with the fungi, is determined by their lack of a nuclear membrane and by the composition of their cell walls. The Actinomycetales are not inhibited by antifungal drugs, but they are susceptible to antibacterial antibiotics. They are closer in size to bacteria than to fungi, and some are partially acid fast. An excellent description of the properties of the two groups, the prokaryotes and the eukaryotes, is given by Stanier in *The Microbial World* (1970).

SUBDIVISIONS AND CLASSES OF THE FUNGI (EUMYCOTA)

The fungi are placed in the taxonomic division called the Eumycota (Table 2A and B). The organization of fungal species within this division has undergone many changes and is still not entirely settled. Ainsworth et al., in *The Fungi* (volumes IVA and IVB), have divided the Eumycota into four subdivisions, ranging from aquatic motile saprophytes through the terrestrial yeasts and molds to the mushrooms. These subdivisions are the Mastigomycotina, the Zygomycotina, the Ascomycotina, and the Basidiomycotina. The placing of a fungus in one of these subdivisions is determined by its sexual spore. A form division called the Fungi Imperfecti (or Deuteromycotina) has been established to accommodate those fungi that do not have a sexual form. Most of the medically significant fungi are in this form division.

Table 2
TAXONOMIC PLACE OF MEDICALLY SIGNIFICANT FUNGI
EUMYCOTA

A. Perfect Fungi (Sexual Forms Present)			
Subdivision	Classes	Orders	Genera and Species
Mastigomycotina Sexual cells: Oospores Motile cells	Chytridiomycetes Hyphochytridiomycetes Oomycetes		*Rhinosporidium seeberii*?
Zygomycotina Sexual cells: Zygospores	Zygomycetes	Mucorales	*Absidia* sp. *Mucor* sp. *Rhizopus* sp. *Syncephalastrum* sp. *Mortierella* sp. *Cunninghamella* sp. *Circinella* sp.
		Entomophthorales	*Basidiobolus* sp. *Entomophthora* sp.
	Other classes		
Ascomycotina Sexual cells: Ascospores	Hemiascomycetes (yeasts with free asci)		*Saccharomyces* sp. *Endomyces* sp. *Hansenula* sp. *Pichia* sp. *Lodderomyces* sp. *Kluyveromyces* sp.
	Plectomycetes (asci in gymnocarp)		*Anthroderma* sp. *Nannizzia* sp.
	(asci in cleisto- thecium)		Perfect forms of: *Aspergillus* sp. *Penicillium* sp.
	Pyrenomycetes (asci in perithecium)		*Chaetomium* sp. *Petriellidium* sp.
	Other classes		Morels and truffles
Basidiomycotina Sexual cells: Basidiospores	Teliomycetes (no basidiocarp)		*Filobasidiella neoformans*
	Other classes (basidiocarps)		Mushrooms

Table 2
TAXONOMIC PLACE OF MEDICALLY SIGNIFICANT FUNGI
EUMYCOTA

B. Imperfect Fungi (Sexual Forms Absent)		
Form Subdivision	Classes	Genera and Species
Fungi Imperfecti (Deuteromycotina)	Coelomycetes (conidia in pycnidium or acervulus)	*Phoma* sp.
Sexual cells: Absent	Blastomycetes (budding cells)	*Candida* sp. *Cryptococcus* sp. *Rhodotorula* sp. *Torulopsis* sp. *Trichosporon* sp.
	Hyphomycetes[1] (mycelium well developed with conidia absent or borne on conidiophores, or directly on hyphae)	*Acremonium* sp. *Alternaria* sp. *Arthrinium* sp. *Aspergillus* sp. *Aureobasidium* sp. *Beauveria* sp. *Blastomyces dermatitidis* *Botrytis* sp. *Chrysosporium* sp. *Cladosporium* sp. *Coccidioides immitis* *Curvularia* sp. *Doratomyces* sp. *Drechslera* sp. *Epicoccum* sp. *Epidermophyton floccosum* *Exophiala* sp. *Fonsecaea pedrosoi* *Fusarium* sp. *Geotrichum* sp. *Gliocladium* sp. *Helminthosporium* sp. *Histoplasma capsulatum* *Madurella* sp. *Microsporum* sp. *Neurospora* sp. *Nigrospora* sp. *Paracoccidioides brasiliensis* *Paecilomyces* sp. *Penicillium* sp. *Phialophora* sp. *Scopulariopsis* sp. *Scytalidium* sp. *Sepedonium* sp. *Sporothrix schenckii* *Torula* sp. *Trichoderma* sp. *Trichophyton* sp. *Trichothecium* sp. *Verticillium* sp. *Wangiella dermatitidis*

[1] Most medically significant fungi are in this class.

Reference:
Ainsworth, Sparrow, and Sussman IV A, IV B.

The four subdivisions and the Fungi Imperfecti are further divided into classes (Table 2A and B). The Mastigomycotina do not contain medically significant fungi, with the possible exception of *Rhinosporidium seeberi,* which is thought to belong to the class Chytridiomycetes (Emmons et al., p. 256). The Zygomycotina are characterized by the production of zygospores. In this division is the class Zygomycete in which are placed several medically significant fungi. The Zygomycetes are further divided into the Mucorales and the Entomophthorales, on the basis of asexual structures. In the Mucorales, which include the opportunistic pathogens *Rhizopus, Mucor,* and *Absidia* species, sporangia containing one or more, or many sporangiospores (endospores) are produced. The hyphae are *coenocytic,* containing many nuclei and few septae. In the Entomophthorales, conidia are produced at the end of hyphal tips and are ejected into the surrounding area. *Basidiobolus* species and *Entomophthora* species, which may be agents of fungal disease, are placed in this group.

The subdivision Ascomycotina, which is divided into six classes, is characterized by the presence of ascospores contained in an ascus. The asci may be free or may be enclosed within a structure called an *ascocarp.* Three classes of the Ascomycotina contain medically significant fungi. The Hemiascomycetes contain the perfect (i.e., sexual) form of many of the yeasts. The asci containing ascospores occur individually. These are not contained within an ascocarp. Figure 12 illustrates the ascospores and asci of *S. cerevisiae.* In the Plectomycetes, the asci and ascospores of medically significant fungi are contained within either a gymnothecium or a cleistothecium. A gymnothecium is a loose mesh of hyphae through which the asci and ascospores are easily sifted. These are seen in the perfect form of the dermatophytes (fungi that cause skin disease), *Nannizzia* species and *Arthroderma*

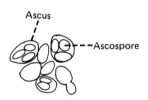

Figure 12. Asci and ascospores.

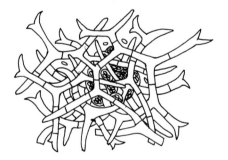

Figure 13. Gymnothecium (from Swatek, p. 414).

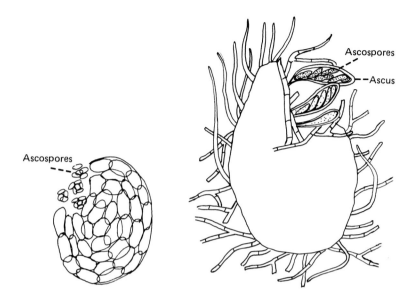

Figure 14. Cleistothecium.   **Figure 15.** Perithecium.

species. Figure 13 is a diagrammatic drawing of a gymnothecium. Cleistothecia or closed ascocarps containing asci and ascospores are seen in a medical laboratory in the perfect form of some of the common molds of the *Aspergillus* and *Penicillium* species. Figure 14 illustrates a cleistothecium seen in *A. glaucus*. In the Pyrenomycetes, the asci and ascospores are generally seen in an ascocarp called a perithecium. A perithecium has an opening at one end through which asci may be released. These are seen in *P. boydii* (which may be an agent in fungal disease) and in *Chaetomium* species, which is more often encountered as a laboratory contaminant. Figure 15 shows a perithecium found in a laboratory contaminant. The three other classes of the Ascomycotina do not contain medically significant fungi.

In the Basidiomycotina, basidiospores are produced. The Basidiomycotina are divided into three classes. In two of the classes the basidiospores are borne on basidiocarps, as in the mushrooms. Occasionally, in unique cases, one of these may be isolated as a human pathogen. In the third class, the Teliomycetes, the basidiospores are borne on a probasidium. (See Fig. 16.) The one major pathogen of the Basidiomycotina, *Filobasidiella neoformans,* is placed here. This is a yeast, known in its imperfect form as *Cryptococcus neoformans,* that causes systemic fungal disease.

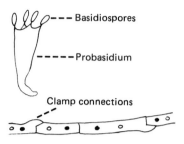

Figure 16. Basidiospores and
clamp connection.

FUNGI IMPERFECTI (DEUTEROMYCOTINA)

In the absence of a sexual stage, fungi that produce only vegetative spores (conidia), or no spores, are artificially placed within the Fungi Imperfecti. Several classification systems of the fungi within this form division have been devised; none is entirely satisfactory. Major proposed systems are those of Saccardo (1886), Vuillemin (1911), Barron [1968, following Hughes (1953) and Tubaki (1963)], Kendrick (1971, report of Kananaskis conference), and Kendrick and Carmichael (1973).

Saccardo's System

This system, first proposed by Saccardo in 1886, is based to a great extent on the color of hyphae and spores, and on the appearance of fungi in nature. Saccardo divided the Fungi Imperfecti into four groups: the Sphaeropsidales, the Melanconiales, the Mycelia Sterilia, and the Moniliales (or Hyphomycetes). The Sphaeropsidales are those fungi in which the conidia and conidiophores are borne within a saclike structure called a pycnidium. (See Fig. 17.) A pycnidium, bearing free conidia, is similar in appearance to a perithecium containing asci and ascospores. This group contains the common mold *Phoma* sp. Ainsworth includes these in a new class, the Coelomycetes. The Melanconiales of Saccardo's system are fungi in

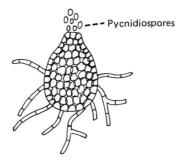

Figure 17. Pycnidium.

which the conidia and conidiophores rise from a saucer-shaped mass of hyphae known as an acervulus. This structure is seen embedded in plant tissues and is rarely seen in laboratory cultures. Because it is often difficult, even for experts, to agree on the presence or absence of an acervulus, Barron includes the fungi formerly placed here within the Hyphomycetes. Ainsworth places the fungi with acervuli along with those that bear pycnidia in the Coelomycetes. Mycelia Sterila are those fungi in which no spore form is produced. Most workers, including Barron, now include this group with the Hyphomycetes. The Moniliales of Saccardo's system are the group in which the majority of medically significant fungi is placed. They correspond to the Hyphomycetes of current systems. This group includes the Fungi Imperfecti that have exogenous conidia, are borne freely, and do not fit into the other groups. Saccardo further divided the Moniliales into four families: the Moniliaceae, the Dematiaceae, the Tuberculariaceae, and the Stilbaceae. The Moniliaceae are those with light-colored conidia and conidiophores. The Dematiaceae are those with dark-colored conidia and conidiophores. This method of dividing fungi by color has not worked well as a primary classification characteristic. As new fungi have been discovered, it has often been difficult to determine in which group a particular fungus should be classified. The Tuberculariaceae are those fungi in which the conidia and conidiophores rise from a cushion-shaped mass of hyphae, called a sporodochium. A sporodochium is similar to, and sometimes indistinguishable from, an acervulus. It may be absent in laboratory cultures, making this an impractical system of differentiating fungi. The Stilbaceae are those fungi in which the conidiophores occur in long, tightly fused masses known as synemata or coremia. Many fungi are not consistent in the production of these structures, making this also an impractical basis for primary classification. Saccardo divides each of these families into sections and subsections based on color and septation of conidia. These include the Amerosporae with nonseptate conidia; the Didymosporae with one-septate conidia; the Phragmosporae, which are multiseptate; the Dictyosporae, which are longitudinally and transversely septate; the Scolecosporae with threadlike (filiform) conidia; the Staurosporae with stellate conidia; and the Helicosporae with conidia that occur in a spiral form.

Workers after Saccardo have developed a system based primarily on methods of conidium production. The first of these was proposed in 1911 by Vuillemin. He divided the Fungi Imperfecti into two groups of spore types. Thallospores are those conidia that are formed from hyphal cells. *Conidia vera* are those conidia that are formed as separate entities, either directly from the hyphae or from specialized hyphal structures.

In 1953, Hughes introduced a system that was subsequently modified by Barron in 1968. Barron's modification of Hughes's system was used as the basis of the deliberations at the Kananaskis conference, the proceedings of which were published by Kendrick in 1971. At this time, substantial decisions and changes were made in the terminology to be used in describing the Fungi Imperfecti.

Following is a description of Barron's system, with changes as introduced at the Kananaskis conference.

Barron's System

Barron divided the Hyphomycetes into 11 groups, which include all of the Fungi Imperfecti except the Sphaeropsidales of Saccardo (now classified as Coelomycetes). Ten distinct forms of conidium production form the basis of classification of the first ten groups. These he called the Aleuriosporae, the Annellosporae, the Arthrosporae, the Blastosporae, the Botryoblastosporae, the Meristem Arthrosporae, the Meristem Blastosporae, the Phialophorae, the Porosporae, and the Sympodulosporae. Mycelia Sterila, with no spores, is the eleventh group. At the Kananaskis conference it was agreed to use the term *conidium* exclusively for spores of the Fungi Imperfecti.

Aleuriospores (aleurioconidia) are usually borne singly, either directly (sessile) on the hypha, on short hyphal projections (pedicels), or on longer, usually undifferentiated, conidiophores. Aleuriospores are produced by a blowing out of the terminal portion of the hypha or conidiophore. They often break off from the parent hypha with difficulty and Barron observed a "frill" that may be present on the free aleuriospore at the attachment point. Major pathogenic fungi included in this group are *B. dermatitidis*, *H. capsulatum*, and the dermatophytes (*Microsporum*, *Epidermophyton*, and *Trichophyton* species). Figure 18 shows (*a*) microaleurioconidia of *T. rubrum*, (*b*) macroaleurioconidia of *M. canis*. The use of the term *aleurioconidium* was rejected at the Kananaskis conference because it de-

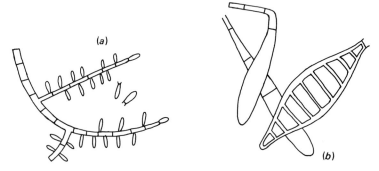

Figure 18. Aleurioconidia: (*a*) microaleurioconidia, (*b*) macroaleurioconidia.

scribes the method of conidium separation rather than the method of development.
It was determined at this conference that conidium production is either *thallic*
(septating walls of conidium are developed before swelling of the conidium occurs),
or *blastic* (swelling and formation of conidium takes place before septating walls
are formed). The aleurioconidia of the dermatophytes are thallic. The aleurioconidia of *H. capsulatum* and of *B. dermatitidis* are probably blastic (McGinnis,
1979). Conidia may be separated from the parent cell by fission (a natural break occurs at a double septum between the walls of the conidium and the conidiogenous
cell), or by fracture (the wall of the cell adjacent to the conidium is ruptured by
some mechanical stress to release the conidium). Aleurioconidia are separated by
fracture. The remnants of the adjacent cell form the frill described by Barron.
Medical mycologists are finding it convenient to retain the term aleurioconidium.

Annellospores (annelloconidia) are produced, with the youngest at the base
(basipetal), in balls or chains from the apex of a flask-shaped or cylindrical sporogenous cell (annellide). (See Fig. 19.) This cell increases in length as successive
spores are produced, leaving an elongated scarred tip (annellated apex). The following fungi, which may be pathogenic, are included in this group: *Exophiala* (*Cladosporium*) *werneckii, E.* (*Phialophora*) *jeanselmei, E.* (*Phialophora*) *spinifera,* and
Scopulariopsis species (illustrated). The noun *annelloconidium* has been replaced
by the descriptive phrase "blastic conidium produced on an annellated conidiogenous cell (annellide)."

Arthrospores (arthroconidia) are produced by septations and breakup, or round-
ing off of simple or branched sporogenous hyphae, or by basipetal budding to form
a chain. The major pathogenic fungus, *C. immitis,* is characterized in culture by the
production of arthroconidia. Also included in this group are the possible oppor-

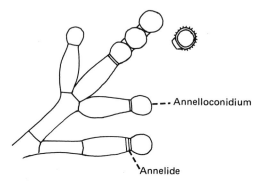

Figure 19. Annelloconidia.

tunists of the *Geotrichum* species (shown in Fig. 20) and the *Trichosporon* species. The term *arthroconidium* is retained and is now defined as a *thallic arthric conidium. Arthric* is defined as a form of conidium production characterized by the breaking away of a preexisting determinate hyphal element. The word *determinate* is used to describe a hyphal element that has ceased extension growth.

Blastospores (blastoconidia) are blown out from another cell, from a hypha, or from a conidiophore. Blastoconidia may produce either other blastoconidia by simple budding or germ tubes that develop into hyphae and that may, in turn, produce new blastoconidia. Pathogenic fungi included in this group by Barron are *Fonsecaea pedrosoi* and the *Cladosporium* species. Barron also included the asporogenous yeasts in this group. These yeasts are now placed by Ainsworth in a separate class, the Blastomycetes, which consist, mainly, of simple blastoconidia that may elongate into pseudohyphae. *Candida* species (shown in Fig. 21), *Cryptococcus* species, *Rhodotorula* species, and *Torulopsis* species are significant yeasts that are

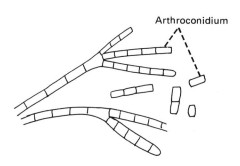

Figure 20. Arthroconidia.

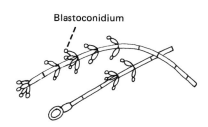

Figure 21. Blastoconidia.

now placed in the class Blastomycetes. In place of the term *blastoconidium,* the Kananaskis conference recommended the term *blastic conidium,* for yeasts that are produced synchronously or in acropetal chains. The term *acropetal* is descriptive of chains of conidia in which the youngest conidium is produced at the tip, that is, each conidium is produced by the preceding one.

Botryoblastospores (botryoblastoconidia) develop simultaneously from the swollen apex (ampulla) of a sporogenous cell, on short denticles, borne singly or in acropetal chains. No major pathogens are included in this group. *Botrytis* species (shown in Fig. 22) and *Oedocephalum* species may, on occasion, be implicated as opportunists. Blastoconidia are released by *fission* (a natural break occurring at a double septum between the walls of the conidium and the conidiogenous cell). No remnants of the adjacent cell are seen.

Meristem arthrospores (meristem arthroconidia) are conidia produced in basipetal (youngest at the base) chains from a conidiophore that increases in length by meristematic growth at the base. The common mold *Trichothecium roseum* (shown in Fig. 23) is placed in this group. The group does not include major pathogens. The Kananaskis conference replaces the term *meristem arthrospore* with the terms *thallic meristem conidia* or *blastic retrogressive conidia.* The term *meristematic* is used to define any place on a hypha, conidiogenous cell, or conidium where growth occurs that results in an increase in volume. The term *retrogressive* defines a conidiogenous cell or hypha that may be converted into a conidium. By contrast, the term *stable* is used to define those conidiogenous cells that remain as they are.

Meristem blastospores (meristem blastoconidia) are conidia that are produced in whorls on conidiophores that elongate from the base. Major pathogens are not

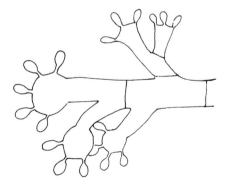

Figure 22. Botryoblastoconidia.

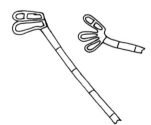

Figure 23. Meristem arthroconidia.

recognized in this group. Figure 24 illustrates the common mold *Arthrinium* (*Papularia*) sp.

Phialospores (phialoconidia) are abstricted from within a conidiogenous cell called a phialide. This is a rounded, or elongated, vaselike structure, which is not altered as conidia are produced. In a chain of phialoconidia, the youngest will be at the base (basipetal). Many fungi commonly encountered in a medical laboratory are included in this group. *Aspergillus* species, *Acremonium* (*Cephalosporium*) species, *Ph. verrucosa* (shown in Fig. 25), other *Phialophora* species, *Penicillium* species, *Paecilomyces* species, and *Wangiella dermatitidis* all may be pathogens. The term *phialoconidium* is now defined as a *blastic phialidic conidium*. The term *phialidic* indicates that the wall of the new conidium is entirely new and is not derived from the inner wall of the conidiogenous cell. The term *tretic* is used to describe those blastic conidia in which the inner wall of the conidiogenous cell develops into the outer wall of the new conidium. (See Fig. 28.)

Porospores (poroconidia) are produced through minute pores in the outer wall of the conidiophore or previously formed conidium. These conidia may be septate, pigmented, solitary or in chains with the youngest at the tip (acropetal). All of those recorded have brown septate conidia. The following genera of common molds, which have been implicated as opportunistic pathogens, produce poroconidia: *Alternaria* species (shown in Fig. 26), *Curvularia* species, *Drechslera* species, *Helminthosporium* species. The term *poroconidium* has been rejected by the Kananaskis conference. Most of these are now determined to be *blastic tretic conidia* or, more simply, *tretoconidia.* These are tretic because they have been shown to be formed from the inner wall of the conidiogenous cell, rather than from both cell walls, or from entirely within the conidiogenous cell.

Sympodulospores (sympodioconidia) are conidia that are blown out successively from a conidiophore that enlarges as each new conidium is produced. The primary conidium is produced at the tip of the conidiophore. Successive conidia are pro-

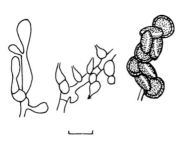

Figure 24. Meristem blastoconidia.

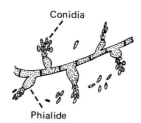

Conidia

Phialide

Figure 25. Phialoconidia.

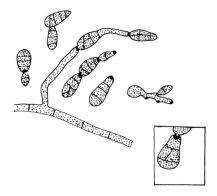

Figure 26. Poroconidia.

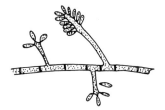

Figure 27. Sympodioconidia.

duced to the side and below each preceding conidium. As these conidia break away, scars are seen at the growing points on the conidium. This kind of sporulation has been described as an acrothecal, or rhinocladiella, type of sporulation and is now described as sympodial. Chains of conidia may be produced on the primary conidium, with the youngest at the tip (acropetal). The two major pathogens included in this group are *F. pedrosoi* and *S. schenckii* (illustrated in Fig. 27). Also included are *Beauveria* species and *Rhinocladiella* species. The term *sympodioconidium* has been replaced by the descriptive term *blastic conidium produced on a sympodial conidiogenous cell.*

In the Mycelia Sterila, conidia are lacking. Units of reproduction consist of irregular groups of cells (bulbils) or hard masses of hyphae or pseudoparenchyma (sclerotia). No major pathogens are included in this group. Those that may be considered common molds are *Papulaspora, Rhizoctonia,* and *Sclerotium* species.

Kendrick and Carmichael's System

In Ainsworth's *The Fungi,* volume IVA, the Fungi Imperfecti have been divided into three classes: (*1*) the Coelomycetes, (*2*) the Blastomycetes, and (*3*) the Hyphomycetes. The Coelomycetes include those fungi with conidia that are borne within a pycnidium or an acervulus. The Blastomycetes include the yeasts commonly seen in a medical laboratory, and the Hyphomycetes are those in which the conidia are borne on hyphae, on specialized conidiophores, or in which there are no conidia.

In their chapter (in Ainsworth's *The Fungi*) on the Hyphomycetes (pp. 323–509), Kendrick and Carmichael list, with synonyms, 566 genera. They divide these genera using, as a key, Saccardo's spore types (amerosporous, dictyosporous, etc.) as primary divisions. Within each division the species are next divided according to the color of the cell wall of the conidium, *hyalo,* meaning light-colored or transparent, and *phaeo,* meaning dark-colored. Next is the arrangement of the conidia: arthrocatenate (chains of arthroconidia), blastocatenate (conidia in chains with the youngest at the tip), basocatenate (conidia in chains with the youngest at the base), gloiosporae (conidia produced in slimy heads), and ceteri (conidia not in chains or slime). The final criterion is the character of the conidiogenous (conidium-producing) cell: *nonspecialized* indicating hyphallike cells, with *phiali-form* referring to phialides as previously defined, *annelliform* referring to annellides as previously defined, *rachiform* being narrow, zigzag sympodial cells, *raduliform* being wide sympodial cells, *ampulliform* being swollen conidiogenous cells, and *miscellaneous* being everything else.

Kananaskis Conference

The classification and terminology proposed at the 1969 Kananaskis conference (Kendrick 1971), is being used with increasing frequency in mycological publications. Ellis, in *Dematiaceous Hyphomycetes* (1971), and McGinnis, in his 1978 paper given at the Fourth International Conference on the Mycoses, describe classification systems using this new terminology. A review of these works and of the descriptions already given in this section gives us the following system for dividing the Hyphomycetes.

Conidia are described, first of all, as *thallic* (with the septating wall of the conidium occurring before the conidium is developed and before any swelling occurs) or as *blastic* (descriptive of a conidium that forms before the septating wall is formed).

The origin of the conidium wall is next defined. Blastic conidia with walls derived from the inner wall of the parent cell are *tretic.* Those with walls derived entirely from within the parent cell, with no involvement of the inner wall, are *phialidic.*

The conidiogenous cell is next examined. This may be *determinate* (i.e., ceasing extension growth at or before the onset of conidium production) or *indeterminate* (i.e., continuing to grow as successive conidia are produced). A determinate conidiogenous cell may be *stable* (not converting into a conidium) or *retrogressive* (converting into a conidium). Indeterminate conidiogenous cells may be *sympodial, annellidic,* or *basauxic.* Sympodial conidiogenous cells grow beneath or beside a previously formed conidium. Annellidic conidiogenous cells elongate at the top, producing a basipetal chain of conidia. Basauxic conidiogenous cells elongate from a basal point. The term *percurrent* describes annellidic and other indeterminate conidiogenous cells that continue to grow through the opening from which a conidium has been released. Figure 28 illustrates some of these kinds of conidium development:

a. Thallic, arthric conidia, retrogressive conidiogenous cell (after Kendrick, p. 161).

b. Blastic conidium formation (drawn from electron micrograph of *Stemphylium botryosum,* Carroll and Carroll, in Kendrick, p. 83).

c. Blastic conidia, retrogressive conidiogenous cell (*Tricothecium* sp. drawn after Barron, p. 49).

d. Blastic conidia, indeterminate sympodial conidiogenous cell (development of *Tritirachium album,* drawn after Cole GT, p. 153 in Kendrick, 1971).

e. Blastic basipetal conidia, indeterminate annellidic conidiogenous cell (conidium formation in *S. brevicaulis,* drawn after Cole GT, in Kendrick, 1971, p. 152).

f. Blastic phialidic conidium formation (development of conidia in *Neurospora crassa,* drawn from electron micrograph of Lowry, Durkee, and Sussman, 1967).

g. Blastic phialidic conidium formation, basipetal arrangement of conidia (*A. niger* conidium formation after Subramanian CV in Kendrick, 1971, p. 104).

h. Blastic tretic conidium formation of *Alternaria* sp. (drawn with reference to Campbell R, 1969).

After this chapter was completed, the proceedings of the second Kananaskis conference, held in 1977, became available in two volumes, entitled *The Whole Fungus* and *The Sexual-Asexual Synthesis,* also edited by Bryce Kendrick. Mycologists at both conferences contributed excellent descriptions of and comments on the capricious ways of fungi, based on observations obtained through the use of the scanning electron microscope, the electron microscope and time-lapse photography. These data, which include historical as well as modern observations, may seem to present more problems than they solve; nevertheless we cordially invite our readers to study these fascinating proceedings. To sum up, we offer these comments from the Introduction to *The Whole Fungus,* page 13.

> *We are still far from agreement about the ultimate shape of our taxonomic scheme (and about the nomenclature with which to express it). . . . The facts still do not of themselves or by themselves create a system for us. . . . There must still . . . be room for the intuition born of experience, and the often rather divergent ideas expressed in this book show that the boredom born of unanimity and uniformity has not yet set in among mycologists.*

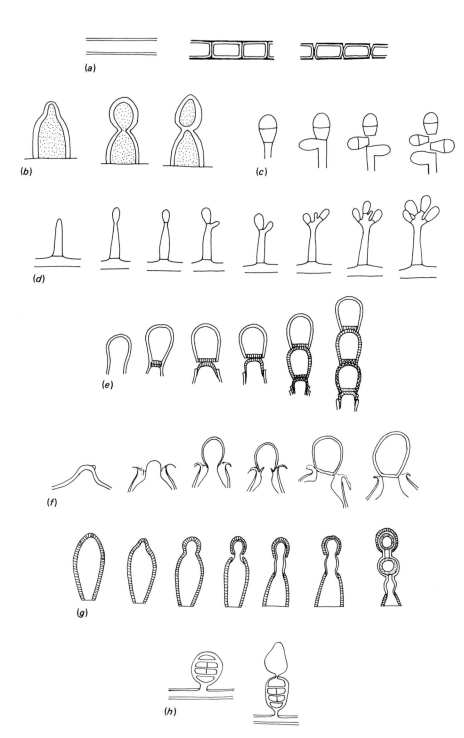

Figure 28. Conidium ontogeny.

BIBLIOGRAPHY

Ainsworth GC, Sparrow FK, Sussman AS (eds): *The Fungi, an Advanced Treatise,* vol IVA. Ascomycetes and Fungi Imperfecti. New York: Academic Press, 1973.

Ainsworth GC, Sparrow FK, Sussman AS (eds): *The Fungi, an Advanced Treatise,* vol IVB. Basidiomycetes and Lower Fungi. New York, Academic Press, 1973.

Barron GL: *The Genera of Hyphomycetes From the Soil.* Huntington, NY: Robert E Krieger Publishing Co, 1968.

Campbell R: An electron-microscopic study of spore structure and development in *Alternaria brassicola. J Gen Microbiol* 54:381, 1969.

Carroll FF, Carroll GC: Fine structural studies on "Poroconidium" formation in *Stemphylium botryosum,* in Kendrick (ed): *Taxonomy of Fungi Imperfecti,* Proceedings of the First International Specialists' Workshop Conference on Criteria and Terminology in the Classification of Fungi Imperfecti. Toronto: University of Toronto Press, 1971, p 75.

Cole GT: The sympodula and sympodioconidum, in Kendrick B (ed): *Taxonomy of Fungi Imperfecti,* Proceedings of the First International Specialists' Workshop Conference on Criteria and Terminology in the Classification of Fungi Imperfecti. Toronto: University of Toronto Press, 1971, p 141.

Davis BD, Dulbecco R, Eisen HN, et al: *Microbiology Including Immunology and Molecular Genetics,* ed 2. Hagerstown: Harper and Row, 1973.

Ellis, MB. *Dematiaceous Hyphomycetes.* Kew, Surrey, England: Commonwealth Mycological Institute, 1971.

Hughes SJ: Conidiophores, conidia and classification. *Can J Bot* 31:577, 1953.

Hughes SJ: Annellophores, in Kendrick B (ed): *Taxonomy of Fungi Imperfecti,* Proceedings of the First International Specialists' Workshop Conference on Criteria and Terminology in the Classification of Fungi Imperfecti. Toronto: University of Toronto Press, 1971, p 132.

Joklik WK, Willett HP (eds): *Zinsser Microbiology,* ed 16. New York: Appleton-Century-Crofts, 1976.

Kendrick B (ed): *Taxonomy of Fungi Imperfecti,* Proceedings of the First International Specialists' Workshop Conference on Criteria and Terminology in the Classification of Fungi Imperfecti, Held at the Environmental Sciences Center of the University of Calgary, Kananaskis, Alberta, Canada. Toronto: University of Toronto Press, 1971.

Kendrick B (ed): *The Whole Fungus, The sexual-asexual synthesis.* Proceedings of the second International Mycological Conference held at the Environmental Sciences Centre of the University of Calgary, Kananaskis, Alberta, Canada. Ottowa. National Museum of Natural Sciences, National Museums of Canada and the Kananaskis Foundation, 1979.

Kendrick WB, Carmichael JW: Hyphomycetes, in Ainsworth GC, Sparrow FK, Sussman AS (eds): *The Fungi, An Advanced Treatise,* vol IVA. New York: Academic Press, 1973, p 323.

Lowry RJ, Durkee TL, Sussman AS: Ultrastructural studies of microconidium formation in *Neurospora crassa. J Bacteriol* 94:1757, 1967.

McGinnis MR: Human pathogenic species of *Exophiala, Phialophora,* and *Wangiella.* Proceedings of Fourth International Conference on the Mycoses. Pan-American Health Organization Scientific Publication No. 356, 1977, p 37.

McGinnis MR, Katz B: *Ajellomyces* and its synonym *Emmonsiella. Mycotaxon* VIII: 157–164, 1979.

Saccardo PA: *Sylloge fungorum,* vol IV. Padua: Italy, 1886.

Stanier RY, Dourdoff M, Adelberg EA: *The Microbial World,* ed 3. Englewood Cliffs NJ: Prentice-Hall Inc, 1970.

Swatek FE: *Textbook of Microbiology.* Saint Louis: CV Mosby Company, 1967.

Subramanian CV: The Phialide, in Kendrick B (ed): *Taxonomy of Fungi Imperfecti,* Proceedings of the First International Specialists' Workshop Conference on Criteria and Terminology in the Classification of Fungi Imperfecti. Toronto: University of Toronto Press, 1971, p 92.

Tubaki K: Taxonomic study of Hyphomycetes. *Ann Rep Inst Fermentation* Osaka 1:25, 1963.

Vuillemin P: Les Conidiosporés, *Bull Soc Sci Nancy* 11:129, 1910.

Vuillemin P: Les Aleuriosporés, *Bull Soc Sci Nancy* 12:151, 1911.

3. Fungal Disease

FUNGAL TOXINS

Medical mycology has, traditionally, been confined to a study of the fungi that are known to invade human tissue. Toxins produced by poisonous mushrooms or by fungi growing on grains or other food, are not a part of this study. Sections on mycotoxicosis are included in Rippon, pp. 499–597, and in Emmons, et al., pp. 45–47.

FUNGAL ALLERGIES

The lines become less clearly drawn when fungal allergies are considered. Some hypersensitive people develop asthma as a result of an allergy to mold spores in house dust. Agricultural workers exposed to repeated inhalation of mold spores may develop severe asthma. The asthma can be followed by a chronic respiratory condition, which may develop into a fatal disease, as in bronchopulmonary aspergillosis. Allergic dermatitis may develop in workers handling moldy materials such as old mattresses or moldy animal fodder. An inflammatory skin response known as an *id* reaction may be triggered by a benign fungal infection in one area of the body, usually the feet, and may occur in another area, usually the hands. The site of fungal invasion, therefore, may be far removed from the inflammatory reaction.

FUNGAL INFECTION

Fungal infection is caused by molds or yeasts that happen to find the right set of conditions for growth in the human body. These infections are caused most frequently by fungi that are found in the soil. Those that have only been isolated from a human host are thought to be mutants of soil fungi that have become adapted to conditions in the human body. Fungi are not a part of the resident flora of most individuals (except for *C. albicans,* which is found in the oropharynx or gastrointestinal tract of many individuals, and *C. parapsilosis* and *Pityrosporum orbiculare,* which commonly occur as transient skin flora). Fungi are known, in some instances, to dwell in a symbiotic relationship with the tissue of the host. There may be no inflammatory response. There may be occasional flare-ups, usually associated with some change of the environment either within or around the host, or there may be an allergic reaction in some area of the body removed from the primary fungal infection. Some fungal diseases are confined to specific geographical areas, others are worldwide in distribution. Some are seen only in certain populations, relating to age, sex, race, occupation, or general physical condition.

Fungal infections are usually divided into four categories: (*1*) superficial, (*2*) cutaneous, (*3*) subcutaneous, and (*4*) systemic. In superficial fungal disease, only the outer surface of the skin is invaded and there is no cellular response of the host. Infected individuals are often unaware of this invasion. Cutaneous fungal disease involves the keratinized tissues of the body (the outer epidermal cells of the skin, the hair, and the nails.) Subcutaneous fungal invasion occurs in the deeper layers of the skin (the dermis), extending into the muscles, sometimes into the bone, and may involve the lymphatic system. This group of infections is caused by direct implantation of a soil fungus into the affected area. Systemic fungal infection is most often initiated by inhalation of fungal spores into the lungs. From here the infection may disseminate to all organs of the body and may sometimes result in the death of the host. These diseases may not be recognized until they are manifested in areas of the body away from the lungs, such as in the skin or the central nervous system.

The fungi that are able to invade human tissue are divided into two groups: (*1*) the primary pathogens, and (*2*) the opportunists. The primary pathogens are capable of producing specific kinds of fungal infection in healthy individuals, given the appropriate strain and dosage of the fungus, and the appropriate host response. These diseases have specific clinical characteristics that are recognized by physicians and are well described in the medical mycology texts.

The opportunistic fungi will only invade the tissue of a compromised host. Any mold or yeast, as well as any of the primary pathogens, may be able to produce fungal invasion of human tissue in an individual whose resistance is lowered by disease or other conditions. Diabetes, leukemia, lymphosarcoma, other malignancies, and chronic or preexisting lung disease are well recognized as diseases that predispose to fungal infection. Many new therapies are causing an increase in fungal disease by a lowering of normal body defenses. Steroid treatment for certain inflammatory conditions, administration of immunosuppressive drugs after organ transplants, cytotoxic drugs used in the treatment of malignancies, and the administration of antibiotics, which eliminate competing bacterial flora, all predispose an individual to fungal infection. Predisposing conditions are also found in patients with indwelling catheters, burn patients, heroin addicts (from infected syringes), and in people living in areas where malnutrition and poor hygiene prevail. It is often difficult to determine the significance of a fungus that is not a primary pathogen when it is isolated from a clinical specimen. *C. albicans* isolated from the sputum and *C. parapsilosis* isolated from the skin are known to be normal residents of these areas and, from these sources, are rarely pathogens. Other common molds, such as *Geotrichum, Aspergillus,* or *Mucor* are not normally found in clinical specimens. When they are isolated repeatedly from the same source, the physician must determine if they are present as simple colonizers or if they are causing fungal disease.

ANTIFUNGAL DRUGS IN CLINICAL USE

One of the difficulties in developing antifungal (antimycotic) drugs is that drugs that are toxic to fungi are also toxic to animals. (Both fungi and animals have eukaryotic cells.) There are, presently, only a few drugs that are established as effective in the treatment of fungal disease. These are: griseofulvin for cutaneous fungal disease caused by dermatophytes (dermatomycoses), nystatin for cutaneous and mucocutaneous yeast infections, and amphotericin B, a highly toxic drug, which is, nonetheless, the drug of choice for all systemic fungal diseases. For some systemic yeast infections 5-fluorocytosine is used. Potassium iodide is the treatment for a subcutaneous fungal disease called sporotrichosis. Other antimycotic drugs are either of limited effectiveness or are still in the experimental stage. These include miconazole and clotrimazole, which are reported to be useful in the treatment of cutaneous and systemic fungal disease, pimaricin and candicidin for cutaneous fungal infections, tolnafate for dermatomycoses, and hydroxistilbamidine, which is of limited usefulness in the treatment of the systemic fungal disease, blastomycosis. The diseases caused by the Actinomycetes, (*Actinomyces* and *Nocardia* species), are treated with penicillin or sulfonamides, or, more recently, a combination drug containing trimethoprim and sulfamethoxazole. These diseases are not affected by antimycotic drugs. More information about antimycotic drugs can be found in the references given in the bibliography: texts by Emmons et al. and by Rippon, and review articles by Kobayashi in 1977 and by Hoeprich in 1978.

Table 3 lists the fungal diseases, areas of the body affected, and the primary pathogens and opportunistic fungi that are established as agents of these diseases. Also listed are the Actinomycetes (*Nocardia, Streptomyces,* and *Actinomyces* species) that cause fungal-like diseases. The organisms listed will become familiar to a worker in a medical mycology laboratory, along with the many common molds and yeasts that may be opportunists and that are described in Chapter 5.

BRIEF DESCRIPTIONS OF INFECTIOUS FUNGAL DISEASE

The following descriptions of fungal disease are given to aid the laboratory worker. Reference is made, with all of these descriptions, to the detailed texts of Conant, Smith, Baker, and Callaway; of Emmons, Binford, Utz, and Kwon-Chung; of Rippon; and of Wilson and Plunkett. Excellent color plates are found in Wilson and Plunkett's book, but not always in the same section where the disease is being discussed; however, page references are given. Additional color photographs are provided by Beneke in the *Scope Monograph,* and these are duplicated in Beneke and Rogers's *Manual of Medical Mycology.* References to these are also given. A complete bibliography is given at the end of this chapter.

Table 3
MEDICALLY SIGNIFICANT FUNGI LISTED ACCORDING TO DISEASE CLASSIFICATION

Classification	Disease	Affected Area	Fungus
Superficial mycoses	Tinea versicolor	Smooth body skin	*Pityrosporum orbiculare*
	Tinea nigra	Thick stratum corneum, palms, and feet	*Exophiala (Cladosporium) werneckii, Cl. (Wangiella?) mansonii*
	White piedra	Beard, scalp, pubic hair	*Trichosporon beigelii*
	Black piedra	Scalp and beard	*Piedraia hortai*
	Trichomycosis axillaria (bacterial infection)	Axillary and pubic hair shaft	*Corynebacterium tenuis*
Cutaneous mycoses	Dermatomycoses	Keratinized layers of body; skin, hair, and nails	*Epidermophyton, Microsporum, and Trichophyton sp.*
	Tinea capitis	Scalp	*M. canis, M. audouinii, T. tonsurans,* and other *Trichophyton* and *Microsporum* sp.
	Tinea favosa	Scalp, skin, and nails	*T. schoenleinii,* and other *Trichophyton* and *Microsporum* sp.
	Tinea barbae	Beard and coarse body hair	*T. verrucosum, T. mentagrophytes,* and other *Trichophyton* and *Microsporum* sp.
	Tinea corporis	Smooth body skin	*T. rubrum, T. mentagrophytes,* all dermatophytes
	Tinea imbricata	Smooth body skin	*T. concentricum*

Table 3 (continued)

Classification	Disease	Affected Area	Fungus
Cutaneous mycoses	Tinea cruris	Groin	*T. rubrum, T. mentagrophytes, E. floccosum*
	Tinea pedis	Feet, interdigital spaces, and soles	*T. rubrum, T. mentagrophytes, E. floccosum* and other *Trichophyton* sp.
	Tinea manuum	Palms and fingers	*T. rubrum, T. mentagrophytes, E. floccosum* and other *Trichophyton* sp.
	Tinea unguium	Nails	*T. rubrum, T. mentagrophytes, E. floccosum,* and other *Trichophyton* sp.
	Intertriginous candidosis	Moist skin areas: groin, glans penis, scrotum, folds of buttocks, under the breast, axilla, interdigital spaces	*Candida albicans*
	Candida diaper rash	Diaper area	*C. albicans*
	Candidal granuloma	Hands, feet, face, and scalp	*C. albicans*
	Other cutaneous mycoses	Skin	*Aspergillus* sp., any yeasts or molds.
	Candida paronychia and onychomycosis	Nail and skin around nail	*C. albicans*
	Onychomycosis	Nails	*C. albicans, Candida* sp., *Scopulariopsis* sp., *Aspergillus* sp., other common yeasts and molds.

Disease	Location	Organism
Mucocutaneous candidosis	Mucocutaneous areas	*C. albicans*
Thrush	Mouth and tongue	*C. albicans*
Perleche	Corners of mouth	*C. albicans*
Vaginal candidosis	Vagina	*C. albicans*
Candida balinitis	Glans penis	*C. albicans*
Esophageal candidosis	Esophagus	*C. albicans*
Perianal candidosis	Anal area	*C. albicans*
Chronic mucocutaneous candidosis	All mucocutaneous areas	*C. albicans*
Keratomycosis	Eye	*Aspergillus* sp., *Candida* sp., *Fusarium* sp., *Acremonium* sp., other common molds. Systemic fungi may disseminate to eye.
Otomycosis	Ear	*C. albicans*, other *Candida* sp., *Aspergillus* sp., other common yeasts and molds.
Subcutaneous mycoses Chromomycosis	Skin surface, mostly lower extremities	*Fonsecaea pedrosoi, Fonsecaea compactum, Phialophora verrucosa, Cladosporium carrionii, Wangiella dermatitidis*
Mycetoma	Skin surface, mostly lower extremities	Various soil fungi, actinomycetes, and bacteria

Table 3 (continued)

Classification	Disease	Affected Area	Fungus
Subcutaneous mycoses	Maduromycetoma		*Petriellidium (Allescheria), boydii, Exophiala jeanselmei, Wangiella dermatitidis, Acremonium* sp. and other molds specific to geographic areas.
	Actinomycetoma		*Nocardia* sp., *Streptomyces* sp., *Ac. israelii*
	Botryomycosis		Bacteria
	Sporotrichosis	Skin, primarily hands, arms and legs.	*Sporothrix schenckii*
	Phaeomycotic Cyst	Smooth skin	*Exophiala (Phialophora) jeanselmei, Exophiala (Phialophora) spinifera, Ph. parasitica, Ph. repens, Ph. richardsiae,* and *Phoma* sp.
Rare subcutaneous mycoses	Entomophthora basidiobolae	Smooth skin	*Basidiobolus* sp.
	Entomophthoromycosis conidiobolae	Nasal tissue and face	*Entomophthora (Conidiobolus) coronata*
	Rhinosporidiosis	Nasal mucosa	*Rhinosporidium seeberi*
	Lobomycosis	Smooth skin	*Loboa loboi*
Systemic mycoses	Coccidioidomycosis	Primary infection in lung, may spread to other organs of body. Skin lesions may be produced.	*Co. immitis*
	Histoplasmosis	Primary infection in lung. Reticuloe₁ ¹othelial system is invaded. Bone	*Histoplasma capsulatum (H. duboisii* in Africa)

		and kidney and other organs, including the skin may be involved.	
Blastomycosis	Primary infection in lung, may spread to all organs, skin lesions are common	Blastomyces dermatitidis
Paracoccidioidomycosis	Subclinical infection in lung, mucous membranes, and skin are involved.	Paracoccidioides brasiliensis
Cryptococcosis	Lung, central nervous system, skin, any organ of body	Cryptococcus neoformans
Opportunistic Systemic mycoses		
Aspergillosis	Lung, skin, mucocutaneous tissue, any of the body organs	A. fumigatus and other Aspergillus sp.
Systemic candidosis	Blood, heart tissue, kidney, bladder, mucocutaneous tissue. (Lungs are colonized, but rarely invaded.)	C. albicans and other Candida sp.
Mucormycosis	Face, sinuses, gastrointestinal tract, lungs	Rhizopus sp., Absidia sp., Mucor sp., Mortierella sp., Cunninghamella sp., Syncephalastrum sp.
Cerebral chromomycosis	Brain or central nervous system	Cladosporium trichoides, Wangiella (Phialophora) dermatitidis, Fonsecaea pedrosoi
Systemic opportunistic fungal disease	Lungs, deep tissue, body organs, blood	Any yeast or fungus Acremonium sp., Alternaria sp., Aureobasidium pullulans, Beauveria bassiana, Cercospora apii, Chaetoconidium sp., Chrysosporium parvum, Curvularia geniculata

Table 3 (continued)

Classification	Disease	Affected Area	Fungus
Opportunistic Systemic mycoses			*Drechslera hawaiiensis* *Fusarium* sp. *Geotrichum candidum* *Helminthosporium* sp. *Paecilomyces* sp. *Penicillium* sp. *Petriellidium boydii* *Phialophora parasitica* *Phoma hibernica* *Pneumocystis carinii* (not a fungus) *Prototheca* sp. (algae, not fungi) *Scopulariopsis brevicaulis* *Torulopsis glabrata*
Bacterial infections (similar to systemic mycoses)	Actinomycosis	Jaw, face, neck, lung, intestine, and may spread to any organ	*Actinomyces israelii, A. bovis*
	Nocardiosis	Lung, central nervous system, other body organs and skin	*Nocardia asteroides*, and occasionally *N. brasiliensis*

Superficial Mycoses

The words *tinea* or *ringworm* were originally used to describe ringlike skin infections that were thought to be caused by a worm but have subsequently been shown to be caused by a fungus. *Tinea* is a Latin word meaning *worm* or *moth*. *Tinea* is still used, because of familiarity, to describe some of the superficial mycoses and the dermatomycoses.

Tinea Versicolor

AGENT: *Pityrosporum orbiculare* (*Malasezzia furfur*) is a lipophilic yeast that is a normal inhabitant of the skin.

CLINICAL CHARACTERISTICS: Multiple dark brown or hypopigmented scaly patches, which do not tan, occur primarily on the upper trunk and back. These may vary in color, but are mainly described as fawn colored. There may be itching, and those patches that itch may be inflamed.

GEOGRAPHY: Disease occurs throughout the world.

POPULATION: Tinea versicolor is primarily seen in young adults.

PREDISPOSING FACTORS: Poor nutrition, poor hygiene, excessive sweating, pregnancy, and Addison's disease are thought to be factors.

THERAPY: Sodium thiosulfate (Tinver) or selenium sulfide (Selsun) are recommended.

For more complete information see

Conant et al., pp. 644-651
Emmons et al., pp. 174-180
Rippon, pp. 84-87
Wilson and Plunkett, pp. 252-258

Color plates are found in

Beneke and Rogers, following p. 62, plate III, nos. 73 and 74
Scope Monograph, p. 25, nos. 73 and 74

Tinea Nigra

AGENT: *Exophiala* (*Cladosporium*) *werneckii, Cl. castellani* in the Western Hemisphere and *Cl.* (*Wangiella?*) *mansonii* in the Orient are soil fungi.

CLINICAL CHARACTERISTICS: Irregular brown to black patches occur, usually on the thick skin of the palm. Hyphae and arthrospores are seen in skin scrapings.

GEOGRAPHY: This is classed, primarily, as a tropical disease.

POPULATION: Cases most often reported are in females under 18, but the disease can affect both sexes of all ages. No known cases have been reported in patients with black skin.

PREDISPOSING FACTORS: Familial disease has been recorded, but little is presently understood about the mechanism that allows infection to occur.

THERAPY: Whitfield's ointment and tincture of iodine are most effective.

For more complete information see

Conant et al., pp. 494–502
Emmons et al., pp. 168–173
Rippon, p. 88
Wilson and Plunkett, pp. 259–263

Color plates are found in

Beneke and Rogers, following p. 62, plate II, nos. 71 and 72
Scope Monograph, p. 24, nos. 71 and 72

White Piedra

AGENT: *Trichosporon beigelii* is a yeastlike fungus. In culture it is identical to the common *Tr. cutaneum,* which is found in the soil and in the general environment. The species name *beigelii* denotes that the isolate was from a case of white piedra.

CLINICAL CHARACTERISTICS: Irregular, white, light brown or cream-colored nodules occur on the hair shaft. The nodules contain hyphae, arthrospores, and blastospores. The fungus grows into the hair shaft, swelling, weakening, and breaking it. The nodules are easily stripped off the hair. These nodules are seen primarily on the beard. The scalp and pubic hair are sometimes infected. Recurrence of the disease is common, suggesting possible individual susceptibility.

GEOGRAPHY: White piedra occurs in temperate climates, but rarely is seen in the United States.

POPULATION: Cases are reported in all ages and both sexes.

PREDISPOSING FACTORS: Not known.

THERAPY: Removal of the infected hairs by shaving or by cutting is the most effective therapy. Topical fungicides may be applied.

For more complete information see

Conant et al., pp. 632–638
Emmons et al., p. 183
Rippon, pp. 91–94
Wilson and Plunkett, pp. 264–266

Color plates are found in

Beneke and Rogers, following p. 54, nos. 3 and 4
Scope Monograph, p. 8, nos. 3 and 4

Black Piedra

AGENT: *Piedraia hortai (Trichosporon hortai)* is a black Ascomycete.

CLINICAL CHARACTERISTICS: The hair shaft is surrounded by brown or black nodules, containing masses of hyphae and ascospores cemented together. These grow into the hair shaft, weakening and breaking them. They are difficult to remove. The infection occurs primarily in the scalp. The beard may also be infected.

GEOGRAPHY: Black piedra occurs in tropical climates.

POPULATION: Cases are reported in all ages and both sexes.

THERAPY: Removal of infected hairs by shaving or by cutting is the easiest way of curing the disease. Topical fungicides may be applied.

For more complete information see

Conant et al., pp. 632-636
Emmons et al., p. 181
Rippon, pp. 91-94
Wilson and Plunkett, pp. 264-266

Color plates are found in

Beneke and Rogers, following p. 54, nos. 1 and 2
Scope Monograph, p. 8, nos. 1 and 2

Trichomycosis Axillaris (Bacterial Disease)

AGENT: *Corynebacterium tenuis.*

CLINICAL CHARACTERISTICS: Soft nodules (red, yellow, or black) surround the pubic or auxillary hair shafts in an irregular soft film. These nodules are easily distinguished from those of piedra by microscopic examination.

GEOGRAPHY: Worldwide distribution is reported, with most cases occurring in tropical areas.

POPULATION: Cases are reported in all ages and both sexes.

PREDISPOSING FACTORS: Poor hygiene and excessive sweating are probably factors.

THERAPY: Removal of hairs is helpful. Daily application of 2% formalin, 1% bichloride of mercury, or 3% sulfur may prevent recurrence.

For more complete information see

Conant et al., pp. 639-643
Emmons et al., pp. 183-184
Rippon, p. 42

Color plates are found in

Beneke and Rogers, following p. 54, no. 5
Scope Monograph, p. 9, no. 5

Cutaneous Mycoses

DERMATOMYCOSES

AGENTS: The dermatophytes are a group of fungi that are able to break down and utilize keratin (nonliving body tissue) found in the skin, hair, and nails. These are classified into three genera, based on the appearance of macroconidia. In the genus *Microsporum,* the macroconidia are rough and thick-walled. Microspora will infect the hair or skin. In the genus *Trichophyton,* the macroconidia are smooth and thin walled. These may be cigar shaped or quite irregular. Trichophytons will infect the hair, skin, or nails. In the genus *Epidermophyton,* which contains only one species, *E. floccosum,* the macroconidia are club shaped and thin walled and may occur both singly and in bunches. This species infects the skin, especially that of the groin and the feet, and occasionally the nails. It is not known to invade the hair.

SEXUAL FORMS: In recent years, by proper matching of different strains, complete sexual forms of some of the dermatophytes have been discovered, all of which belong in the Ascomycotina. Species classified asexually as *Microsporum* and *Trichophyton* belong to the genera *Nannizzia* and *Arthroderma,* respectively when classified as perfect fungi.

OCCURRENCE OF DERMATOPHYTES: Some species of dermatophytes are widespread throughout the world. Others are limited to certain geographic or climatic areas. (See tinea capitis, geographical distributions.) Some are found in soil (geophilic). Some are adapted to certain animals (zoophilic) and others to humans (anthropophilic). Different species may produce different clinical types of disease or diseases of different severity. Even different strains of the same species may differ in the severity and chronicity of the disease produced. Zoophilic and geophilic strains of dermatophytes usually produce more inflammation than anthropophilic strains. The clinical characteristics of dermatophyte diseases are well established. These diseases are classified according to the body area invaded.

Tinea Capitis

AGENT: *Microsporum* and *Trichophyton* species (see geographical distribution).

CLINICAL CHARACTERISTICS: Tinea capitis is a scalp infection caused by a dermatophyte. Both the skin on the scalp and the hair may be involved. The fungal hyphae grow into the hair follicle and down along or into the keratinized zone. As the hair grows, the hyphae are brought back with it to the skin surface, and spores are produced within or around the hair shaft. In ectothrix invasion, the spores surround the hair shaft. In endothrix invasion, the spores are formed within the hair shaft. Under ultraviolet light (Wood's light) certain *Microsporum*-induced infections fluoresce with a bright green color.

GEOGRAPHY: Worldwide incidence of *M. canis, M. audouinii, M. gypseum, M. fulvum, M. nanum, T. tonsurans, T. mentagrophytes, T. violaceum,* and *T. verrucosum* infection is reported. Isolated and infrequent incidents of *M. distortum* and *M. vanbreuseghemii* are reported. *M. ferrugineum* is reported primarily in Asia and Africa. *T. megninii* is reported in Europe and Africa. *T. soudanense, T. yaoundei,* and *T. gourvilii* are reported from Africa.

POPULATION: Although tinea capitis is seen primarily in prepuberal children, all ages may be infected.

PREDISPOSING FACTORS: Conditions existing in prepuberal children, possibly the absence in the skin of certain fatty acids known to be fungicidal, predispose to tinea capitis. Proximity to infected animals, poor hygiene, and poor nutrition also play a role.

THERAPY: Oral griseofulvin is the most effective therapy.

For more complete information see

Conant et al., pp. 573–578
Emmons et al., p. 127
Rippon, pp. 110–116
Wilson and Plunkett, pp. 216-221

Color plates are found in

Beneke and Rogers, following p. 62, plate II
Scope Monograph, pp. 22 and 23
Wilson and Plunkett, following p. 222, plates 34, 35, and 36

Tinea Favosa (Favus)

AGENT: *Trichophyton schoenleinii* causes the majority of cases of favus. *T. violaceum* and *M. gypseum* have also been reported. *M. gallinae* is reported in birds. *T. equinum* produces favus in horses. *T. mentagrophytes* (*quinckeanum*) and *M. persicolor* are also agents of mouse favus.

CLINICAL CHARACTERISTICS: Dense masses of hyphae and epithelial debris form a cuplike structure called a scutulum around the hair follicle. Hairs are invaded by the hyphae. Skin and nails may also be infected. A characteristic mousy odor is described.

GEOGRAPHY: Favus occurs in Europe, the Middle East, the Orient, Greenland, Africa, and also in isolated areas of North America (Kentucky and Quebec).

POPULATION: Onset of disease is usually in childhood and may last through a lifetime. All ages and both sexes may be affected.

PREDISPOSING FACTORS: Poor hygiene and constant association with infected individuals are recognized as factors conducive to favus.

THERAPY: Griseofulvin and improved hygiene are the recommended treatment.

For more complete information see

Conant et al., pp. 579-586
Emmons et al., p. 125
Rippon, pp. 116-118
Wilson and Plunkett, pp. 214 and 229

Color plates are found in

Beneke and Rogers, following p. 62, plate II, nos. 57 and 58
Scope Monograph, p. 22, plate nos. 57 and 58
Wilson and Plunkett, following p. 222, plate 36

Tinea Barbae

AGENT: *T. verrucosum* and *T. mentagrophytes* are the most common causes. *M. canis* is also reported. *T. rubrum* is being isolated with increasing frequency as the agent of folliculitis of the beard.

CLINICAL CHARACTERISTICS: Beard and coarse body hair are invaded in a manner similar to tinea capitis.

GEOGRAPHY: Distribution is worldwide in rural areas.

POPULATION: Cases are reported in men who are in close contact with animals, particularly cattle.

PREDISPOSING FACTORS: Proximity to infected animals is the most widely recognized predisposing factor.

THERAPY: Griseofulvin therapy is usually effective.

For more complete information see

Conant et al., pp. 570–573
Emmons et al., pp. 123, 125, and 136
Rippon, p. 131
Wilson and Plunkett, pp. 221 and 222

Color plates are found in

Beneke and Rogers, following p. 62, plate III, nos. 69 and 70
Scope Monograph, p. 24, nos. 69 and 70
Wilson and Plunkett, following p. 222, plate 37

Tinea Corporis (Tinea Glabrosa)

AGENT: All species of dermatophytes are able to cause tinea corporis. *T. rubrum* is the most consistently isolated species. *T. mentagrophytes* is also frequently seen.

CLINICAL CHARACTERISTICS: Initial site of infection, characteristically, spreads in a circular fashion, producing rings of inflammation. The most active infection is always in the outermost ring. Spontaneous healing occurs at the center. Lesions may be scaly or they may occur as small blisters (vesicles). These are confined to the stratum corneum (outer nonliving layer of skin). The infection may also occur as a scaly rash indistinguishable from many other skin diseases. Fungal hyphae are easily observed in most wet mount preparations. In patients with immunodeficiencies, a more serious kind of infection may occur, in which the dermis (deeper layers of living tissue) is invaded. This is called Majocchi's granuloma.

GEOGRAPHY: Tinea corporis is seen throughout the world.

POPULATION: It is seen more often in adults than in children.

PREDISPOSING FACTORS: Factors that predispose to tinea corporis are not well understood. Poor nutrition and poor hygiene can play a role. Underlying diseases and immunodeficiencies are also implicated.

THERAPY: Spontaneous healing is usually seen in patients who are otherwise healthy. Topical treatment is sufficient for solitary patches in most uncomplicated cases. Griseofulvin therapy is necessary for chronic or widespread cases.

For more complete information see

Conant et al., pp. 563-568
Emmons et al., p. 114
Rippon, p. 118
Wilson and Plunkett, p. 222

Color plates are found in

Beneke and Rogers, following p. 62, plate II, nos. 61 and 62, plate III, nos. 63-70
Scope Monograph, pp. 22-24, nos. 61-70
Wilson and Plunkett, following p. 222, plates 37 and 38

Tinea Imbricata (Tokelau)

AGENT: *T. concentricum*

CLINICAL CHARACTERISTICS: Fungal invasion of the glabrous skin is seen in elaborate circular lesions that do not heal at the center.

GEOGRAPHY: Disease is reported in rural areas in the South Pacific, Southeast Asia, and Central and South America.

POPULATION: There is no predilection of sex or age for this disease.

THERAPY: Griseofulvin administered over a long period of time is reported to be effective. Relapses may occur.

For more complete information see

Conant et al., pp. 568-570

Emmons et al., pp. 123 and 128, Figure 10-7
Rippon, p. 123
Wilson and Plunkett, p. 223

Tinea Cruris

AGENT: *T. rubrum, T. mentagrophytes, E. floccosum* are agents of tinea cruris. *C. albicans,* which causes a similar disease called candidosis, is discussed separately.

CLINICAL CHARACTERISTICS: Invasion of the groin is characterized by an acute or chronic inflammation. *E. floccosum* invasion is usually confined to this area. *T. rubrum* and *T. mentagrophytes* may spread to the buttocks and upper trunk. The scaling lesions tend to spread in a typical annular fashion along the upper and inner thighs and often into the pelvic area and buttocks. The border is relatively sharp and raised, while the central area tends to clear. The scrotum and the glans penis are not invaded. The feet and the intertriginous areas are often invaded by the same fungus.

GEOGRAPHY: Disease is seen throughout the world, but most often in tropical areas.

POPULATION: This disease is most commonly seen in males and particularly where groups of men are together, as on shipboard, in locker rooms, or in institutions.

PREDISPOSING FACTORS: Heat and high humidity, perspiration, irritation of clothes are definite contributing factors. According to Emmons et al., invasions may also be spread by continued contact with contaminated clothing or towels.

THERAPY: Topical treatment with antifungal agents (see antifungal section) is usually successful. Griseofulvin therapy may be necessary for *T. rubrum* infections.

For more complete information see

Conant et al., pp. 560–563
Emmons et al., p. 125
Rippon, pp. 125–127
Wilson and Plunkett, p. 224

Color plates are found in

Beneke and Rogers, following p. 62, plate III, nos. 78, 79, and 87
Scope Monograph, pp. 24 and 25, nos. 78, 79, and 87
Wilson and Plunkett, following p. 222, plate 39

Tinea Pedis (Athlete's Foot)

AGENT: *T. mentagrophytes, T. rubrum, Ep. floccosum* cause the majority of cases. Dermatophytes endemic to specific geographic areas may be involved (see tinea capitis).

CLINICAL CHARACTERISTICS: Dermatophyte invasion of the feet, particularly the soles and toe webs, is the most common type of fungal disease. Lesions may be mild or chronic and scaling, or they may be acute with vesicles and inflammation. Infections that are not apparent may occur, with no inflammation.

GEOGRAPHY: Tinea pedis occurs throughout the world, but particularly in warm areas when shoes are worn.

POPULATION: All ages and both sexes may contract tinea pedis, but the incidence increases in adult years and is extremely rare in children under 10 years old.

PREDISPOSING FACTORS: Moisture and warmth and anatomical problems that occur between the toes when shoes are worn predispose to tinea pedis. Repeated exposure to floors of locker rooms or showers contaminated with dermatophytes apparently plays a role.

THERAPY: Topical therapy is usually sufficient. Griseofulvin is administered in chronic *T. rubrum* infections which may resist even this treatment.

For more complete information see

Conant et al., pp. 548-557
Emmons et al., p. 118
Rippon, pp. 135-139
Wilson and Plunkett, pp. 225-227

Color plates are found in

Beneke and Rogers, following p. 62, plate III, nos. 77, 80, 81, 82, 84, 85, 86, 87, and 90

Scope Monograph, p. 24, nos. 77, 80, 81, 82, 84, 85, 86, 87, and 90
Wilson and Plunkett, following p. 222, plates 40 and 41

Tinea Manuum (Hand Invasion)

AGENT: All dermatophytes may cause tinea manuum. T. *rubrum* and T. *menta-grophytes* are common. *Ep. floccosum* is reported.

CLINICAL CHARACTERISTICS: Tinea manuum is a dermatophyte infection of the palms and the areas between the fingers. Lesions may vary from mild to scaly to vesicular. Often only one hand is infected. An *id* (allergic) reaction with no fungal invasion may occur on the hand, resulting from a dermatophyte infection in another part of the body, usually in both feet. This is known as the *two-feet, one-hand disease.*

GEOGRAPHY: Distribution is worldwide.

POPULATION: All ages and both sexes may be infected, with a higher incidence in adults than in children.

PREDISPOSING FACTORS: Dermatophyte infection in another area of the body, particularly the feet, predisposes to tinea manuum.

THERAPY: Topical therapy with antifungal agents is usually sufficient.

For more complete information see

Emmons et al., p. 119
Rippon, p. 134
Wilson and Plunkett, p. 225

Color plates are found in

Beneke and Rogers, following p. 62, plate III, nos. 75 and 76
Scope Monograph, p. 24, nos. 75 and 76
Wilson and Plunkett, following p. 222, plates 40, 41, and 43

Tinea Unguium (Nail Invasion by Dermatophytes)

AGENT: T. *rubrum* and T. *mentagrophytes* are most often reported in nail invasion. *E. floccosum* is frequently seen. Species of dermatophytes that invade the nail may often be those invading other areas of the body. Nondermatophytes that may invade the nail are discussed under onychomycosis.

CLINICAL CHARACTERISTICS: Two types of nail invasion are recognized. In one, known as white onychomycosis, which is superficial and usually caused by *T. mentagrophytes,* patching and pitting occur and only the surface of the nail is involved. In the second type, the invasion, most often by *T. rubrum,* occurs underneath the nail plate. There is an increasing accumulation of debris, which causes a characteristic thickening of the underside of the nail. This debris is often secondarily invaded with bacteria and nondermatophyte fungi. The nail bed is not invaded. Fungal hyphae may be seen invading the undersurface of the nail, although it is not always possible to demonstrate them. Often only a single nail may be involved in a chronic infection that lasts many years. Slight inflammation may occur. Such inflammation seen around the nail bed is called paronychia.

GEOGRAPHY: Tinea unguium occurs throughout the world.

POPULATION: Cases are reported in all ages and both sexes.

THERAPY: Tinea unguium is extremely resistant to treatment. Griseofulvin is effective in some cases. Nail removal is sometimes necessary.

For more complete information see

Conant et al., pp. 557-559
Emmons et al., p. 119
Rippon, p. 127
Wilson and Plunkett, p. 227

Color plates are found in

Beneke and Rogers, following p. 62, plate III, no. 90
Scope Monograph, p. 25, no. 90
Wilson and Plunkett, following p. 222, plate 42

Cutaneous Candidosis

AGENT: *C. albicans* and the *Candida* species are budding yeast-type fungi that produce mycelium on continued growth. *C. albicans* is found in small numbers of normal people in the mouth, gastrointestinal tract, vagina, and at mucocutaneous junctions. *C. parapsilosis* is frequently found as a normal part of the skin flora. *Candida* species (other than *C. albicans*) may be found in the soil, particularly where there is a large amount of organic debris. *C. albicans* is rarely isolated outside of an animal host. When candidosis occurs in any form, there will almost always be an underlying disease or other compromising condition present.

Intertriginous Candidosis

Candida invasion of the moist areas of the skin most often occurs in the groin, on the glans penis, and on the scrotum. It also occurs in the folds of the buttocks (intergluteal), under the breast (inframammary), in the umbilicus, in the axillae, and in interdigital spaces. Characteristic lesions have a red "scalded skin" appearance and a scalloped border. Satellite pustular lesions surround the primary lesion and aid in the differentiation of a *Candida* invasion from a dermatophyte invasion. Dry, scaly lesions may also occur. Budding cells and pseudohyphae may be seen and are characteristic of *C. albicans*. Hyphae, which are indistinguishable from dermatophyte hyphae, may also be seen in skin scrapings. It is not possible to distinguish dermatophyte from *Candida* invasion by observing the presence of hyphae in tissue.

PREDISPOSING FACTORS: Compromising of the body by diabetes, obesity, antibiotics, steroids or chronic alcoholism is given as the predisposing factor. Environmental factors that lead to increased moisture, such as tight clothing worn in a hot climate or continued immersion of hands in water, contribute to cutaneous candidosis by compromising the tissue.

THERAPY: Topical treatments are used. Nystatin is the drug of choice.

Candida Diaper Rash

CLINICAL CHARACTERISTICS: *Candida* diaper rash is initiated by a colonization of *C. albicans* in the diaper area. An allergic reaction is seen first, followed by invasion of the epidermis. Invasion may spread to other areas of the body, including the eyes and the intertriginous areas.

PREDISPOSING FACTORS: Poor hygiene, including constant exposure to unclean diapers, may lead to *Candida* diaper rash. Preexisting mucocutaneous candidosis (oral or perianal) also may precede diaper rash. Underlying diseases and immune deficiencies that may be undetected before the onset of candidal granuloma are also factors.

THERAPY: Proper hygiene and nystatin are described. It is important to keep the area dry. The use of cornstarch as dusting powder is not recommended because corn meal is a good medium for growing the organism.

Candidal Granuloma
   Candidal granuloma is a rare and fatal kind of skin invasion that is reported in children with immune deficiencies and with diabetes. Unlike previously described kinds of cutaneous candidosis, where moist areas of the body are invaded, the hands, the feet, the face, and the scalp are most often invaded. Inflammation occurs in the deeper layers of the skin, with invasion only in the outer layers. Lesions develop encrustations that may form into hornlike protrusions up to 2 cm in length. Successful treatment of the underlying condition will often give the best results.

For further information see

Conant et al., pp. 328–331
Emmons et al., p. 187
Rippon, pp. 186 and 187
Wilson and Plunkett, pp. 167 and 170

Color plates are found in

Wilson and Plunkett, following p. 158, plate no. 30

Candida **Paronychia**

CLINICAL CHARACTERISTICS: Invasion of the soft tissue around the nail and invasion of the nail itself is initiated by a *Candida* colonization of the moist folds around the nail. A red swelling occurs and extends into the tip of the finger or toe involved. As this swelling (paronychia) becomes chronic, the nail is invaded (onychomycosis), producing a characteristic brownish color and striations. (Paronychia may also be caused by bacteria and, in *Candida* paronychia, bacteria are often present as secondary invaders.) *Candida* onychomycosis may occur without paronychia.

PREDISPOSING FACTORS: Continued immersion of hands in water is the most frequent cause. Mechanical irritation is also described.

THERAPY: Mechanical therapy, which includes a drying of the area involved, and various topical and mechanical treatments are described as effective by Wilson and Plunkett. Nystatin ointment, topical amphotericin, gentian violet, 10% resorcin in 70% alcohol, 1% iodine in chloroform, 15% sulfacetamide, 4% thymol in chloroform are also described as possibly effective.

For more complete information see

Conant et al., p. 329
Emmons et al., pp. 187, 189, and 190
Rippon, p. 187
Wilson and Plunkett, pp. 169 and 176

Color plates are found in

Beneke and Rogers, following p. 62, plate III, no. 89
Scope Monograph, p. 25, no. 89
Wilson and Plunkett, following p. 222, plate no. 42

Mucocutaneous Candidosis

Mucocutaneous *Candida* infections are so common that often the word "fungus disease" brings to mind only these infections.

AGENT: These are almost entirely caused by *C. albicans,* although other *Candida* species may be involved in seriously compromised patients.

CLINICAL CHARACTERISTICS AND PREDISPOSING CONDITIONS: Thrush (oral candidosis) is characterized by white-to-gray membranous patches that may cover the tongue and all of the mucous membranes of the mouth and pharynx. In newborn infants, *C. albicans* in the vagina of the mother may cause a primary oral *Candida* infection before competing flora are established. In older children, and in adults, poor nutrition, diabetes, and other underlying disease contribute. Ill-fitting dentures can play a part.

Perlêche is a *Candida* infection of the corners of the mouth.

Vaginal candidosis is common and is characterized by a yellow, milky or cheesy discharge and either a mild redness or inflammation with pustules and ulcers and severe itching. The incidence of *Candida* vaginitis increases in pregnancy, in diabetes, and following antibiotic therapy.

Candida balinitis (*Candida* infection of the glans penis) is rare, most often occurs in uncircumcized males, and is usually associated with vaginal candidosis in the spouse.

Esophageal candidosis is evidenced by a destruction of the esophageal membranes and by characteristic x-ray film findings. Underlying compromising conditions are always present.

Perianal candidosis is seen in infants, usually where oral thrush is also present. Lesions are dull red in irregular patches, which may spread to other areas of the body. In adults there is severe itching and intense inflammation.

Chronic mucocutaneous candidosis is seen primarily in children with genetic defects and in common with other genetic diseases.

THERAPY: Topical treatment includes gentian violet, nystatin, and amphotericin washes. Haloprogin, miconazole nitrate, and candicidin may be effective.

For more complete information see

Conant et al., pp. 325-328
Emmons et al., pp. 188
Rippon, pp. 181-186
Wilson and Plunkett, pp. 116-169

Color plates found in

Wilson and Plunkett, following p. 158, plate 30

Cutaneous Invasion by Other Yeasts and Common Molds

These are rare but have been reported. *Aspergillus* species are most often the molds responsible in these diseases. Cutaneous invasion by *Alternaria* sp. has been proven in the dermatology clinic at the University of Oregon Health Sciences Center. A case of primary cutaneous phaeohyphomycosis caused by *Drechslera spicifera* has recently been described by Estes. *Hendersonula toruloidea* has also been implicated (Mariat et al.). In compromised patients and patients with multiple burns, any yeast or fungus may cause invasion of the skin. Lesions caused by subcutaneous and systemic fungi are discussed under the specific diseases.

THERAPY: Topical miconazole nitrate, haloprogin, and nystatin may be effective in the treatment of these diseases. For systemic treatment, amphotericin B is the drug of choice.

For more complete information see

Rippon, p. 130
Estes et al., pp. 813–815
Kobayashi and Medoff, pp. 292–306

Onychomycosis (Nail Invasion by Fungi)

AGENT: *C. albicans* and the dermatophytes are the leading agents in fungal nail invasion. In addition, many fungi that exist primarily as common molds may become invasive. *Scopulariopsis brevicaulis* is well established as a nail invader. Various species of *Aspergillus* (particularly *A. terreus*) have been recognized in nail invasion, as well as *Acremonium* (*Cephalosporium*) sp., *Fusarium oxysporum,* and a black yeast, *Hendersonula toruloidea* (Mariat et al.). Many common molds may colonize diseased nails, and it is not always easy to determine if invasion is present.

THERAPY: See *Candida* paronychia and onychomycosis.

For further information see

Onsberg (1978)
Rippon, p. 130
Zaias (1972)

Keratomycosis (Eye Invasion)

AGENTS: *Aspergillus* species (including *A. fumigatus, A. flavus, A. niger*), *C. albicans, Fusarium solani, Acremonium* (*Cephalosporium*) sp., *Petriellidium boydii,* and many other common soil fungi have been implicated as secondary invaders in eye infections following damage to the cornea by trauma or by disease. Fungal invasion by systemic fungi may disseminate through the central nervous system to the orbit of the eye. These are discussed under the specific disease.

CLINICAL CHARACTERISTICS: Fungal eye invasion may be evidenced by the presence of corneal ulcers, conjunctivitis, red and painful eyes, or orbital involvement.

PREDISPOSING FACTORS: Infection by trauma in individuals and exposure to large masses of fungal spores can predispose an individual to fungal infection.

THERAPY: Pimaricin is the drug that gives the most promise of effective therapy in ocular fungal disease.

For more complete information see

Beneke and Rogers, pp. 215 and 216
Emmons et al., pp. 485 and 486
Rebell and Forster, pp. 481 and 486
Wilson and Plunkett, pp. 272-274

Color plates are found in

Beneke and Rogers, following p. 108, plate XI
Scope Monograph, p. 47

OTOMYCOSIS (FUNGAL INFECTION OF THE EAR CANAL)

AGENTS: *C. albicans, Aspergillus* species, *Rhizopus* species, *Mucor* species, *Penicillium* species, and other common molds and yeasts may invade the ear canal.

CLINICAL CHARACTERISTICS: When the tissues of the ear canal are invaded, large masses of fungal hyphae and epithelial debris will collect. Often the hearing is impaired. Bacterial infection is almost always associated with fungal infection of the ear. While fungi are frequently isolated from ear infections, they are only responsible for a small percentage of actual ear invasions.

GEOGRAPHY: Worldwide incidence of fungal ear infection is reported.

POPULATION: All ages and both sexes may be infected.

PREDISPOSING FACTORS: The wax and debris that collect in the ear canal provide a good medium for growth of fungi that will often colonize the ear, particularly where bacterial infection already exists.

THERAPY: Cleansing of the ear canal and removal of the epithelial and fungal debris are the first methods of treatment recommended. The ear is to be kept as dry as possible (swimming is prohibited). The administration of antibacterial antibiotics to cure the bacterial infection will often eliminate the conditions that allow fungal invasion.

For more complete information see

Conant et al., pp. 657–663
Emmons et al., pp. 287 and 483
Rippon, p. 489
Wilson and Plunkett, p. 269

Subcutaneous Mycoses

CHROMOMYCOSIS

AGENTS: Closely related, but variable, pigmented (dark brown to grayish black) soil fungi, most frequently *Fonsecaea pedrosoi*, but also *Fonsecaea compactum, Phialophora verrucosa, Wangiella (Phialophora) dermatitidis,* and *Cl. carrionii.*

CLINICAL CHARACTERISTICS: Chromomycosis is a percutaneous infection, mostly occurring below the knee in workers in contact with the soil, especially when shoes are not worn. Lesions often exist for many years and remain localized. Early ulcerated nodules develop into cauliflowerlike masses. These are often secondarily infected with bacteria. *Sclerotic bodies* (brown septate spores) are seen in tissue examination. Hematogenous spread to the brain has been reported in rare instances (see cerebral chromomycosis).

GEOGRAPHY: Chromomycosis is most commonly seen in Cuba and Brazil and in subtropical countries.

POPULATION: Men between 30 and 50 working in agricultural areas are most often infected.

PREDISPOSING FACTORS: Close contact with the soil is the single most prevalent predisposing condition.

THERAPY: Oral 5-fluorocytosine, local amphotericin, and surgical excision are all current modes of therapy.

For more complete information see

Conant et al., pp. 503-526
Emmons et al., pp. 386-405
Rippon, pp. 232-237
Wilson and Plunkett, pp. 179-187

Color plates are found in

Beneke and Rogers, following p. 108, plate XI
Scope Monograph, p. 47
Wilson and Plunkett, following p. 190, plates 32 and 33

Mycetoma (Maduromycetoma, Maduromycosis)

AGENTS: The agents of mycetoma may be fungi (maduromycetoma), actinomycetes (actinomycetoma), or bacteria (botryomycosis). Different organisms are involved in different geographical areas. Lists of these agents are given in the major texts. (See also Table 18, Chap. 4.) The organisms include *Petriellidium boydii, Exophiala (Phialophora) jeanselmei, Madurella mycetomi,* and *Acremonium (Cephalosporium)* species. *Nocardia brasiliensis, N. asteroides,* and *Actinomyces israelii* may cause actinomycetoma. Staphyloccal and streptococcal organisms, *Eschericia coli,* and *Pseudomonas aeruginosa* may be agents of botryomycosis.

CLINICAL CHARACTERISTICS: *Mycetoma* is a term applied to any tumor produced by a fungus. The term is used here to describe a chronic, indolent infection, usually of the foot, hand, or arm that produces a markedly deforming swelling with draining sinuses that discharge pus containing granules that are microcolonies of the invading organism. These granules are of a size and color characteristic of the agent involved. Local fascia and bone are usually affected. The route of infection is through the injured skin. Hematogenous spread is rare but has been reported.

GEOGRAPHY: Cases are most often seen in tropical and subtropical countries.

POPULATION: Because this disease is related to occupation, it is most often seen in male agricultural workers.

PREDISPOSING FACTORS: The disease is caused by direct inoculation of the organism into the skin, where there has been an injury, particularly in bare feet that are in contact with the soil. Poor nutrition and poor hygiene are important factors.

THERAPY: In maduromycetoma, lesions remain localized. Surgical removal may be necessary. Poor results are obtained with antifungal drugs. Actinomycetoma responds to sulfonamides and antibacterial antibiotics. Botryomycosis responds to antibacterial antibiotics.

For more complete information see

Conant et al., pp. 458-481
Emmons et al., pp. 437-463
Rippon, pp. 48-69
Wilson and Plunkett, pp. 150-159

Color plates are found in

Beneke and Rogers, following p. 108, plate IX
Scope Monograph, p. 47
Wilson and Plunkett, following p. 158, plates nos. 28 and 29

Sporotrichosis

AGENT: *Sporothrix (Sporotrichum) schenckii* is isolated from soil, vegetable debris, and moist wood.

CLINICAL CHARACTERISTICS: Sporotrichosis is primarily a percutaneous infection. An ulcerated papular lesion develops at the site of inoculation. Ulcerated nodules and abscesses develop along draining lymphatics in about 75% of reported infections. In individuals previously infected, as indicated by positive skin tests (sporotrichin), skin lesions may occur without lymphatic involvement. Sporotrichosis is now known to occur also as an opportunistic infection accompanied by acute pneumonitis and bronchitis, that becomes chronic and is characterized by nodular masses and cavities. Enlargement of tracheobronchial lymph nodes may cause bronchial obstruction. Hematogenous dissemination is rare. The infection spreads to the skin, to the oral mucosa, to bones and joints, and, rarely, to the viscera. Lowered resistance is a factor.

GEOGRAPHY: Worldwide distribution is reported. Sporotrichosis is commonly seen in Central and South America.

POPULATION: All ages and both sexes may be infected.

PREDISPOSING FACTORS: Little is known about the factors that lead to the development of percutaneous sporotrichosis in healthy individuals. Reports of outbreaks that are attributed to inoculation from a common source give evidence that environmental conditions play a role. Pulmonary sporotrichosis is often related to alcoholism.

THERAPY: Potassium iodide taken orally in water or milk is the specific and effective treatment for percutaneous sporotrichosis. Spontaneous healing may often occur. Amphotericin B is used in the treatment of systemic sporotrichosis.

For more complete information see

Conant et al., pp. 417–457

Emmons et al., pp. 406–423

Rippon, pp. 251–255

Wilson and Plunkett, pp. 49–62

Color plates are found in

Beneke and Rogers, following p. 108, plate IX

Scope Monograph, p. 47

Wilson and Plunkett, following p. 54, plates nos. 5–8

Rare Subcutaneous Mycoses

PHAEOMYCOTIC CYST (SUBCUTANEOUS INFECTION BY BLACK, BROWN, OR DARK GREEN FUNGI)

AGENTS: Many fungi with brown hyphal walls may cause this subcutaneous infection. Those described include *Exophiala (Phialophora) jeanselmei (Ph. gougerotii), Exophiala (Phialophora) spinifera, Ph. parasitica, Ph. repens, Ph. richardsiae,* and *Phoma* species.

CLINICAL CHARACTERISTICS: As defined by Emmons, "A phaeomycotic cyst is a subcutaneous granuloma (rarely involving the muscle and bone) caused by fungi with brown hyphal walls." These lesions are usually solitary. Brown hyphae and budding cells may be seen easily in microscopic preparations of invaded tissue. This is a disease entity distinctly different from chromomycosis, mycetoma, and sporotrichosis.

GEOGRAPHY: Infections are reported throughout the world.

POPULATION: The disease occurs primarily in people in agricultural or other occupations that allow contact with the soil or moist wood.

PREDISPOSING FACTORS: A lowering of body defenses by preexisting chronic disease or by steroid therapy appears to predispose individuals to infection by these agents.

THERAPY: Surgical excision is the only successful therapy reported.

For more complete information see

Conant et al., pp. 527-540
Emmons et al., pp. 425-436
Nielsen, pp. 528-540
Rippon, p. 235

Entomophthoromycosis Basidiobolae

AGENT: *Basidiobolus* species are reported as agents of this disease. These organisms belong to the class Zygomycete, of the order Entomophthorales.

CLINICAL CHARACTERISTICS: Infection starts as a subcutaneous nodule, which develops into a movable mass that may involve a whole section of the body.

GEOGRAPHY: This disease is reported from Africa and Southeast Asia.

POPULATION: It is seen primarily in male children.

PREDISPOSING FACTORS: Little is known about predisposing factors, but initial inoculation is thought to be through insect bite.

THERAPY: Potassium iodide is helpful.

For more complete information see

Conant et al., pp. 407-408
Emmons et al., p. 261

Rippon, pp. 273-276
Wilson and Plunkett, pp. 191 and 192

Entomophthoromycosis Conidiobolae
(Rhinophycomycosis Entomophthorae)

AGENT: *Conidiobolus coronatus* is the name given by Emmons. Rippon describes the fungus as *Entomophthora coronata.* These fungi belong to the class Zygomycete, of the order Entomophthorales.

CLINICAL CHARACTERISTICS: The disease starts in nasal tissues. A painless, swollen mass develops, which may disfigure the entire face.

GEOGRAPHY: Most cases are reported from Nigeria. All are reported from warm climates.

POPULATION: Most cases are reported in males. All ages are susceptible.

PREDISPOSING FACTORS: Exposure to soil seems to be a factor.

THERAPY: Spontaneous clearing may occur. Potassium iodide is helpful.

For more complete information see

Emmons et al., p. 262
Herstoff et al. (1978)
Rippon, p. 268

Rhinosporidiosis

AGENT: *Rhinosporidium seeberi* is only seen in tissue and has not been isolated successfully in culture.

CLINICAL CHARACTERISTICS: Primary infection is in the nasal mucosa. The lesion develops into a tumor that may enlarge, leading to gross disfigurement of the nasal area. Bloody discharge and mild itching are reported. This is a chronic disease of long duration. Large spherules containing many endospores are seen in tissue.

GEOGRAPHY: The disease is reported primarily from India but is seen in all parts of the world.

POPULATION: Cases are reported in all age groups, but adult males are primarily affected.

PREDISPOSING FACTORS: The disease occurs mainly in people who work or play in the water. Ocular disease is reported more often in dry areas.

THERAPY: Surgical removal of tissue is the only effective treatment described.

For more complete information see

Conant et al., pp. 482–493
Emmons et al., pp. 464–465
Rippon, pp. 286–290
Wilson and Plunkett, pp. 205–209

Lobomycosis

AGENT: *Loboa loboi* has not been isolated in culture, but it is clearly seen in tissue in chains of budding cells.

CLINICAL CHARACTERISTICS: Lesions begin as small, hard nodules that may spread by trauma to other areas of the body. These nodules may become wartlike and will often last for many years. There is little discomfort.

GEOGRAPHY: The majority of cases are reported from Brazil.

POPULATION: Male agricultural workers account for almost all cases.

PREDISPOSING FACTORS: Exposure to soil is the only factor suggested.

THERAPY: Surgical excision of the affected area is the only effective treatment reported.

For more complete information see

Conant et al., pp. 161–168
Emmons et al., p. 382
Rippon, pp. 278–284
Wilson and Plunkett, p. 106

Systemic Mycoses

Coccidioidomycosis (Valley Fever)

AGENT: *Coccidioides immitis* is found in the dry, arid, alkaline soil of the Lower Sonora life zone (in southwestern United States and in Mexico.) It grows well after a heavy winter rainfall followed by a hot, dry summer. It does not survive in moist climates where there are competing fungal flora.

CLINICAL CHARACTERISTICS: In the majority of cases, coccidioidomycosis occurs as a mild respiratory infection or is completely asymptomatic. All individuals who are or who have been infected with *C. immitis* will have a positive delayed-type skin reaction (except for those in whom the disease is progressing rapidly and fatally due to a lack of cell-mediated immunity). In a minority of cases acute pneumonitis occurs. Allergic skin reactions known as erythema nodosum may be seen, particularly in adult white women. Some pneumonitis may progress to tuberculosislike disease with consolidation and cavity formation. Rarely, in less than 0.5% of cases and most often in males, particularly Filipinos, blacks, American Indians, and Orientals, dissemination occurs to various organs and tissues, including the skin and central nervous system. Laboratory workers, particularly people of Filipino extraction and pregnant women, are extremely susceptible to this disease by inhalation of spores from the mold phase, which may be produced in great abundance on culture media. Percutaneous infection is rare. In the few known instances of skin infection, chancrelike lesions and regional adenitis developed and healed in a few weeks.

GEOGRAPHY: The majority of cases are reported from southwestern United States and from Mexico.

POPULATION: All ages and both sexes may be infected, with serious disease developing in a minority of cases, as described above.

PREDISPOSING FACTORS: Inhalation of masses of spores is the single factor that leads to coccidioidomycosis. Race and sex seem to play a role in serious disease.

THERAPY: In the majority of cases, no treatment is necessary. Amphotericin B is the drug of choice for disseminated disease.

For more complete information see

Conant et al., pp. 171–217
Emmons et al., pp. 230–253
Rippon, pp. 356–388
Wilson and Plunkett, pp. 25–44

Color plates are found in

Beneke and Rogers, following p. 108, plate XI
Scope Monograph, p. 47
Wilson and Plunkett, following p. 30, plates nos. 1–4

Histoplasmosis (Mississippi Valley Fever)

AGENT: *Histoplasma capsulatum,* now known in its perfect stage as *Ajellomyces (Emmonsiella) capsulata,* is a fungus associated with bats, starlings, and chickens. African histoplasmosis is caused by a similar fungus called *Histoplasma capsulatum var. duboisii.*

CLINICAL CHARACTERISTICS: The majority of cases of histoplasmosis occur as unnoticed or mild respiratory infections that are self-limited and recognized later by the presence of a positive skin test and calcification of the lungs. In the initial infection, lesions occur throughout the lung with lymph-node enlargement. These lesions are usually unnoticed and mostly self-limited. When dissemination occurs, calcified lesions are seen in many organs and tissues. Reticuloendothelial cells are always involved. Lowered resistance is probably always involved in dissemination, which is often associated with leukemias, lymphoma, and other diseases. Percutaneous infections are rare. Self-healing ulcerated nodules are seen with regional adenitis. This disease resembles tuberculosis in many of its manifestations. African histoplasmosis may occur in any part of the body, but the skin, lymph nodes, and bone are the areas most often invaded. The primary inoculum appears to be through the skin by abrasion.

GEOGRAPHY: Histoplasmosis is seen primarily in North America, in the central part of the United States, particularly in the Mississippi valley. African histoplasmosis is seen only in Africa.

POPULATION: All ages are susceptible to histoplasmosis. Serious disease is most often reported in children and elderly people. African histoplasmosis is seen in twice as many males as females, and more often in dark-skinned than in light-skinned people.

PREDISPOSING FACTORS: Inhalation of large quantities of spores in infected areas, which include bat caves, chicken coops, and starling nests leads to the onset of histoplasmosis. African histoplasmosis is associated with the same kinds of sources, that is, bats and chickens.

THERAPY: In histoplasmosis, spontaneous resolution usually occurs. Amphotericin B is administered in severe cases. In African histoplasmosis, infections may be treated by excision and drainage. Amphotericin B is also effective.

For more complete information see

Conant et al., pp. 218-287
Emmons et al., pp. 305-341
Rippon, pp. 321-347
Wilson and Plunkett, pp. 67-71

Color plates are found in

Beneke and Rogers, following p. 108, plate XI
Scope Monograph, p. 47
Wilson and Plunkett, following p. 54, plates nos. 9-12

Blastomycosis (North American Blastomycosis)

AGENT: *Blastomyces dermatitidis* is now recognized in its perfect stage as *Ajellomyces dermatitidis.* Attempts to isolate it from natural settings have been unsuccessful. It is probably a soil fungus, found in the central United States and the central eastern seacoast states.

CLINICAL CHARACTERISTICS: Primary infection is pulmonary. It may occur as a mild respiratory infection that heals with or without leaving a small scar (dissemination may have occurred before healing). It may progress to bronchopneumonia or lobar pneumonia, which can become chronic or disseminate rapidly. When dissemination to skin and other organs occurs, skin lesions, chronic and spreading, are prominent. Percutaneous infection is rare. It occasionally occurs as the result of laboratory accidents. Ulcerated nodules with regional adenitis are seen. These nodules are self-healing.

GEOGRAPHY: The majority of cases are reported in the central United States and in the central eastern sea coast states. An African form of blastomycosis has been reported.

POPULATION: Cases are reported from all ages and both sexes, but the majority of those affected are middle-aged men, with three times as many infections in dark-skinned races. (Dogs are frequently infected.)

THERAPY: Amphotericin B is the most effective treatment. Hydroxystilbamidine is described as being of limited usefulness.

For more complete information see

Conant et al., pp. 84–133
Emmons et al., pp. 342–364
Rippon, pp. 297–320
Wilson and Plunkett, pp. 84–99

Color plates are found in

Beneke and Rogers, following p. 108, plate XI
Scope Monograph, p. 47
Wilson and Plunkett, following p. 94, plates 13–16

Paracoccidioidomycosis (South American Blastomycosis)

AGENT: *Paracoccidioides brasiliensis* has been isolated from the soil, most often in Brazil. However, the natural habitat of this organism is not fully understood.

CLINICAL CHARACTERISTICS: Although the mucocutaneous membranes are those most prominently infected, it is now accepted that the primary inoculation is by inhalation into the lungs. The pulmonary infection is usually subclinical. Dissemination often occurs early, with little evidence of lung involvement, along a hematogenous and lymphatic route, especially to mucous membranes and mucocutaneous junctions. Papules develop into vesicles and then into ulcers, becoming encrusted and granulomatous. Deeper destruction follows, with spread to adjacent tissues. Regional nodes ulcerate and develop draining sinuses. Dissemination occurs to the lymphatic system, spleen, intestine, and liver. Other organs are more rarely invaded. This disease is rarely progressive. When it occurs, there is marked loss of pulmonary function. Percutaneous infection is rare. There is a possibility that isolated skin lesions have been observed.

GEOGRAPHY: The majority of cases are reported in South America, primarily in Brazil.

POPULATION: Cases are reported in all ages from 10 to 70, but the majority are in males 20 to 50 years old.

PREDISPOSING FACTORS: Underlying disease and malnutrition play a role. Exposure to soil or plants where fungus is thought to exist is certainly a factor.

THERAPY: Many cases are self-limiting. Amphotericin B is now the drug of choice.

For more complete information see

Conant et al., pp. 134–160
Emmons et al., pp. 365–378
Rippon, pp. 389–403
Wilson and Plunkett, pp. 101–110

Color plates are found in

Beneke and Rogers, following p. 108, plate XI
Scope Monograph, p. 47
Wilson and Plunkett, following p. 94, plates 17–20

Cryptococcosis

AGENT: *Cryptococcus neoformans* has now been demonstrated in its perfect form to be a Teliomycete in the subdivision Basidiomycotina, *Filobasidiella neoformans*. It is found particularly in association with pigeon droppings. It also may be isolated from the soil and from decaying vegetables and fruits.

CLINICAL CHARACTERISTICS: The primary pulmonary infection may occur as a subclinical or mild respiratory infection, which may heal and may leave an actual fungal mass in the lungs. Progressive fatal disease may occur. No satisfactory skin test has been developed. This disease may disseminate to the skin and many organs, especially the meninges and the brain. Unless meningitis or brain abscess occurs, cryptococcosis is often not considered, and cryptococcal respiratory infection may be ascribed to other causes. Serious cryptococcosis is often associated with resistance-lowering factors, such as leukemia, diabetes, and ingestion of corticosteroids. Percutaneous infection occurs rarely.

GEOGRAPHY: Infections are reported throughout the world, in urban as well as rural areas.

POPULATION: All ages and both sexes are infected, with more cases reported in males than females.

PREDISPOSING FACTORS: Exposure to pigeon excreta predisposes to initial infection. Underlying deficiencies, as described above, may lead to serious disease.

THERAPY: Amphotericin B is the drug of choice; 5-fluorocytosine is helpful in some cases.

For more complete information see

Conant et al., pp. 288-324
Emmons et al., pp. 206-229
Rippon, pp. 205-228
Wilson and Plunkett, pp. 111-125

Color plates are found in

Beneke and Rogers, following p. 108, plate XI
Scope Monograph, p. 47
Wilson and Plunkett, following p. 134, plates 21-24

Opportunistic Systemic Mycoses

Aspergillosis

AGENT: *A. fumigatus* is the most common and invasive species. Other species of *Aspergillus* are also able to cause disease. The aspergilli occur in the soil and in nature throughout the world.

CLINICAL CHARACTERISTICS: Aspergillosis is most commonly seen as a pulmonary disease, of which three kinds are recognized:

1. Allergic aspergillosis may occur as asthma, from inhalation of spores. The most severe form is known as bronchopulmonary aspergillosis, with fungal growth on the bronchial membrane. Asthma becomes severe. Sputum is bloody.
2. Aspergilloma is the second kind of aspergillosis, also known as *fungus ball* or *mycetoma.* A massive growth of the fungus occurs in a lung cavity, often formed

by a previous disease such as tuberculosis. This is the colonizing form of the disease.

3. The invasive form of aspergillosis is the most serious. There may be acute or chronic lung infection with necrosis and cavitation. This may be fatal. The disease may spread hematogenously to the viscera, the skin, bone, and central nervous system.

Other forms of aspergillosis are caused by direct implantation. Organs involved may be the eye (keratitis), nasal and sinus membranes, the ear (otitis) with growth on wax or exudate, and rarely, and in compromised patients, the skin.

GEOGRAPHY: Worldwide distribution is reported.

POPULATION: All ages and both sexes may be infected.

PREDISPOSING FACTORS: Humans are constantly exposed to *Aspergillus* spores, which are produced in tremendous numbers and spread widely. Lowered resistance is always involved in aspergillosis. Patients with malignant diseases, particularly leukemia and lymphoma, are especially susceptible to invasion by *Aspergillus.* Immunosuppression and immunodeficiencies play a leading role.

THERAPY: Treatment of underlying disease may be effective. Surgical removal of fungus ball may be necessary. Nystatin is sometimes effective. Amphotericin B is the drug of choice.

For more complete information see

Conant et al., pp. 377–402
Emmons et al., pp. 285–304
Raper and Fennell, pp. 82–126
Rippon, pp. 406–429
Wilson and Plunkett, pp. 197–203

Color plates are found in

Beneke and Rogers, following p. 108, plate XI
Scope Monograph, p. 47

Systemic Candidosis

AGENT: *Candida* species, particularly *C. albicans,* which may be a resident of the oropharynx or gastrointestinal tract, are implicated in candidosis.

CLINICAL CHARACTERISTICS: In normal hosts, *Candida* species may cause a temporary systemic infection resulting from a heavy inoculation of *Candida* cells. *Candida* colonization at a catheter tip may lead to a *fungemia,* resulting in the isolation of *Candida* species from the blood stream. When the catheter is removed, the disease usually clears. A bladder or kidney infection in an otherwise normal host is easily treated. When there is a chronic debilitating condition, often combined with long-term treatment, the body defenses are broken down and *Candida* can disseminate, unchecked, throughout the whole body into any organ. Because the *Candida* species so frequently colonize debilitated body tissues, it is often difficult to determine whether invasion is actually occurring. When it does occur in a seriously compromised patient, the result is almost always fatal. *Candida* septicemia (invasion of the blood stream) and *Candida* meningitis (invasion of the central nervous system) may occur. Pulmonary candidosis is extremely rare. *Candida* endocarditis (invasion of the heart tissue) may occur in drug addicts from contaminated syringes, in patients with heart disease following long-term anti- biotic treatment and colonization of damaged tissue, and, following heart surgery with artificial valve replacement. *Candida* species other than *C. albicans* are often responsible for *Candida* endocarditis.

PREDISPOSING FACTORS: In the normal host, various factors including general good health, competing bacterial flora, and competent immune systems, appear to keep down the number of *Candida* organisms. When this balance is disturbed, excessive growth of the fungus occurs and disease production is possible. The following factors may predispose to excessive growth of *C. albicans* or other *Can- dida* species: elimination of competitive flora by antibiotics; *Candida* colonization of membranes in the newborn before competitive flora are established; factors causing general lowering of resistance (such as hypoparathyroidism, diabetes, other endocrine diseases, late malignancy, chronic disease, genetic deficiencies, and drugs injuring the immune system (immunosuppressives, cytotoxins, cortico- steroids). Various local factors (skin maceration by perspiration or immersion in water), poor mouth hygiene, and ill-fitting dentures predispose to *Candida* coloniza- tion and subsequent invasion of the whole body system.

GEOGRAPHY: Candidosis has a worldwide incidence.

POPULATION: All ages and both sexes may be infected.

THERAPY: Amphotericin B and nystatin are used in treatment of systemic candidosis.

For more complete information see

Conant et al., pp. 325-364
Emmons et al., pp. 185-201
Rippon, pp. 187-189
Wilson and Plunkett, pp. 165-177

Color plates are found in

Beneke and Rogers, following p. 108, plate XI
Scope Monograph, p. 47

Mucormycosis (Zygomycosis, Phycomycosis)

AGENTS: Various genera and species of the class Zygomycete, order Mucorales are involved.* Organisms include *Rhizopus* species, *Absidia* species, *Mortierella* species, and *Mucor* species. These are found principally in the soil and in decaying vegetables. Cutaneous infection by *Syncephalastrum* has been reported (Kamalam and Thambiah 1980).

CLINICAL CHARACTERISTICS: The organisms infect and invade arterial vessels. The disease is usually acute and often fatal. Depending on the portal of entry, the disease may affect the face and cranium, lungs, gastrointestinal tract, or skin. Diagnosis is often made without culture, by detection of nonseptate, wide hyphae in tissues taken at autopsy. Infection of the nose, palate, or pharynx may spread to the central nervous system. Such an infection will often be fatal within a few days and is often found in uncontrolled diabetes in children. Pulmonary mucormycosis may occur from inhalation of spores or from aspiration of exudate from nasal lesions, producing bronchitis and pneumonia, followed by invasion of the arteries. Often fatal in a few days, dissemination may occur hematogenously to the central nervous system or to the gastrointestinal tract. Cutaneous and subcutaneous mucormycosis occurs by direct implantation and also by dissemination.

GEOGRAPHY: Worldwide distribution is reported.

---

*The genera and species of Zygomycetes were formerly lumped together with all the lower fungi in one class called the Phycomycetes. The fungi that were placed in the Phycomycete class are now placed in the two subdivisions, the Mastigomycotina and the Zygomycotina. The Zygomycetes are a class of the Zygomycotina. (See Chap. 2, Taxonomy.)

POPULATION: Individuals with underlying diseases or other compromised conditions are affected.

PREDISPOSING FACTORS: Lowered resistance is always a factor. Predisposing conditions include diabetes, malnourishment, severe burns. Leukemia, other malignancies, and other debilitating disease or drugs affecting the immune system are often involved.

THERAPY: Treatment of the underlying disease is often the most effective method of controlling mucormycosis. Amphotericin B offers some possible help.

For more complete information see

Conant et al., pp. 403–416
Emmons et al., pp. 254–259
Rippon, pp. 430–447
Wilson and Plunkett, pp. 189–194

Cerebral Chromomycosis

AGENT: *Cladosporium trichoides* (*bantianum*) is the most frequently isolated agent. *Fonsecaea pedrosoi* and *Wangiella* (*Phialophora*) *dermatitidis* have also been reported.

CLINICAL CHARACTERISTICS: Initial infection is usually pulmonary with dissemination either to the brain, where an abscess may form, or to the meninges, without a localized brain lesion.

THERAPY: Surgical drainage and excision are the only reported treatment.

For more complete information see

Conant et al., pp. 527–540
Emmons et al., pp. 471–482
Nielsen, p. 535
Rippon, pp. 234–235
Wilson and Plunkett, p. 182

OPPORTUNISTIC FUNGAL DISEASE

AGENT: Any mold or yeast may be responsible for opportunistic fungal invasion. Diseases caused by the fungi listed below are described by Rippon and by Emmons.

Fungi	*Disease*
Acremonium (Cephalosporium) sp.	Cephalosporiosis
Alternaria sp.	Alternariosis
Aureobasidium pullulans	Aureobasidiomycosis
Beauveria bassina	Beauveriosis
Cercospora apii	Cercosporomycosis
Chaetoconidium sp.	Chaetoconidiosis
Chrysosporium (Emmonsiella) parvum	Adiasporosis
Curvularia geniculata	Phaeohyphomycosis
Drechslera hawaiiensis	Drechsleriosis
Fusarium sp.	Fusariomycosis
Geotrichum candidum	Geotrichosis
Helminthosporium sp.	Helminthosporiosis
Paecilomyces sp.	Paecilomycosis
Penicillium sp.	Penicillosis
Petriellidium (Allescheria) boydii	Petriellidiosis (Allescheriosis)
Phialophora parasitica	Phaeohyphomycosis
Phoma hibernica	Phomamycosis
Pneumocystis carinii (not a fungus)	Pneumocystosis
Prototheca sp. (alga, not a fungus)	Protothecosis
Scopulariopsis brevicaulis	Scopulariopsosis
Torulopsis glabrata	Torulopsosis

CLINICAL CHARACTERISTICS: As invasion by a specific fungus is recognized, the clinical disease can be described. Descriptions of the above-named diseases may be found in the references given below, and new ones are being described in the literature with increasing frequency as they are recognized.

PREDISPOSING CHARACTERISTICS: Any condition that compromises a patient, either by disease or by altering the immune system, by long-term therapy, or by environmental conditions can lead to opportunistic fungal infection. The list of compromising conditions given for systemic candidosis applies to any opportunistic fungal disease.

For more complete information see

Beneke and Rogers, pp. 147–150, 163, and 164
Conant et al., pp. 365–376, 677–698
Emmons et al., pp. 202–205, 488–517, 511–534
Rippon, pp. 205–228, 448–474

Bacterial Infections (Similar to Systemic Mycoses)

Actinomycosis

AGENTS: *Actinomyces israelii* is the usual cause of human actinomycosis. *Actinomyces bovis* is the usual cause of actinomycosis in cattle (lumpy jaw). Occasionally other species are involved. *Actinomyces* species are anaerobic or microaerophilic, gram-positive, nonacid-fast bacteria of the order Actinomycetales that produce filaments that branch and also break up readily into diphtheroidlike bacilli. No aerial hyphae or spores are produced. *Actinomyces* species exist endogenously on the mucous membranes of humans and animals. They are found in the mouth, in tonsillar crypts, in tartar on teeth, and in the alimentary tract. *Actinomyces israelii* is not recovered exogenously from the soil.

CLINICAL CHARACTERISTICS: The disease is characterized by suppurative to granulomatous lesions, which spread peripherally through any tissue, often involving the bone and producing draining sinuses with discharges containing characteristic grains called sulfur granules. Depending on the origin of the infection, the lesions may be: cervicofacial, involving the jaw, the face, and neck; thoracic, involving the lung, and often extending through the chest wall; abdominal, involving the intestine, sometimes spreading to other viscera and the vertebral column. The disease is produced only in injured tissue and then only in symbiosis with other bacteria; anaerobic streptococci, anaerobic gram-negative bacilli, and many others.

GEOGRAPHY: Actinomycosis is reported throughout the world.

POPULATION: Cases are reported most frequently in people aged 20 to 40, but all ages and both sexes may be infected.

PREDISPOSING FACTORS: Tooth extraction, ill-fitting dentures, and chronic injury to cheek or tongue can initiate cervicofacial infections. Thoracic actinomycosis may be initiated by inhalation of drainage from upper lesions; abdominal disease, by intestinal injury from swallowed sharp objects or from knife or gunshot wounds.

THERAPY: Clindomycin is the drug of choice, and penicillin is often administered with other antibiotics.

For more complete information see

Conant et al., pp. 1–37
Emmons et al., pp. 89–102
Rippon, pp. 13–30
Wilson and Plunkett, pp. 130–142

Color plates are found in

Beneke and Rogers, following p. 108, plate IX
Scope Monograph, p. 47
Wilson and Plunkett, following p. 134, plates 25–27

Nocardiosis

AGENT: *Nocardia asteroides* and, occasionally, *N. brasiliensis* are the organisms responsible for nocardiosis. These organisms are found in the soil, with some slim evidence that they may exist as transient flora of the oropharynx.

CLINICAL CHARACTERISTICS: The pulmonary infection may be benign, acute, or chronic. The disease often resembles tuberculosis. When there is dissemination, frequent abscesses occur in subcutaneous tissues and in the central nervous system. The disease is often fatal, even with treatment. Primary lung infection must be ruled out when subcutaneous abscesses are due to *N. asteroides.* Nocardial lesions, occasionally occuring in the mouth or intestine, may be due to dissemination or to the swallowing of infected sputum. The percutaneous infection that may be caused by various *Nocardia* species is described under mycetoma.

GEOGRAPHY: Worldwide incidence is reported.

POPULATION: All age groups may be infected. Incidence is higher in the age groups 30 to 50, and higher in males than in females. No relationship to agricultural workers is noted.

PREDISPOSING FACTORS: Nocardiosis is considered to be an opportunistic infection, secondary to other diseases. Rippon lists pulmonary alveolar proteinosis, Cushing's syndrome, diabetes mellitus, and the use of corticosteroids, immuno-suppressive agents, and, perhaps, antibiotics.

THERAPY: With early diagnosis, antibacterial agents are effective.

For more complete information see

Conant et al., pp. 38–61
Emmons et al., pp. 103–116
Rippon, pp. 31–39
Wilson and Plunkett, pp. 143–149

Color plates are found in

Beneke and Rogers, following p. 108, plate XI
Scope Monograph, p. 47
Wilson and Plunkett, following p. 134, plates 26 and 27

BIBLIOGRAPHY

Beneke ES, Rogers AL: *Medical Mycology Manual,* ed. 3. Minneapolis: Burgess Publishing Co, 1970.

Conant NF, Smith DT, Baker RD, et al: *Manual of Clinical Mycology,* ed. 3. Philadelphia: W.B. Saunders Co, 1971.

Emmons CW, Binford CH, Utz JP, et al: *Medical Mycology,* ed 3. Philadelphia: Lea and Febiger, 1977.

Estes SA, Merz WG, Maxwell LG: Primary cutaneous phaeohyphomycosis caused by *Drechslera spicifera. Arch Dermatol* 113:813, 1977.

Hoeprich PD: Chemotherapy of systemic fungal diseases. *Ann Rev Pharmacol Toxicol* 18:205, 1978.

Herstoff JK, Bogaars H, McDonald CJ: Rhinophycomycosis entomophthorae. *Arch Dermatol* 114:1674, 1978.

Kamalam A, Thambiah AS: Cutaneous infection by *Syncephalastrum. Sabouraudia* 18:19, 1980.

Kobayashi G, Medoff G: Antifungal agents: Recent developments. *Ann Rev Microbiol* 31:291, 1977.

Mariat F, Liautaud B, Liautaud M, et al: *Hendersonula toruloidea,* agent d'une dermatite verriqueuse mycosique observee en Algerie. *Sabouraudia* 16:133, 1978.

Nielsen HS, Conant NF: Practical evaluation of antigenic relationships of yeast-like dematiaceous fungi. *Sabouraudia* 5:283, 1968.

Onsberg P, Stahl D, Veien NH: Onychomycosis caused by *Aspergillus terreus. Sabouraudia* 16:39, 1978.

Raper KB, Fennell DI: *The Genus Aspergillus.* Huntington NY: Robert E Krieger Publishing Co, 1973.

Rippon JW: *Medical Mycology.* Philadelphia: WB Saunders Co, 1974.

Scope Monograph on Human Mycoses. Kalamazoo, Upjohn Company, 1968.

Wilson JW, Plunkett OA: *The Fungous Diseases of Man.* Berkeley: University of California Press, 1974.

Zalas N: Onychomycosis. *Arch Dermatol* 105:263, 1972.

PART II
DOING IT

4. How It Is Done: Clinical Laboratory Methods

In this chapter a way to do medical mycology procedures in a clinical laboratory is outlined, based primarily on the methods used at the University of Oregon Health Sciences Center. Frequent references are made to methods used in other medical centers. For convenience these other methods are cited simply by author and page number. A complete bibliography is given at the end of the chapter.

FOR PEACE OF MIND: SAFETY MEASURES

Working in the fascinating field of medical mycology will be more enjoyable if the suggested measures for personal safety are followed.

1. Never smell a fungal culture.
2. Never examine a fungal culture in an open Petri dish, except under a hood.
3. Use a safety hood for working with all molds isolated from respiratory secretions, deep body tissues, urine, blood, and other body fluids, as well as for processing specimens submitted for both mycobacterial and fungal isolation.
4. Autoclave all cultures before discarding, and do not allow old, unneeded cultures to accumulate.

5. Use agar slants in screw-capped tubes or bottles for subcultures of all stock cultures and fungal isolates.

6. Disinfect all bench tops and working areas daily. Do not allow accumulation of dust in corners or crevices where fungal spores may gather and germinate.

7. Do not keep potted plants in the laboratory. Plants could become a culture medium for a major systemic pathogenic fungus, particularly *Coccidioides immitis,* which produces infectious spores when grown in the soil. Also, plants may attract mites, plant pathogens, and soil fungi that can contaminate fungal cultures.

8. Dark-skinned people, and pregnant women are advised not to handle cultures of *C. immitis,* because these people are extremely susceptible to spores of this fungus.

GETTING READY: EQUIPPING A MYCOLOGY LABORATORY

A mycology laboratory is relatively inexpensive to equip and to maintain. Most of the needed instruments, tools, glassware, and miscellaneous items will be found in any bacteriology laboratory.* A laminar flow safety hood will be needed for work with systemic pathogenic fungi. (Yeast and dermatophyte identification can be done without a safety hood.) A stiff, sharp-pointed blade on a long handle is used for subculturing molds. We prefer a Bard-Parker #11 blade on a #7 handle. Dissecting needles are helpful in making microscopic mounts.

Reagents for making preparations used in microscopy (10% KOH, India ink, and lactophenol cotton blue or aniline blue) and media for primary inoculation of specimens (without antibiotics, with antibacterial antibiotics, and with a combination of an antibacterial and a selective antibiotic) are basic requirements for any laboratory that accepts requests for fungal isolation. Additional staining reagents and a battery of media for differential tests used in yeast and mold identification procedures will be added as needed by individual laboratories.

The media may be used in one of several containers. The safest method is to

*For the convenience of a person setting up a mycological unit, a list of needed items and formulae for reagents and media is given the Appendix.

use screw-capped tubes or bottles with agar slants. This allows less chance of infection by dissemination of spores to laboratory personnel and also reduces contamination by airborne molds. Prescription bottles, particularly the 4-ounce size, are preferable to test tubes because they provide a wider surface for the isolation of separate fungal colonies. However, prescription bottles are more expensive than test tubes. Screw caps are to be kept loose to allow for adequate aeration. For maximum isolation, Petri dishes provide the largest agar surface and the best aerobic conditions. These are to be used only where safety precautions are practiced by experienced workers, including the use of a safety hood for inoculation of media and for examination of all mold isolates. A double quantity of agar (36 to 40 ml) is poured into standard Petri dishes to eliminate dehydration over the long incubation period, and the humidity of the incubator is maintained at 60 or higher. Incubators are cleaned weekly with disinfectant solution.

APPROACHING THE JOB: GENERAL DISCUSSION

Specimens are collected, transported to the laboratory, examined microscopically, and inoculated onto appropriate media, as outlined in Table 4 and as described in the Procedures for Processing of Individual Specimens and the Procedures for Microscopic Examination of Specimens.

Fungal elements that may be recognized in microscopic preparations of specimens are described in Tables 5A and 5B and are illustrated in Plates 1 and 2. Most specimens will be observed in a KOH wet-mount preparation. This is a rapid method for clearing away cellular debris and observing undistorted fungal elements. An India ink preparation will be made when *Cr. neoformans* is to be isolated. A Gram stain may also be done, even though it is not a satisfactory stain for fungi. For a rapid stain, a Giemsa, Wright, or plain methylene blue stain are better choices. The rapid methenamine silver nitrate stain gives the most satisfactory results and provides a good permanent preparation. While it is theoretically a 20-minute procedure, we have found that in practice this staining procedure takes about an hour from start to finish. A periodic acid–Schiff stain takes a little longer and is almost as satisfactory as the methenamine silver nitrate stain. The hematoxylin-eosin (H&E) stain is useful for demonstrating the wide hyphae of the Zygomycetes.

Table 4
SETTING UP OF CLINICAL SPECIMENS

	Procedure	Blood	Bone Marrow	Cerebro-spinal Fluid	Body Fluids	Tissue (Biopsy or Autopsy Specimen)
				Systemic or Opportunistic — Sterile		
Microscopic preparations	India ink			x		
	Gram's stain			x	x	x
	Wet mount (potassium hydroxide)				x	
	Giemsa or Wright stain[1]	x	e			
	Methenamine silver nitrate (MSN) stain[2]		x	e	e	x
	Mucicarmine stain[3]	e	e	e	e	e
Media incubated at 30°C (Optional: 22° to 25°C room temperature)	Sabouraud (Emmons) agar		x	x	x	x
	Brain-heart infusion agar		x	x	x	x
	Enriched agar with antibacterial antibiotics[4]				x	x
	Cycloheximide agar with antibacterial antibiotics[5]				x	x
	Yeast extract phosphate agar with ammonia[6]					
	Biphasic medium[7]	x	e		e	

Explanation:

"x" means procedure is routinely performed; "e" means procedure is performed only in special situations.

[1] Giemsa or Wright stain is done when *Histoplasma capsulatum* is strongly suspected, and as a rapid fungal stain.

[2] Methenamine silver nitrate stain (MSN) is done in special instances when fungal elements have not been observed in routine preparations.

[3] Mucicarmine stain is done to demonstrate the capsules of *Cryptococcus neoformans,* which stain a deep rose diffuse color.

[4] Inhibitory mold agar (IMA) (BBL) contains chloromycetin. Antibiotics may also be added to Sabhi agar (Difco), Sabouraud (Emmon's) agar or other enriched agars. All yeasts and molds are able to grow on these agars. Other recommended antibiotics include gentamycin and tetracycline.

Table 4
SETTING UP OF CLINICAL SPECIMENS

Systemic or Opportunistic				Dermatophytes Opportunists or Superficial			Candida albicans Isolation
Nonsterile				Nonsterile			Nonsterile
Bronch-oscopy, Trans-tracheal Aspirate	Sputum (Expect-orated) Nasotracheal Aspirate Tracheostomy	Pus Drainage Exudate	Voided Urine	Eye	Ear	Skin Hair Nails	Nasal Mouth Throat Rectal Swab Stool Vaginal
x	x	x	x	x	x		x
x	x	x				x	
				x			
e	e	e	e	e	e		
e	e	e	e	e	e		
x		x		x			
x		x		x			
x	x	x	x	x	x	x	x
x	x	x	x		x	x	x
e	e						

[5] Mycosel agar (BBL) and Mycobiotic agar (Difco) both contain cycloheximide and chloromycetin. Cycloheximide inhibits some molds and yeasts, and allows most primary pathogenic fungi to grow. Significant pathogens which are inhibited are: *Cryptococcus neoformans*, *Aspergillus fumigatus*, and *Petriellidium boydii*. Also inhibited are *Candida tropicalis*, *Candida parapsilosis*, *Candida krusei*, *Trichosporon cutaneum*, and *Nocardia* species.

[6] Yeast extract phosphate agar with ammonia is designed to inhibit the growth of *Candida albicans* and bacteria, and to allow the growth of fastidious fungi, particularly *Blastomyces dermatitidis* and *Histoplasma capsulatum*.

[7] Biphasic medium is a combination of brain-heart infusion agar and brain-heart infusion broth, designed to encourage the growth of fastidious fungi.

Table 5A
COMPARATIVE SIZES OF FUNGAL HYPHAE AND SPORES IN SPECIMENS OTHER THAN HAIR

10	20	30	40	50	60

μm

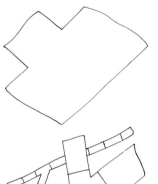

Aseptate hyphae, 10 to 20 μm
(Zygomycete)

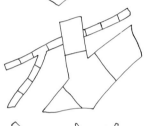

Septate hyphae, 2 to 10 μm
Fungus present

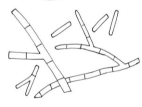

Branching filaments, 0.5 to 2.0 μm
Modified acid-fast positive
Probable *Nocardia* species

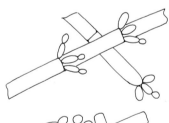

Pseudohyphae and budding cells 3 to 4
  μm
Probable *Candida albicans*

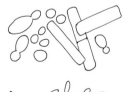

Nonbranched hyphae, 2.5 to 4.0 μm
Budding cells 2 to 8 μm
Probable *Pityrosporum orbiculare*

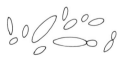

Narrow budding cells, 1–3 μm × 3–10
  μm
Possible *Sporothrix schenckii*

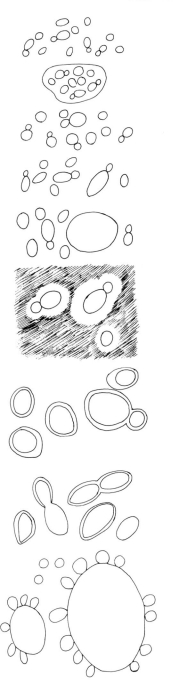

Budding cells, 2 to 4 μm
Possible *Histoplasma capsulatum*

Budding cells, 2 to 4 μm intracellular[a]
Probable *Histoplasma capsulatum*

Budding cells, 2 to 5 μm
Possible *Torulopsis glabrata*

Budding cells, 3 to 8 μm
Possible *Candida albicans*

Budding cells, 4 to 20 μm
Possible *Cryptococcus neoformans*

Capsule surrounding narrow necked
  budding cell, 4 to 20 μm
Presumptive *Cryptococcus neoformans*

Double-contoured, broad-based budding
  cells, 8 to 15 μm
Presumptive *Blastomyces dermatitidis*

"Hour-glass" budding cells, 8 to 15 μm
Possible *Histoplasma capsulatum* var.
  duboisii

Single and multiple budding cells 2 to
  30 μm
Presumptive *Paracoccidioides brasiliensis*

(continued)

Table 5A (continued)

Nonbudding cells and hyphae

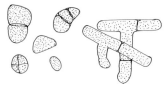

Branched, brown-walled hyphae 2 to 5 μm
Septate cells (sclerotic bodies) 4 to 12 μm
Agent of chromomycosis

Single cells only

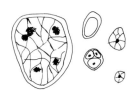

Cells 2 to 5 μm^b
Possible *Pneumocystis carinii* (with silver stain in lung tissue)

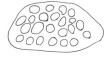

Cells 2 to 30 μm
Cytoplasmic cleavage
Prototheca species

Intracellular cells, 2 to 4 μm^a
Possible *Histoplasma capsulatum*

Cells 2 to 5 μm^b
Possible *Torulopsis glabrata*

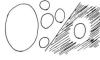

Cells 3 to 8 μm^b
Possible *Candida albicans*

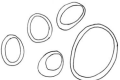

Cells 4 to 20 μm^b
Possible *Cryptococcus neoformans* (look for capsule with India ink)

Cells 8 to 15 μm^b
Possible *Blastomyces dermatitidis*

92

Table 5A (continued)

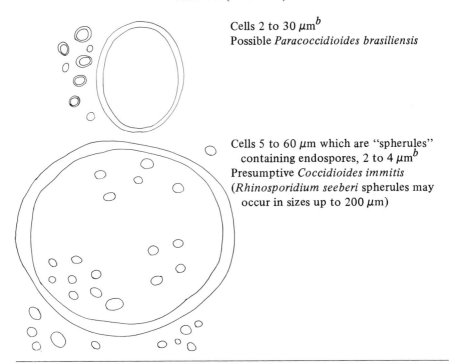

Cells 2 to 30 μm[b]
Possible *Paracoccidioides brasiliensis*

Cells 5 to 60 μm which are "spherules"
   containing endospores, 2 to 4 μm[b]
Presumptive *Coccidioides immitis*
   (*Rhinosporidium seeberi* spherules may
   occur in sizes up to 200 μm)

---

[a] Leishmania may occur intracellularly.
[b] Possible pollen grains.

A modified acid-fast stain will be done when *Nocardia* sps. are suspected. Mayer's mucicarmine process stains the capsules of *Cr. neoformans*. The Papanicolaou stain, used by cytologists, turns out to be excellent for demonstrating fungal elements, and fluorescent antibody stains have been developed for the diagnosis of specific fungi. The Swartz-Medrek stain described in the appendix is a useful rapid stain for observing fungal elements in skin, hair, and nails.

Basically one must use four kinds of media for fungal isolation from a clinical specimen: one medium for the general support of fungal growth, an enriched medium for isolation of fastidious fungi, and two types of media containing antibiotics. One medium should have an antibiotic to inhibit bacteria. The other should have both an antibiotic to inhibit bacteria and an antibiotic to inhibit saprophytic fungi. An additional medium to inhibit *C. albicans* has been developed and is now in use in many medical centers. If aerobic actinomycetes are to be isolated, it must be done on media without antibiotics.

Table 5B
EXAMINATION OF SPECIMENS OF PARASITIZED HAIR

Ultraviolet light (Wood's light)
Bright yellow-green fluorescence
M. canis
M. audouini
M. distortum
M. ferrugineum
M. gypseum
Dull fluorescence
T. schoenleinii
No fluorescence
All other dermatophytes

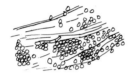

Ectothrix hair invasion (spores surround the hair shaft)
Spores 2–3 μm, in masses
M. canis
M. audouini
M. ferrugineum
M. distortum
Spores 3–5 μm, in a sheath
T. mentagrophytes
Spores 5–8 μm, in a sheath or in isolated chains
T. equinum
T. rubrum (rare)
Spores 5–8 μm, in chains or irregular masses
M. fulvum
M. gypseum
M. nanum
M. (T.) gallinae
M. vanbreuseghemii
T. megninii
Spores 8–10 μm, in a sheath or isolated chains
T. verrucosum

Endothrix invasion (spores within the hair shaft)
Spores 4–8 μm, in chains
T. tonsurans
T. soudanense
T. violaceum
T. yaoundei
T. rubrum (rare)
T. gourvilii

Table 5B (continued)

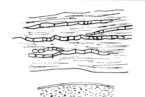	Favic hair invasion (hyphae within the hair shaft) *T. schoenleinii*
	No hair invasion *T. concentricum* *E. floccosum* *M. persicolor*

References:
Rebell and Taplin (1974), p. 12
Rippon (1974), p. 110
Ajello and Padhye in Lennette et al., p. 473

The media that may be used for specimens taken from normally sterile sites are Sabouraud's agar, Emmons modification (pH 7.0), or Sabouraud's dextrose agar (pH 5.0). These are general support media for the growth of all fungi. The higher pH of Sabouraud's (Emmons) is more supportive of the growth of fastidious fungi. The lower pH of Sabouraud's dextrose agar was designed to discourage the growth of bacteria. For specimens that are normally sterile the lower pH is not necessary, making the Sabouraud (Emmons) the medium of choice.

For an enriched medium, brain-heart infusion agar is excellent, with or without the addition of sheep blood. Eugonagar (available from BBL) with 5% to 10% defibrinated sheep blood, described by Wolf, Russell, and Shimoda, p. 357, and Sabhi agar (available from Difco), described by Haley and Callaway, p. 189, are also used for this purpose. In addition to these media, a biphasic medium combining brain-heart infusion broth and brain-heart infusion agar is an excellent enriched medium used for the isolation of fungi from blood. It is also useful in instances when a fastidious fungus is suspected in a normally sterile site, such as bone marrow or spinal fluid.

When bacterial contamination may be present, a medium with an antibacterial antibiotic, such as streptomycin, penicillin, gentamycin, tetracycline, chloromycetin, neomycin, or a combination of any of these, is used. None of these antibiotics will inhibit fungi. Antibiotics may be added to any of the media described above for this purpose. Excellent results are obtained with an enriched agar containing chloromycetin available from BBL and inappropriately named Inhibitory Mold Agar (IMA). For a medium to inhibit both bacteria and saprophytic molds and yeasts, cycloheximide is added to any of the above antibiotic-containing media, or it may be obtained commercially under the name of Mycosel (BBL) or Mycobiotic Agar (Difco). The dermatophytes (fungi that invade the skin, hair, and nails) grow well on this medium. Many pathogenic yeasts and molds will be inhibited. While this is a useful medium for fungal isolation, noncycloheximide medium must always be used at the same time.

C. albicans, which may be present as part of the normal flora in some respiratory secretions, may overgrow a fastidious fungus that is to be isolated. A yeast extract phosphate medium with ammonia has been developed at the University of Kentucky by Smith and Goodman (1975) for the isolation of *H. capsulatum* and *B. dermatitidis* from such specimens. It has been found that *Cr. neoformans* also grows on this medium. The growth of *Aspergillus* and *Penicillium* species is suppressed (Haley and Callaway, p. 189).

For the isolation of the aerobic actinomycetes, Middlebrook 7H10 is the medium of choice (Haley and Callaway, p. 190). This isolation is an appropriate part of the routine bacteriology procedure. These organisms will grow on the nonantibiotic mycology media. None will be isolated on the antibiotic-containing media.

Cultures for the primary isolation of fungi are incubated at room temperature (22° to 25°C) or in a 30°C incubator with a humidity of 60 or more, for a period of four to six weeks. Incubation at 35° to 37°C is no longer considered necessary for the primary isolation of fungi in a medical laboratory. It has been recognized that, if a significant fungus is present, it will grow well at 30°C or at room temperature (Koneman et al., p. 17). The characteristic growth at 35° to 37°C can be shown on subculture after the initial isolation. On occasion, when *H. capsulatum* is strongly suspected, a primary incubation temperature of 35° to 37°C may be justified (always in addition to a 22°-to-30°C culture), because the conversion of *H. capsulatum* from a mold form at room temperature to a yeast form at 37°C may be difficult. Cultures for the isolation of aerobic actinomycetes are incubated at 35° to 37°C for seven days, and cultures for the isolation of *A. israelii* are incubated anaerobically at 35° to 37°C for seven days.

Agar media are observed for visual growth at least twice during the first week and at least once a week thereafter, for a total of four weeks, or longer, if it seems indicated. Blood cultures on biphasic medium are examined for growth and gently mixed daily for a total of four weeks, or longer if indicated.

Reports are sent after the initial microscopic reading and at regular intervals during the incubation period. When cultures are negative, a final report is sent at the end of the incubation period. When fungal growth (yeast or mold) occurs, it is reported immediately, without waiting for the identification to be completed. Subsequent reports are made at appropriate intervals during the identification process and when the identification is complete. A final report is sent at the end of the incubation period or as soon thereafter as the identification is complete. (A final report of a fungal identification is not sent before the end of the incubation period, because it is always possible that more than one fungus will be isolated.)

Steps in Identification

The steps discussed below are outlined in Tables 6 through 19. Detailed procedures for microscopic preparations and differential tests used in fungal identifications are given at the end of this chapter. Formulae for reagents and media and suggestions for quality control are given in the Appendix.

Table 6
DIFFERENTIAL TESTS

Yeast Identification Tests

Ascospore production
Bromcresol green agar with neosporin for differentiation of yeasts by colony color
Carbohydrate assimilation (Wickerham tubes or auxonographic plate)
Carbohydrate fermentation (infusion broth with Durham tubes, or fermentation
   tablets.)
Cycloheximide sensitivity
Corn meal agar or chlamydospore agar plate for demonstration of yeast morphology
Eosin methylene blue agar with tetracycline for *Candida albicans* identification
Germ-tube tests for *Candida albicans* identification
Nitrate-Zephiran swab test for reduction of nitrate to nitrite
Sabouraud broth for film production
Seed agar for *Cryptococcus neoformans* identification
Urease production on Christensen's urea agar for screening of *Cryptococcus* sp.
Commercial test kits are available including API 20C, Corning Uni-yeast-Tek and
   BBL Mini-tek

Dermatophyte Identification Tests

Boiled rice for identification of *Microsporum audouini*
Corn meal agar with 0.2% dextrose for pigment production by *Trichophyton rubrum*
Dermatophyte Test Medium
Lactophenol cotton blue microscopic mount
Hair-pentration tests
Potato dextrose agar slant or cover-slip culture
Trichophyton vitamin agars for differentiation of some *Trichophyton* species
Urease production on urea dextrose agar slant for identification of *Trichophyton
   mentagrophytes*

(continued)

Table 6 (continued)

Dimorphic Fungus Identification

Animal inoculation
Conversion (in vitro) of arthroconidia to spherules of *Coccidioides immitis*
Conversion of mold form to yeast form of other dimorphic systemic pathogenic
fungi
Conversion of yeast form to mold form, to confirm dimorphism
Cycloheximide tolerance (screening tests)
Growth at 37°C (screening tests)
Lactophenol cotton blue microscopic mount

Mold Identification

Corn meal agar cover slip or slide culture
Growth at 37°C (screening test)
Lactophenol cotton blue microscopic mount
Löeffler's slant, or gelatin deep for demonstration of proteolytic activity
Potato dextrose agar cover slip or slide culture

Aerobic Actinomycete Identification

0.4% gelatin for liquefaction test
Hydrolysis tests, casein, xanthine, and tyrosine

When growth is first observed on any of the primary isolation media, the initial steps outlined in Table 7 are taken. Moist or pasty colonies are possible yeasts, early mold growth, aerobic actinomycetes, or bacteria. These colonies are examined microscopically with a Gram stain or lactophenol cotton blue mount. Yeast colonies are inoculated onto appropriate yeast identification media (Table 8). Bacteria are identified as part of routine bacteriology procedures. Those that appear as thin branching filaments are stained with a modified acid-fast preparation and the procedure outline in Table 15A is followed for the identification of aerobic actinomycetes. When a mold (a waxy, velvety, powdery, or cottony colony) grows from skin scrapings, hair, or nails, the procedure for dermatophyte identification (Table 10) is followed. When molds are isolated from other specimens, precautions are immediately taken to rule out dimorphic systemic pathogens, as described in Tables 13A, 13B, and 13C.

YEAST IDENTIFICATION

The identification of yeasts (Tables 8 and 9) may range from a few simple tests to identify *C. albicans* and *Cr. neoformans* to a large battery of tests to identify

Table 7
FLOW CHART OF INITIAL STEPS

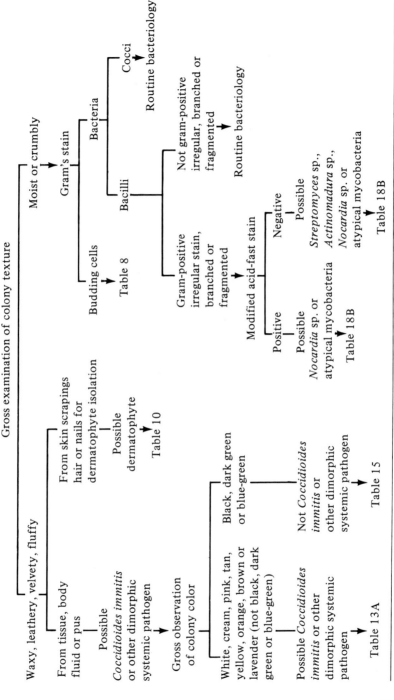

99

Table 8
FLOW CHART OF YEAST IDENTIFICATION

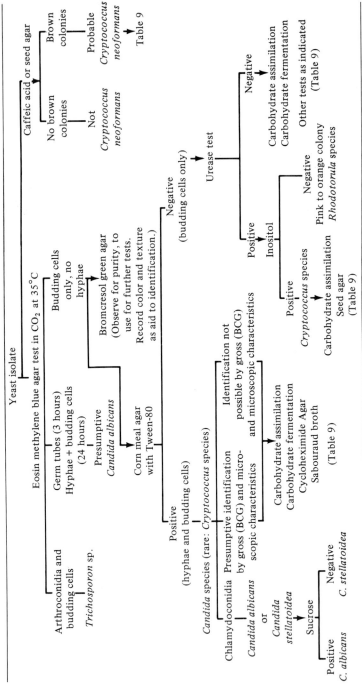

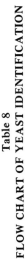

References:

Silva-Hutner and Cooper in Lennette et al. (1974).

UOHSC, Department of Clinical Pathology, Clinical Microbiology Division, Procedure No. 0318 (1979)) p. 29.

all yeasts that are commonly isolated in medical laboratories. Several commercial systems are now available that make it possible for smaller laboratories to do these identifications without maintaining a large inventory of media. We can recommend the BBL Mini-Tek system, the Corning Uni-Yeast-Tek system, and the Analylab API 20C system. Basically all systems follow the same general procedure of: (1) ruling out C. albicans and Cr. neoformans; (2) obtaining a pure culture; (3) observation of microscopic morphologic characteristics on corn meal or rice agar; (4) observing patterns of carbohydrate assimilations and reactions in a few other tests. Our own system is outlined in Table 8 and is discussed with some other possible choices in the paragraphs that follow.

The most rapid identification of C. albicans is done by observing the formation of germ tubes within three hours, either on serum at 35° to 37°C or on eosin-methylene blue agar (EMB) with tetracycline, incubated at 35° to 37°C in CO_2. At 24 hours on EMB, C. albicans can be identified by the production of hyphae and budding cells (Plate 4). Isolates not so identified on these media that must be further identified are next inoculated onto corn meal agar or rice agar, for observation of microscopic morphologic characteristics, and onto bromcresol green agar plates or other agar plates such as blood agar or Sabouraud agar, for obtaining isolated colonies in pure culture. When Cr. neoformans is strongly suspected, a seed agar or caffeic agar plate is inoculated to demonstrate the brown colonies of Cr. neoformans (Plate 3). Candida species will produce hyphae and budding cells on corn meal or rice agar, each having distinct morphologic characteristics (Plate 5). Other yeasts (Cryptococcus sp., Torulopsis sp., and Saccharomyces cerevisiae) produce only budding forms (blastoconidia).

Bromcresol green agar with Neosporin is used primarily as a screening test for obtaining a pure culture (see Plate 3). In a mixed culture, species of yeasts are differentiated by color, which is a function of pH, and by the morphologic characteristics of the colony. A laboratory worker will quickly learn to recognize the characteristic color and texture of each of the commonly isolated yeasts. These, together with the microscopic morphologic characteristics, seen on the corn meal or rice agar, may often lead to an early presumptive identification. For a definitive identification, carbohydrate assimilation and other tests must be done (Table 9). Yeasts that produce only budding cells on corn meal agar could be Cr. neoformans. The most specific screening test for Cr. neoformans is the production of brown colonies on seed agar (Plate 3). The most generally used screening test is the positive urease test. A negative urease test from a pure culture of yeast rules out Cryptococcus species. We have had some problems in detecting a positive urease reaction from strains of Cr. neoformans mixed with C. albicans, but we have had no problem in obtaining brown colonies on seed agar from the same mixtures.

The ability of a yeast to assimilate (use) carbohydrates is determined by the observation of growth when only a carbohydrate is provided in a simple yeast

Table 9
YEAST IDENTIFICATION CHART

Species	Eosin Methylene Blue (24 hours, 35°–37°C)	Bromcresol Green Agar (3 days, room temp.)	Corn Meal Tween-80 (1 week, room temp.)	Cycloheximide (Mycosel) (3 days, room temp.)
Candida albicans		White, pale yellow, or light green		+ (few are 0)
Candida stellatoidea		Pale yellow or light green		+
Candida pseudotropicalis	Metallic	Medium to deep blue-green, yellow border		+
Candida guillermondii		Blue-green; glossy; slow growth		+
Candida tropicalis		Yellow-green or gray-green; dry, fringed edge		0
Candida parapsilosis		Pale yellow or yellow-green reverse, blue-green center, sharp yellow border		0
Candida krusei		Yellow, pale green; flat; dry		0
Cryptococcus neoformans		Blue; moist; slow growth		0
Cryptococcus albidus var. *albidus*		Blue-green		0
Cryptococcus albidus var. *diffluens*		Yellow or blue; slow growth		0

Sabouraud Broth Film and Gas (1 week, room temp.)	Seed Agar (1 week, room temp.)	Urease Production (3 days, room temp.)	India Ink for Capsules	Growth at 37°C	Reduction of Nitrate	Ascospores (room temp.)
0	0	0	0	+	0	0
0	0	0	0	+	0	0
0	0	0	0	+	0	0
0	0	0	0	+	0	0
+ (narrow)	0	0	0	+	0	0
+/0	0	0	0	+	0	0
+ (wide)	0	+ or 0	0	+	0	0
0	+	+	+	+	0	0
0	0	+	+	0	+	0
0	0	+	+	+	+	0

(continued)

Table 9 (continued)

Species	Assimilation								
	Suc-rose	Dex-trose	Galac-tose	Mal-tose	Lac-tose	Raf-finose	Cello-biose	Tre-halose	Xylose
Candida albicans	+	+	+	+	0	0	0	+	+
Candida stellatoidea	0	+	+	+	0	0	0	+/0	+
Candida pseudotropicalis	+	+	+	0	+	+	+	0	+/0
Candida guillermondii	+	+	+	+	0	+	+	+	+
Candida tropicalis	+	+	+	+	0	0	+/0	+	+
Candida parapsilosis	+	+	+	+	0	0	0	+	+
Candida krusei	0	+	0	0	0	0	0	0	0
Cryptococcus neoformans	+	+	weak	+	0	+/0	+	+	+
Cryptococcus albidus var. *albidus*	+	+	0/+	+	+/0	+	+	+/0	+
Cryptococcus albidus var. *diffluens*	+	+	0/+	+	0	+	+	+	+

		Fermentation		
Inositol	Sucrose	Dextrose	Maltose	Lactose
0	0	AG	AG	0
0	0	AG	AG	0
0	AG	AG	0	AG
0	0/AG	0/AG	0	0
0	AG	AG	AG	0
0	A/0	AG/0	A/0	0
0	0	AG	0	0
+	0	0	0	0
+	0	0	0	0
+	0	0	0	0

(continued)

Table 9 (continued)

Species	Eosin Methylene Blue (24 hours, 35°–37°C)	Bromcresol Green Agar (3 days, room temp.)	Corn Meal Tween-80 (1 week, room temp.)	Cycloheximide (Mycosel) (3 days, room temp.)
Cryptococcus luteolus				0
Cryptococcus laurentii		Varied, green or blue		0
Cryptococcus uniguttulatus		Blue-green; slow; raised		0
Cryptococcus terreus				0
Rhodotorula glutinis		Pink or orange		0
Rhodotorula rubra				+/0
Saccharomyces cerevisiae		Deep blue to blue-green		0
Torulopsis glabrata		Bright yellow or deep green		0
Trichosporon cutaneum (beigelii)		Blue, green, or yellow; dry heaped; wrinkled		+
Trichosporon capitatum				+
Trichosporon penicillatum				+
Geotrichum candidum		Blue-green or yellow		0

Cycloheximide (Mycosel): + means growth; 0 means no growth

Sabouraud broth film and gas: + means both film and gas are produced; 0 means both film and gas are not produced

Seed agar: + means a brown colony grows; 0 means a brown colony does not grow

Sabouraud Broth Film and Gas (1 week, room temp.)	Seed Agar (1 week, room temp.)	Urease Production (3 days, room temp.)	India Ink for Capsules	Growth at 37°C	Reduction of Nitrate	Ascospores (room temp.)
0	0	+	0	0	0	0
0	0 (rare +)	+	+	+/0	0	0
0	0	+	+	0	0	0
0	0	+	+	+	+	0
0	0	+	0	0	+	0
0	0	+	0	+/0	0	0
0	0	0	0	+	0	+
0	0	0	0	+	0	0
+	0	+ or 0	0	+	0	0
+	0	0			0	0
+	0	0			0	0
+	0	0	0	+/0	0	0

Urease production: + means urease is produced (a pink color is seen); 0 means urease is not produced
India ink for capsules: + means a capsule is present; 0 means a capsule is not present
Growth at 37°C: + means growth at 37°C; 0 means no growth at 37°C
Reduction of nitrate: + means nitrate is reduced; 0 means nitrate is not reduced

(continued)

Table 9 (continued)

Species	Assimilation								
	Suc-rose	Dex-trose	Galac-tose	Mal-tose	Lac-tose	Raf-finose	Cello-biose	Tre-halose	Xylose
Cryptococcus luteolus	+	+	+	+	0	0/+	+	+	+
Cryptococcus laurentii	+	+	+	+	++	0/+	+	+	+
Cryptococcus uniguttulatus	+	+	0/+	+	0	+/0	+/0	+/0	+
Cryptococcus terreus	+/0	+	+/0	+/0	+/0	0	+	+	+
Rhodotorula glutinis	+	+	+/0	+	0	+	+	+	+
Rhodotorula rubra	+	+	+/0	+	0	+	+/0	+	+
Saccharomyces cerevisiae	+	+	+	+	0	+	0	+/0	0
Torulopsis glabrata	0	+	0	0	0	0	0	+	0
Trichosporon cutaneum (*beigelii*)	+/0	+	+	+/0	+	+/0	+	+/0	+
Trichosporon capitatum	0	+	+	0	0	0	0	0	0
Trichosporon penicillatum	0	+	+	0	0	0	0	0	+
Geotrichum candidum	+	+	0	0	0	0	0	0	+

Ascospores: + means ascospores are produced on ascospore agar; 0 means ascospores are not produced on ascospore agar

Assimilation: + means growth is seen, greater than negative control; 0 means no growth

		Fermentation		
Inositol	Sucrose	Dextrose	Maltose	Lactose
+	0	0	0	0
+	0	0	0	0
+	0	0	0	0
+	0	0	0	0
0	0	0	0	0
0	0	0	0	0
0	AG	AG	AG	0
0	0	AG	0	0
+	AG/0	AG/0	AG/0	AG/0
0	AG	0	0	0
0	0	AG	0	0
0	0	0	0	0

Fermentation: A means acid reaction is seen; G means gas is produced +/0, 0/AG, A/0, AG/0: means strains may vary, either reaction may occur nitrogen base. These tests may be done either in a liquid or a solid medium. The Wickerham tubes, with each individual carbohydrate incorporated into a basal liquid medium, are the most accurate and are easy to read. The API 20C test system is based primarily on the Wickerham tube system. Auxanographic plates, with the carbohydrate absorbed into a paper disc placed on a plate of previously inoculated agar, are almost as accurate as the tubes and are easier to prepare. The BBL Mini-Tek system is a modified auxanographic technique, as is the Corning Uni-yeast-Tek system. For all systems, the inoculum is a suspension of an isolated yeast colony in sterile distilled water or, in the case of the API 20C system, in a specially prepared medium that must be held at a temperature of 50°C during inoculation. These tests are all completed within 72 hours and are often definitive at 24 hours. Table 9 gives the carbohydrate assimilation patterns for many commonly isolated yeasts. Most yeasts will produce acid and gas on certain carbohydrates in anaerobic conditions (fermentation). Two fermentation procedures are described. One uses a liquid medium with indicator dye to detect acid reaction and Durham tubes to detect gas. The other uses fermentation tablets added to a water suspension of yeast with a Vaspar plug for anaerobiasis. A miscellaneous battery of additional tests is helpful. These include cycloheximide sensitivity, production of film and gas on Sabouraud broth, ascospore production, and the nitrate–Zephiran swab test to demonstrate nitrate reduction. Criteria used in these tests are given in Table 9.

Occasionally a yeast whose characteristics do not fit the criteria in the chart will be isolated. A close review of the morphologic characteristics on the corn meal agar plate will usually resolve this difficulty. Such a yeast may turn out to be *Candida* species, an early *Aureobasidium pullulans,* a moist *Trichosporon* species, a *Ustilago* or *Sporothrix* species, or some other yeast or mold. (Individual descriptions of these organisms are given in Chap. 5.) If an identification is not possible, the yeast may be reported simply as "Yeast isolated, not *Candida albicans* or *Cryptococcus neoformans.*" If a definitive identification beyond this is needed, the book by Lodder may be helpful. We are told that a new edition of this book to be edited by Kreger van Rij will soon be published. A useful service is being given by the Analytab Products Division of Ayerst Laboratories (producers of the API 20C test system). This company is developing a computerized data bank with results from many thousands of yeast isolates, and we have found them to be very responsive to requests for help with difficult isolates.

Each laboratory must develop its own policy about the need to do a complete identification on each yeast isolate. Yeasts isolated from blood or from spinal fluid or other normally sterile sites are certainly significant and need to be identified. Yeasts from respiratory secretions are not usually significant, except for *Cr. neoformans.* For this reason many laboratories will only screen for *Cr. neoformans* when a yeast is isolated from these specimens. From mucocutaneous, skin, and nail specimens, *C. albicans* is usually the only significant yeast isolate. Others are considered to be skin contaminants. The exception to this would be when a yeast, not *C. albicans,* is isolated repeatedly from a seriously compromised patient. A good working policy is to screen all yeast isolates for *C. albicans* and *Cr. neoformans.* These tests are within the capabilities of most clinical laboratories. Beyond this, it is important to remember that any yeast isolated from a seriously compromised patient is possibly significant.

DERMATOPHYTE IDENTIFICATION

Dermatophytes (fungi of the *Microsporum, Epidermophyton,* and *Trichophyton* genera that invade skin, hair, and nails) are identified by the recognition of gross and microscopic characteristics, often with the help of a few tests. The battery of media maintained for this purpose will depend on the needs and limitations of each laboratory. Table 10 is a flow chart giving steps that may be followed in these identifications. Table 11 gives the criteria for the identification of the eight most commonly isolated dermatophytes. These, as well as those less commonly seen, are described in greater detail in Chapter 5.

It is often possible to recognize a dermatophyte by gross characteristics alone. However, the fascination as well as the frustration of dermatophyte identification lies in the tremendous variability of isolates of the same species. Surprises are frequent. When mold growth is observed on a medium inoculated for dermatophyte isolation, a lactophenol cotton blue mount is made. Dermatophytes will be recognized, in general, by the presence of microconidia or of macroconidia that are characteristic of one of the dermatophyte genera (*Microsporum, Epidermophyton,* or *Trichophyton*). Many chlamydoconidia may also be present. When identifying structures are not observed, four different media may be inoculated: (*1*) potato dextrose agar for production of spores; (*2*) Dermatophyte Test Medium for a positive (red) reaction by dermatophytes and for inhibition of some saprophytic molds; (*3*) a corn meal agar slant with 0.2% dextrose for production of a red color by *T. rubrum;* (*4*) a Sabouraud agar slant as a control. These media will usually lead to an identification. When these fail, additional tests are done. These tests may include urease production and hair penetration test for *T. mentagrophytes* identification, *Trichophyton* vitamin agars to demonstrate nutritional requirements, and boiled rice for *M. audouini* identification.

A physician may ask a laboratory simply to report whether a dermatophyte is present. Because the therapy for infections by all dermatophytes is essentially the same and because of the time and expense often involved in a complete dermatophyte identification, this seems a reasonable request. However such a determination is often not as simple or as wise as it seems. Even an expert will find it difficult to distinguish the nonpathogenic *Trichophyton* species (i.e., *T. terrestre* and *T.*

Table 10

FLOW CHART DERMATOPHYTE IDENTIFICATION
(Identification of Mold Isolate from Skin, Hair, or Nails)

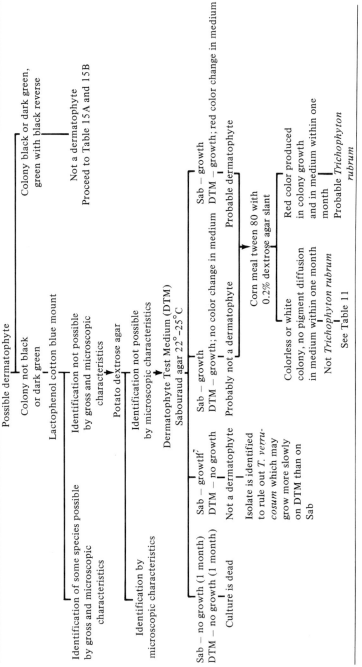

Possible dermatophyte

- Colony not black or dark green
  - Lactophenol cotton blue mount
    - Identification not possible by gross and microscopic characteristics
      - Potato dextrose agar
        - Identification not possible by microscopic characteristics
          - Dermatophyte Test Medium (DTM)
          - Sabouraud agar 22°–25°C

- Colony black or dark green, green with black reverse
  - Not a dermatophyte
  - Proceed to Table 15A and 15B

Identification of some species possible by gross and microscopic characteristics

Identification by microscopic characteristics

Sab – no growth (1 month)
DTM – no growth (1 month)
Culture is dead

Sab – growth
DTM – no growth
Not a dermatophyte

Isolate is identified to rule out *T. verrucosum* which may grow more slowly on DTM than on Sab

Sab – growth
DTM – growth; no color change in medium
Probably not a dermatophyte

Colorless or white colony, no pigment diffusion in medium within one month
Not *Trichophyton rubrum*
See Table 11

Corn meal tween 80 with 0.2% dextrose agar slant

Sab – growth
DTM – growth; red color change in medium
Probable dermatophyte

Red color produced in colony growth and in medium within one month
Probable *Trichophyton rubrum*

Reference:
UOHSC, Department of Clinical Pathology, Clinical Microbiology Division, Procedure No. 0318 (1979), p. 33

fischeri), and some of the *Chrysosporium* species from the pathogenic *Trichophyton* species. Those less experienced have mistaken *Alternaria, Acremonium, Aspergillus, Fusarium, Scopulariopsis* and *Verticillium* species for dermatophytes. All these may be positive on Dermatophyte Test Medium. Also, an increasing number of nondermatophyte molds are being reported as agents of skin and particularly, nail infections. These molds do not respond to dermatophyte therapy. They include *Scopulariopsis* sp., *Aspergillus terreus, A. flavus, A. glaucus, Alternaria* sp., and *Hendersonula toruloidea*. With these considerations in mind, the following criteria have, reluctantly, been established. If (*1*) fungal hyphae are seen in wet-mount (KOH) preparation of the specimen, (*2*) the Dermatophyte Test Medium is positive at one week, (*3*) the gross and microscopic characteristics are consistent with dermatophyte characteristics (hyphae light colored, macroconidia of the *Epidermophyton, Microsporum,* or *Trichophyton* species present, or microconidia borne directly on the sides of the hyphae or on short hyphal projections), the isolate may be reported as "presumptive dermatophyte." If the isolate is clearly not a dermatophyte, as determined by spore arrangements other than those of dermatophytes, or by the inhibition of growth on cycloheximide media, or by gross colony characteristics (blue-green or black colonies), it may be reported as "nondermatophyte mold." For the isolation of subcutaneous or systemic fungi that have disseminated to the skin, the physician should more appropriately submit a biopsy section or pus from draining sinuses and should alert the laboratory to the possibility of one of these infections.

SYSTEMIC FUNGI

Molds isolated from deep body tissues, fluids, or respiratory secretions are possible primary or opportunistic systemic pathogens. The tissue and cultural forms of these are given in Table 14 (dimorphic pathogenic fungi) and Table 16 (monomorphic systemic pathogenic fungi). The steps given in the flow charts, Table 13A, 13B, and 13C, are designed for the safe handling of any mold isolated from these sources.

The dimorphic pathogenic fungi are *Coccidioides immitis, Blastomyces dermatitidis, Paracoccidioides brasiliensis, Histoplasma capsulatum,* and *Sporothrix schenckii*. All these fungi are able to grow in the presence of cycloheximide at room temperature.* The dimorphism (two forms) of *C. immitis* is seen as a spherule form in tissue and an arthroconidium form in culture. The characteristic conidia, which are highly infectious, will usually develop in 7 to 10 days on all media. These organisms can be handled safely by wetting down the colony with sterile distilled water and adding a drop or two of Tween-80 before making a subculture

---

***H. capsulatum* and *B. dermatitidis* are inhibited on cycloheximide agar at 37°C.

Table 11
COMMON DERMATOPHYTE IDENTIFICATION CRITERIA

| Organism | Gross Colony Sabouraud's or Mycosel Agar | | |
| | Color | | |
	Front	Reverse	Texture
Epidermophyton floccosum	Yellow, grey, or grey-green	Tan	Velvety, folded, shaggy border, white tufts
Microsporum audouini	Buff, white, or tan	Pale yellow, tan or brown	Flat, velvety
Microsporum canis	White or tan	Pale yellow to deep lemon or orange-yellow	Velvety to fluffy, flat to folded
Trichophyton mentagrophytes (var. *mentagrophytes*	White to buff to cinnamon	White to tan, to yellow, to brown-red, to red	Powdery to velvety, becoming downy
Trichophyton mentagrophytes (var. *interdigitale*)	White to cream-color to pink	White to tan to yellow, to brown-red	Downy, flat with some powdery areas
Trichophyton rubrum	White	Yellow, to pale brown or deep red	Cottony, velvety or granular
Trichophyton tonsurans	Brown-red, buff, to cream to white	Tan to brown to red-brown	Velvety, flat to folded
Trichophyton verrucosum	White, buff, or yellow	White or pale yellow, deep penetration	Waxy to velvety, heaped
	Slow growth, may be faster at 37°C		

Critical characteristics are indicated in shaded areas.
Urea dextrose: + means urease is produced (a bright pink color is seen); 0

114

Table 11

COMMON DERMATOPHYTE IDENTICATION CRITERIA

Microscopic Characteristics

Microconidia	Macroconidia	Other
Lacking		Numerous chlamydoconidia
Lacking	Lacking on routine media	Chlamydoconidia
Scattered, 2–3 μm	Rough-walled	Few chlamydo- conidia
Abundant		Coiled spirals in some isolates
Less abundant	Infrequent	Spirals infrequent
	Develop at ends of thick hyphae	Conidia may be scarce
Variable	Smooth-walled Seen in few species	Coiled, spirals, rare
Few, 2–3 μm	Lacking	Chlamydoconidia in chains

means urease is not produced, no color change; +/0 means a weak reaction is seen (pale pink).

(continued)

Table 11 (continued)

Organism	Colony Color on Corn Meal Agar with .2% Dext.	Urea Dextrose Agar (5 days)	Hair Penetration (in vitro)
Epidermophyton floccosum	White or yellow	+/0	0
Microsporum audouini	White	+/0	0
Microsporum canis	White or yellow	+/0	0
Trichophyton mentagrophytes (var. *mentagrophytes*)	White	+	+
Trichophyton mentagrophytes (var. *interdigitale*)	White	+	+
Trichophyton rubrum	Red	0 (granular strains +)	0
Trichophyton tonsurans	White	+/0	0
Trichophyton verrucosum	White	0	0

Hair penetration: + means hair is penetrated; 0 means hair is not penetrated.
Trichophyton agars: +++ means good growth, over more than half of

Trichophyton Agars 2 to 3 weeks				
1 Casein (no vit- amins)	3 Thiamine and Inositol	4 Thia- mine only	Rice (boiled)	Source
+++	+++	+++	++	Anthropophilic Groin, feet, nails
+++	+++	+++	+/0	Anthropophilic Scalp, skin
+++	+++	+++	++	Zoophilic Scalp, skin
+++	+++	+++	++	Zoophilic Skin, scalp, nails Inflammatory
+++	+++	+++	++	Anthropophilic Skin, scalp, nails Mild infection
+++	+++	+++	++	Anthropophilic Skin, nails, beard (rarely hair of scalp)
+	+++	+++	++	Anthropophilic Scalp, skin
0	+	+ (50%) 0 (50%)	+	Zoophilic Scalp, skin

slant; + means poor growth, over less than half of slant; 0 means no growth.
Rice (boiled): + means growth; +/0 means poor or no growth.

Table 12

GROWTH PATTERN OF DERMATOPHYTES ON TRICHOPHYTON AGARS

Dermatophyte (Control No.)	Media with Casein Base					Media with Ammonium Nitrate Base	
	Casein Only (1)	Inositol (2)	Inositol Thiamine (3)	Thiamine (4)	Nicotinic Acid (5)	NH$_4$NO$_3$ Only (6)	Histidine (7)
T. verrucosum							
84%	0	+/0	+	0	0		
16%	0	0	+	+	0		
T. schoenleinii	+	+	+	+	+		
T. concentricum							
50%	++	++	++	++	++		
50%	+	+	++	++	+		
T. tonsurans	+ or +/0	+ or +/0	+++	+++	+ or +/0		
T. mentagrophytes	++++	++++	++++	++++	++++		
T. rubrum	++++	++++	++++	++++	++++		
M. ferrugineum	++++	++++	++++	++++	++++		
T. violaceum	+ or +/0	+ or +/0	++++	++++			
T. megninii						0	++++
Microsporum gallinae						++++	++++
T. equinum	0	0	0	0	++++		
T. soudanense	+++	+++	+++	+++	+++	0	0

Key: + = growth;   0 = no growth;   +/0 = weak growth or none

References:

UOHSC, Department of Clinical Pathology, Clinical Microbiology Division Procedure No. 0318 (1979), p. 89

Difco (1972), pp. 76–77

Georg and Camp (1957), p. 74

or a microscopic mount. For added safety, the culture may be completely in-activated by autoclaving or by adding formalin at least eight hours before a micro-scopic mount is made. (Before this is done, another viable culture must be available in case spores are not seen on the first mount.) It is not advisable to inoculate a cover-slip culture, a slide culture, or any kind of a Petri-dish culture until *C. immitis* is ruled out. When arthroconidia in chains are observed there is a strong possibility that the isolate is *C. immitis*. Demonstration of the tissue form (spherules and endospores) confirms the identification. Many molds are grossly and microscopi-cally similar to *C. immitis*. These molds include *Geotrichum* sp., *Trichosporon* sp., *Scopulariopsis* sp., and *Chrysosporium* sp. At high temperatures, *Ch. parvum*

Table 13A
DIMORPHIC SYSTEMIC PATHOGENS
Flow Chart: Initial Steps to Rule Out Dimorphic Systemic Pathogens[a]

ALL WORK IS DONE UNDER THE HOOD

Subculture to:

Sabouraud, (Emmons) agar slant, room temperature (control)
Cycloheximide agar slant, room temperature
Sabouraud, (Emmons) agar slant, 35°–37°C
Brain-heart infusion blood agar, 35°–37°C
Potato dextrose agar, room temperature

After one week, or when good growth is established on Sabouraud Emmons room temperature control slant, the following observations are made and steps are taken:

Cycloheximide agar, room temperature	
Growth	No growth
Possible: *Coccidioides immitis*	Not *Coccidioides immitis*
Histoplasma capsulatum	Not *Histoplasma capsulatum*
Blastomyces dermatitidis	Not *Blastomyces dermatitidis*
Paracoccidioides brasiliensis	Not *Paracoccidioides brasiliensis*
Sporothrix schenckii	Not *Sporothrix schenckii*
Table 13B	Tables 15A and 15B

[a]*Coccidioides immitis, Histoplasma capsulatum, Blastomyces dermatitidis, Paracoccidioides brasiliensis, Sporothrix schenckii*

produces adiaspores that are superficially similar to the spherules of *C. immitis*. These organisms are all described in Chapter 5. Huppert, Sun, and Rice (1978) have compared over 30 additional arthroconidium producing fungi to *C. immitis*.

The dimorphic forms of *B. dermatitidis, H. capsulatum, P. brasiliensis* and *S. schenckii* appear as a mold form on culture media at 22° to 30°C and a yeast form in tissue and on enriched culture media at 35° to 37°C. The identification of these fungi includes demonstrating both forms. When the gross and microscopic morphologic characteristics of an isolate are consistent with one of these pathogenic fungi, a subculture is made on enriched agar and incubated at 35° to 37°C, preferably in a CO_2 atmosphere. Several successive subcultures may be necessary to convert a mold form to a yeast form. It is also possible, particularly in molds isolated from respiratory secretions, that a yeast contaminant may be misinter-

Table 13B
DIMORPHIC SYSTEMIC PATHOGENS
Flow Chart to Rule out *Coccidioides immitis*
Growth on Sabouraud and Cycloheximide Agar at 22°–30°C
Growth on Sabouraud and Brain-Heart Infusion Blood Agar at 35°–37°C

ALL WORK IS DONE UNDER THE HOOD
Gross observation
of colonial morphologic characteristics

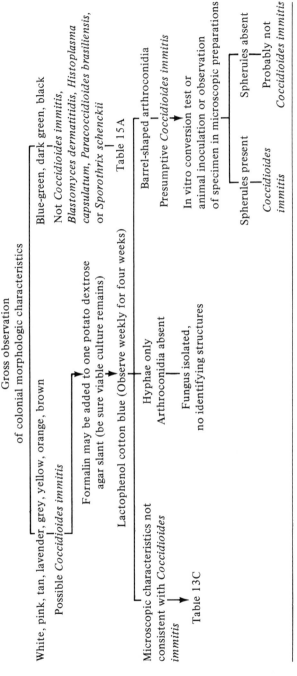

White, pink, tan, lavender, grey, yellow, orange, brown
Possible *Coccidioides immitis*

Formalin may be added to one potato dextrose
agar slant (be sure viable culture remains)

Lactophenol cotton blue (Observe weekly for four weeks)

Hyphae only
Arthroconidia absent

Fungus isolated,
no identifying structures

Microscopic characteristics not
consistent with *Coccidioides
immitis*
Table 13C

Blue-green, dark green, black
Not *Coccidioides immitis*,
Blastomyces dermatitidis, *Histoplasma
capsulatum*, *Paracoccidioides brasiliensis*,
or *Sporothrix schenckii*
Table 15 A

Barrel-shaped arthroconidia
Presumptive *Coccidioides immitis*

In vitro conversion test or
animal inoculation or observation
of specimen in microscopic preparations

Spherules present
*Coccidioides
immitis*

Spherules absent
Probably not
Coccidioides immitis

Reference:
UOHSC, Department of Clinical Pathology, Clinical Microbiology Division, Procedure No.
0318 (1979), p. 37

Table 13C
DIMORPHIC SYSTEMIC PATHOGENS
Flow Chart for Conversion of Mold Form to Yeast Form (Dimorphism)
of *Blastomyces dermatitidis, Histoplasma capsulatum, Paracoccidioides brasiliensis,* and *Sporothrix schenckii*
Growth on Sabouraud and Cycloheximide Agar at 22°-30°C

ALL WORK IS DONE UNDER THE HOOD

Step 1. Lactophenol cotton blue (LCB) from potato dextrose agar slant

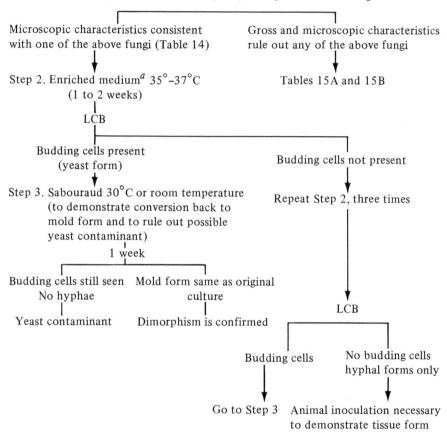

Microscopic characteristics consistent with one of the above fungi (Table 14)

Gross and microscopic characteristics rule out any of the above fungi

Step 2. Enriched medium[a] 35°-37°C (1 to 2 weeks)

Tables 15A and 15B

LCB

Budding cells present (yeast form)

Budding cells not present

Step 3. Sabouraud 30°C or room temperature (to demonstrate conversion back to mold form and to rule out possible yeast contaminant)

Repeat Step 2, three times

1 week

Budding cells still seen No hyphae

Mold form same as original culture

LCB

Yeast contaminant

Dimorphism is confirmed

Budding cells

No budding cells hyphal forms only

Go to Step 3

Animal inoculation necessary to demonstrate tissue form

[a] For *Blastomyces dermatitidis:* Pharmamedia or brain-heart infusion agar
For *Histoplasma capsulatum:* Brain-heart infusion agar with 1% sheep blood
For *Paracoccidioides brasiliensis:* Brain-heart infusion agar with 1% sheep blood
For *Sporothrix schenckii:* Brain-heart infusion agar or Sabouraud agar

Reference:

UOHSC, Department of Clinical Pathology, Clinical Microbiology Division Procedure No. 0318 (1979) p. 38.

121

Table 14
DIMORPHIC SYSTEMIC PATHOGENS

	Tissue Form			Culture Characteristics			
				Primary Isolation at 30°C		Subculture at 35° to 37°C	
Organism and Significant Culture Sites	Microscopic Preparations	Forms Seen (low power)	Other	Colony	Microscopic (high power)	Colony	Microscopic (high power)
Coccidioides immitis Blood Respiratory secretions Lung tissue Cerebrospinal fluid Pus and exudate Body fluids Granulomatous skin lesions	KOH, MSN, PAS, H&E (not seen on Gram's stain or India ink)	5–60 µm	Endospores in tissue form will produce germ tubes in saline. Arthroconidia in culture form are dangerous to inhale.	Waxy to fluffy to granular; white or cream or tan or pink, lavender or yellow No inhibition by antibiotic		Waxy to fluffy to granular; white, cream, tan or pink or lavender or yellow No inhibition by antibiotic	
Blastomyces dermatitidis Blood Respiratory secretions Lung tissue Skin Pus and exudate Bone Body fluids	KOH, MSN, PAS, H&E (not easily seen on Gram's stain or India ink)	8–15 µm	Budding cells of tissue form will produce germ tubes in saline.	Waxy with tufted spikey center, to velvety; white to cream to tan No inhibition by antibiotics at 22°–30°C		Waxy to pasty, heaped Pharmamedia is good medium for conversion Inhibited by cyclo-heximide at 37°C	8–15 µm

Organism / Specimen	Stains	Tissue form (size)	Notes	Mold form culture	Yeast form culture
Histoplasma capsulatum Blood Respiratory secretions Lung tissue Biopsy Bone marrow Urine Cerebrospinal fluid	Giemsa stain, MSN, PAS (not easily seen on Gram's stain or India ink, or KOH)	Intracellular 2–5 μm	Microconidia and tuberculate macroconidia in culture form are dangerous to inhale.	Velvety, cream to tan No inhibition by antibiotics at 22°–30°C 10–25 μm Buds 1–10 μm	Waxy to pasty, heaped Brain heart infusion agar with blood and cysteine is best Inhibited by cycloheximide at 35°–37°C 2–5 μm
Paracoccidioides brasiliensis Mouth, nasal or throat tissue Skin, exudate and drainage biopsy tissue	KOH, MSN, PAS, Giemsa stain	10–25 μm Buds 1–10 μm		Slow-growing, velvety, cream to tan No inhibition by antibiotics at 22°–30°C 2–10 μm	Waxy to pasty, heaped May be inhibited by cycloheximide at 37°C Same as *B. dermatitidis*
Sporothrix schenckii Pus, scrapings, biopsy specimen (subcutaneous form) Respiratory secretions (systemic form)	MSN and PAS, after treatment with malt diastase (not seen on KOH and Gram's stain)	1–3 × 3–10 μm	Asteroid bodies may be seen in tissues from test animals.	Leathery to waxy; cream, brown, or tan No inhibition by antibiotics Sympodioconidia 2–6 μm	Moist to pasty; cream to tan Brain heart infusion agar is best No inhibition by antibiotics 1–3 × 3–10 μm

KOH: 10% Potassium hydroxide wet mount

MSN: Methenamine silver nitrate stain

PAS: Periodic acid-Schiff stain

H&E: Hematoxylin and eosin stain

preted as the yeast form of a dimorphic fungus. This possibility is ruled out by subculturing the yeast colony to Sabouraud agar and incubating at room temperature to demonstrate a return to the mold form. When a mold form appears, dimorphism is confirmed and a final identification can be made. When dimorphism cannot be demonstrated in culture, it must be done by animal inoculation.

Many common molds have gross and microscopic characteristics similar to the dimorphic systemic pathogens. The *Chrysosporium* species may be particularly misleading. In addition, *Petriellidium boydii* has been confused with *B. dermatitidis. Sepedonium* sp. and *Scopulariopsis* sp. have been mistaken for *H. capsulatum.* Some of these species may be inhibited by cycloheximide at room temperature. Some are unable to grow at 37°C. None will convert to a yeast form at 37°C. Immunodiffusion techniques for the rapid identification of the dimorphic pathogenic fungi are now being reported (see references given in individual descriptions of *C. immitis, B. dermatitidis* and *H. capsulatum* in Chapter 5). Such techniques will hopefully reduce the need for tedious conversion procedures.

Monomorphic molds may be identified by following the steps in the flow charts, Tables 15A and 15B. Identifying characteristics of clinically important monomorphic molds and actinomycetes are given in Tables 16 through 18. The first step is to observe the microscopic morphologic characteristics in a lactophenol cotton blue or other microscopic mount. Often no identifying spores are present and the procedure given in Table 15A may be followed. The possibility of an aerobic actinomycete (*Nocardia, Actinomadura,* or *Streptomyces* species) is considered when the "hyphae" are in fact, very thin filaments, less than 2 μm in width. A modified acid-fast stain and hydrolysis tests are carried out and the steps, as outlined in Table 15A are followed. These tests will lead to a presumptive identification of these organisms. For a complete identification, the isolate may be referred to a major research center, such as the National Center for Disease Control in Atlanta, Georgia. When true hyphae (2 μm or wider) are present, identifying spores may be produced on potato dextrose or corn meal agar. When an isolate fails to produce spores on either of these media after four weeks, the possibility that it is a dermatophyte is considered and usually, after that, further efforts to achieve an identification are not justified.*

When spores are produced, the steps given in Table 15B may be followed. It may be necessary to make a cover-slip culture in order to observe the method of attachment of spores to hyphae or conidiophores. Many kinds of molds will be isolated and it is important that a reasonable effort be made to identify them.

---

*Diligent workers may want to experiment with media using other grains or vegetative or organic material. Rich forest soil or decayed bits of bark or leaves could be sterilized by autoclaving in a flask and inoculated with a mold isolate. Some of these isolates have been known to turn out to be mushrooms!

Table 15A
SYSTEMIC OR OPPORTUNISTIC MONOMORPHIC MOLD
ISOLATES FLOW CHART – SPORES ABSENT

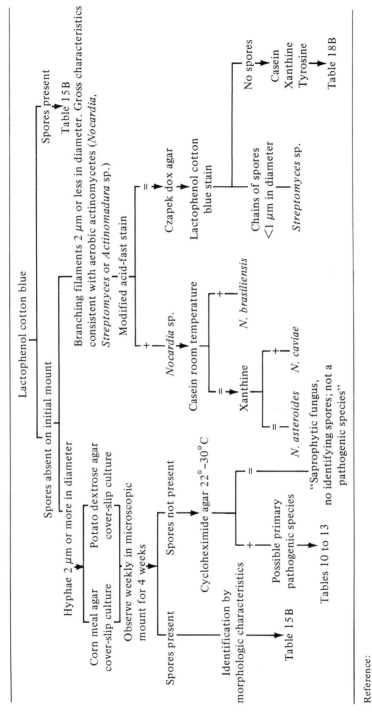

Reference:

UOHSC, Department of Clinical Pathology, Clinical Microbiology Division, Procedure No. 0318 (1979), p. 41

125

Descriptions and drawings of the most common of these molds are given in Chapter 5.

Aspergillus species isolated from clinical specimens, particularly from respiratory secretions, are often significant, the most common one being *A. fumigatus.* The steps given in Table 15B aid in identifying the different *Aspergillus* groups. A discussion of aspergillosis is given in Chapter 4, and the clinical significance of each *Aspergillus* group is briefly described in Chapter 5 as part of the individual descriptions.

Dematiaceous molds (brown, dark green, or black colonies with a black reverse) may be significant as the causative agents of chromomycosis, phaeomycotic cysts, phaeohyphomycosis, and eumycetoma. The most frequently isolated dematiaceous molds are the *Cladosporium* species. These molds are recognized by the presence of conidia with two or three dark connection points (disjunctors). The common species, which are rarely if ever pathogenic, are proteolytic, a characteristic that is demonstrated by liquefaction of Löeffler's serum or of 12% gelatin. The pathogenic species (*C. trichoides, C. carrionii,* and *F. pedrosoi*) are not proteolytic and will not liquefy Löeffler's serum slants or 12% gelatin deeps. Table 17 gives the characteristics of the *Cladosporium* species and some other dematiaceous molds. It may be necessary to use an oil immersion lens to distinguish between the simple budding of *Aureobasidium pullulans* from the short annellides (with roughened scars on the tips) of *E. jeanselmei* and the simple phialides seen in *W. dermatitidis,* or the phialides with flared openings seen in the *Phialophora* species. The most definitive references available on these species are two books by Ellis, *The Dematiaceous Hyphomycetes* (1971), and *More Dematiaceous Hyphomycetes* (1976).

The agents of mycetoma (both eumycetoma and actinomycetoma) occur in tissue form as grains, typical of the causative organism. The agents of eumycetoma are soil fungi; the most common in the United States is *P. boydii.* Table 18A gives the identifying criteria for this group of organisms. The agents of actinomycetoma belong to the genera *Nocardia, Actinomadura,* or *Streptomyces,* which are described in Table 18B.

The agents of mucormycosis are of the Zygomycete class in the order Mucorales and are recognized by rapid woolly or cottony growth, wide, rarely septate hyphae (10 to 20 μm in diameter), and endospore-filled sporangia. These agents usually belong to the genera *Absidia, Mucor,* or *Rhizopus* (Table 16).

Individual descriptions of pathogenic fungi and common molds and yeasts are given in Chapter 5, along with a guide to colony color and texture (Table 20) and a microscopic key (Table 21).

SURVEY OF FUNGI ISOLATED

It is helpful to the clinician when a mycology laboratory keeps a record of all fungi isolated from clinical specimens. The University of Oregon Health Sciences

Table 15B
SYSTEMIC OR OPPORTUNISTIC MONOMORPHIC MOLD ISOLATES FLOW CHART – SPORES PRESENT

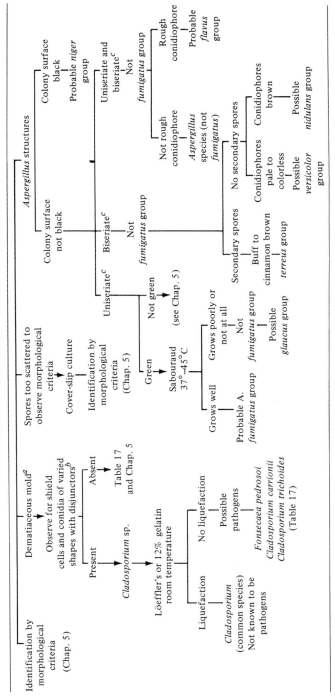

[a] Dark olive-green, grey-green, grey-black, or black mold colonies with black reverse.

[b] Disjunctors are growth points, observed as small dark spots on loose conidia. Shield cells are conidia with two growth points at one end and one growth point at the other end.

[c] *Uniseriate* and *biseriate* are defined for *Aspergillus* sp. in Chapter 5.

Reference:

UOHSC, Department of Clinical Pathology, Clinical Microbiology Division, Procedure No. 0318 (1979), p. 42

Table 16

MAJOR MONOMORPHIC PATHOGENIC FUNGI AND ACTINOMYCETES

Organism and Significant Culture Sites	Tissue Form		Other	Culture Form (growth from 22°–37°C)	
	Microscopic Preparation	Forms Seen		Colony	Microscopic

SYSTEMIC YEASTS

| *Cryptococcus neoformans* Blood Cerebrospinal fluid Lung biopsy tissue Respiratory secretions Pus and exudate Bone marrow Urine | India ink and muci-carmine (to demon-strate capsules); also KOH, Gram's, MSN and PAS, Giemsa stain |
Cells 4–20 μm | Brown colonies on Staib's (birdseed, caffeic acid) agar; urease positive; carbohydrate assimilation tests | Moist, glistening, white to tan

Inhibited by cycloheximide |
4–20 μm |
| *Candida albicans* Blood Urine Skin, nails Mucocutaneous areas Biopsy tissue Stool (Routinely isolated from sputum) | KOH, Gram's stain, MSN, PAS, India ink (no capsules); Giemsa stain |
Cells 3–8 μm | Germ tubes on serum and on EMB at 3 hours; hyphae and budding cells on EMB at 24 hours; chlamy-doconidia, hyphae, budding cells (blastoconidia) on corn meal agar after 3 days | Moist to pasty; white to cream-color, often with fringed border and down growth

1% of isolates inhibited by cycloheximide |
Cells 3–8 μm |

PATHOGENIC MOLDS

| *Aspergillus fumigatus* Blood Respiratory secretions Lung biopsy tissue Ear Scrapings from lesions | KOH, MSN, PAS, Giemsa stain (not easily seen on gram stain or India ink) |
Hyphae 2–10 μm in width | Common soil fungus, not a common resident of respiratory tract or of skin; growth at 56°C | Early cultures may be white, later green-gray, velvety

Inhibited by cycloheximide | |

Specimen	Stains	Microscopic morphology	Characteristics	Colony morphology	
Agents of Mucormycosis Necrotic, purulent material, Draining lesions, Biopsy tissue, Respiratory secretions	H&E, MSN, PAS, KOH (not easily seen on Gram's stain)	Hyphae 10–20 μm in width	Agents include: *Absidia* species, *Mucor* species, *Rhizopus* species; pathogenic species grow well at 37° C or higher	All agents have rapid growth, are white to gray, and fill tube or plate in 3 days; Inhibited by cycloheximide	
Agents of Chromomycosis (Several dark green or brown or black molds) Biopsy tissue, Pus, Skin	KOH, MSN, PAS, H&E, Giemsa stain (not as easily seen on Gram's stain)	12 μm sclerotic bodies 2–5 μm hyphae in width	Greenish-brown sclerotic bodies on Giemsa stain; agents include: *Fonsecaea pedrosoi, Fonsecaea compactum, Phialophora verrucosa, Cladosporium carrionii, Wangiella dermatitidis*	*Fonsecaea pedrosoi*: slow, dark green to brown, velvety; No inhibition by cycloheximide	
Petriellidium boydii Mycetoma, Skin scrapings, pus, biopsy tissue, Opportunistic Respiratory secretions, Cerebrospinal fluid, Body fluids	KOH, MSN, PAS, H&E, Giemsa stain (not as easily seen on Gram's stain)	Hyphae 5 μm in width	Granules seen in pus from draining sinuses; perithecia observed on corn meal agar	Gray, woolly surface with green-gray reverse; Inhibited by cycloheximide	

PATHOGENIC ACTINOMYCETES

Specimen	Stains	Microscopic morphology	Characteristics	Colony morphology	
Nocardia asteroides Blood, Respiratory secretions, Pus from draining sinuses, Aspirated fluid	Modified acid fast stain, Gram's stain, MSN, KOH, PAS, Giemsa	Filaments 0.2–2.0 μm in width	Granules may be seen in pus from draining sinuses	Mealy orange and white chalky colonies; Inhibited by antibiotics	Filaments 0.2–2.0 μm

(continued)

Table 16 (continued)

Organism and Significant Culture Sites	Tissue Form			Culture Form (growth from 22°–37°C)	
	Microscopic Preparation	Forms Seen	Other	Colony	Microscopic
Actinomyces israelii Blood Pus from draining sinuses Aspirated fluid (especially cervicofacial)	Gram's stain, MSN, H&E (not easily seen in other preparations)		Sulfur granules may be seen in pus from draining sinuses or in biopsy tissue; individual filaments resemble diphtheroids	Anaerobic or micro-aerophilic growth at 37°C	

KOH: Potassium hydroxide wet mount preparations

MSN: Methenamine silver nitrate stain

PAS: Periodic acid-Schiff stain

EMB: Eosin methylene blue agar with tetracycline incubated at 35°C in 5%–10% CO_2

H&E: Hematoxylin and eosin stain

130

Table 17
SOME COMMON AND SOME DEMATIACEOUS MOLDS
THAT ARE GROSSLY AND MICROSCOPICALLY SIMILAR

Organism	Pathogenicity	Cultural Characteristics	
		Colony	Microscopic
Initial Growth Is Yeastlike			
Aureobasidium pullulans	Common mold (Rare pathogen)	Early growth cream color, moist, becoming black, leathery, and glistening	
Exophiala (Cladosporium) werneckii	*Tinea nigra palmaris*	Early growth moist or waxy, black to brown, becoming leathery, or velvety	
Exophiala (Phialophora) jeanselmei	Maduromycetoma Common mold	Early growth may be waxy, glistening black or brown, becoming leathery or velvety	
Wangiella (Phialophora) dermatitidis	Chromomycosis Common mold	Early growth moist and runny, black or brown, becoming leathery and velvety; slow growth	
Mold Forms Only			
Cladosporium sp.	Common mold (Rare pathogen)	Velvety dark brown or dark green; moderate rate of growth; Proteolytic	
Cladosporium carrionii	Chromomycosis	Velvety, dark brown or dark green; no growth at 42°C; not proteolytic	
Cladosporium trichoides	Cerebral chromomycosis	Velvety dark brown or dark green; grows well 42°–45°C; not proteolytic	

(continued)

131

Table 17 (continued)

Fonsecaea pedrosoi	Chromomycosis	Velvety dark brown or dark green; slow growth; grows at 37°C; not proteolytic	
Phialophora verrucosa	Chromomycosis	Velvety dark brown or dark green; slow growth; grows at 37°C; not proteolytic	

For further information see individual descriptions in Chapter 5.

Center tally for the years 1976, 1977, and 1978 is given in Table 19. In addition, it is helpful from time to time to identify and keep a record of fungi that grow as contaminants on uninoculated media. These lists will vary from region to region. The isolation from a clinical specimen of a fungus that is rarely found as a laboratory contaminant becomes potentially more significant than the isolation of a mold that frequently occurs as a air-borne contaminant. It is emphasized that even the most common contaminants may, on occasion, become opportunistic pathogens. The laboratory is obligated to report to the physician all fungi isolated from clinical specimens. The physician determines the significance of each isolate. In Chapter 5 the known pathogenicity of each fungus described is briefly stated. We have found that physicians appreciate receiving all this information from a laboratory.

DOING THE JOB: PROCEDURES

This section includes the following specific procedures:

1. Transporting and processing specimens for fungal isolation.
2. Microscopic preparations for examination of fungal elements in specimens.
3. Microscopic preparations for examination of fungal isolates.
4. Differential tests.

Table 18A
IDENTIFICATION CRITERIA OF AGENTS OF MYCETOMA – EUMYCOTA

| Eumycetes | Color of Grain in Pus from Draining Sinus, Size and Texture | Size of Hyphae in Grain, Tissue or Culture | Stain in Tissue | Culture | | Geographical Distribution |
				Gross	Microscopic	
Petriellidium (Allescheria) boydii	White or yellow 0.5–3 mm soft	2 μm	PAS or MSN	White to grey-green, woolly surface, grey-green reverse	Single oval conidia Rare perithecia	U.S.A., Worldwide
Acremonium (Cephalosporium) falciforme Acremonium recifei	White or yellow 1–3 mm	2 μm	PAS or MSN	White, pale pink or tan, waxy or velvety	Slender phialides Conidia single or in clusters	U.S.A., Worldwide, So. America, Africa, India, Europe
Exophiala (Phialophora) jeanselmei	Brownish yellow to dark brown 0.5–2 mm soft to firm	2 μm	PAS or MSN	Dark brown or black to dark green leathery to woolly	Slender annellides Annelloconidia fall on sides of annellides, and are clustered at tip	Worldwide
Madurella grisea	Black 0.5–3 mm firm to hard	2 μm	PAS or MSN	Leathery, grey or black-brown. May have reddish-brown diffusable pigment. Does not assimilate lactose.	No phialides or spores on Sabouraud or corn meal agar	North and South America

(continued)

133

Table 18A (continued)

Eumycetes	Color of Grain in Pus from Draining Sinus, Size and Texture	Size of Hyphae in Grain, Tissue or Culture	Stain in Tissue	Culture		Geographical Distribution
				Gross	Microscopic	
Madurella mycetomi	Dark brown to black 0.5–5 mm hard	2 μm	PAS or MSN	Same as *M. grisea*; assimilates lactose	Slender phialides may be seen on corn meal agar, not on Sabouraud	Madagascar, India, Indonesia
Leptosphaeria senegalensis	Black 0.5–3 mm hard	2 μm	PAS or MSN	Dark greyish-brown to black. Black reverse.	Deep brown to black ascocarps, ascospores multicelled, 6–8	Senegal
Pyrenochaeta romeroi	Black 0.5–2 mm	2 μm	PAS or MSN	Dark greyish-brown to black, black reverse	Black pycnidia	Rare
Neotestudina rosatii	Buff to light 0.3–1 mm soft	2 μm	PAS or MSN	Tan to brown, deep black reverse	Ascocarps, 2-celled ascospores	Rare

For further information see Schneidau JD in Lennette et al. (1974), pp. 522–527.

PAS = Periodic Acid Schiff stain.

MSN = Methenamine Silver Nitrate stain.

Table 18B
IDENTIFICATION CRITERIA OF AGENTS OF MYCETOMA – ACTINOMYCETALES

Organism	Color of Grain	Size of Hypha	Modified Acid-fast[a]	Hydrolysis[b]			Urea[c]	0.4% Gelatin[d]	Colony and Temperature Characteristics
				Casein	Xanthine	Tyrosine			
Nocardia asteroides	White to yellow	1 μm	+ variable	0	0	0	+	0	Orange or white, grows at 46°C
Nocardia brasiliensis	White to yellow	1 μm	+ variable	+	0	+	+	++	Orange or white, no growth at 46°C
Nocardia caviae	White to yellow	1 μm	+ variable	0	+	0	+	0	Orange or white, may or may not grow at 46°C
Actinomadura pelletieri	Deep red	.1 μm	0	+	0	+	0	+	Chalky or granular, deep red. Optimal temperature 37°C
Actinomadura madurae	White to red	1 μm	0	+	0	+	0	+	Leathery or chalky, white to tan, pale orange, pink or red. Optimal temperature 37°C
Streptomyces somaliensis	Yellow to brown	1 μm	0	+	0	+	0	+	Cream or black, leathery to chalky. Optimal temperature 30°C
Streptomyces sp.	Nonpathogen		0	+	+/0	+	+/0	+	Leathery or chalky, white to grey, will grow at 10°C

[a]Modified acid-fast: + means modified acid-fast positive, 0 means not modified acid-fast.

[b]Hydrolysis: + means hydrolysis (clearing) is seen, 0 means hydrolysis is not seen.

[c]Urea: + means urea is split by urease and a red color is seen, 0 means urea is not split, no red color is seen.

[d]0.4% gelatin: 0 means no growth in 10 days, ++ means good growth in 10 days, + means poor or stringy growth in 10 days.

For further information see: Gordon in Lennette et al., pp. 175–188.

135

Table 19
FUNGI ISOLATED IN MYCOLOGY UNIT,
UNIVERSITY OF OREGON HEALTH SCIENCES CENTER

	1976		1977		1978	
	Clinics and Hospitals	Dermatology Clinic	Clinics and Hospitals	Dermatology Clinic	Clinics and Hospitals	Dermatology Clinic
Total Number of Specimens Submitted	2192	690	2188	477	2133	531
Acremonium sp.	4	2	2	5	3	3
Alternaria sp.	7	1	1	3	6	2
Aspergillus flavus[a]	4		2		2	
Aspergillus fumigatus[a]	38		23		22	
Aspergillus glaucus[a]	1		2		1	
Aspergillus nidulans[a]	3		2			
Aspergillus niger[a]	6		2		7	
Aspergillus terreus[a]			1			
Aspergillus versicolor[a]	3		5		2	
Aspergillus sp.	13	5	38	7	37	6
Aureobasidium pullulans	4		3	1	15	1
Beauveria sp.					3	
Botrytis	1		2			
Candida albicans	504	67	338	31	382	32
Candida guillermondii[a]			2			
Candida krusei[a]	9		15		13	
Candida parapsilosis[a]	43		7		12	
Candida pseudo-tropicalis[a]	1					
Candida stellatoidea[a]	1					
Candida tropicalis[a]	58		10		14	
Candida sps.	9		4		9	
Chaetomium sp.		1				2
Chrysosporium tropicum			1			
Chrysosporium pannorum	2	7		1	3	4

136

Table 19 (continued)

	1976		1977		1978	
	Clinics and Hospitals	Dermatology Clinic	Clinics and Hospitals	Dermatology Clinic	Clinics and Hospitals	Dermatology Clinic
Cladosporium sp.	5	9	12	4	19	2
Coccidioides immitis	4		4			
Cryptococcus albidus var. *albidus*[a]					2	
Cryptococcus laurentii[a]					1	
Cryptococcus neoformans[a]	6		1		10	
Cunninghamella sp.	1					
Curvularia sp.					1	1
Drechslera sp.					1	
Epicoccum sp.		1		3	2	
Epidermophyton floccosum		6		7	2	8
Exophiala jeanselmei	2		1	1		
Exophiala werneckii					1	
Fonsecaea pedrosoi	1					
Fusarium sp.	3			1	4	1
Geotrichum sp.	6		7		6	1
Microsporum canis	5	8	1	7	1	7
Mucor sp.	2	2	3	1	2	4
Neurospora sp.				1		
Nigrospora sp.	2					
Paecilomyces sp.		1	2	2	3	2
Penicillium sp.	53	10	25	11	51	14
Petriellidium boydii	2	1	4		2	
Phialophora verrucosa	2		1			
Phoma sp.	3		2	2	5	1
Rhizopus sp.	2				5	
Rhodotorula sp.	12	21	6	5	8	18
Saccharomyces sp.[a]	15		7			
Scopulariopsis sp.	6	4		4	2	7

(continued)

Table 19 (continued)

	1976		1977		1978	
	Clinics and Hospitals	Dermatology Clinic	Clinics and Hospitals	Dermatology Clinic	Clinics and Hospitals	Dermatology Clinic
Torulopsis glabrata[a]	77		36		41	
Trichoderma sp.	1				2	
Trichophyton mentagrophytes	2	19	2	16	3	16
Trichophyton rubrum	5	70	10	38	5	55
Trichophyton tonsurans	1	6		4		9
Trichophyton verrucosum				2		1
Trichosporon sp.	6	3	4	4	3	3
Verticillium sp.				1	3	1
Wangiella dermatitidis		2				9
Yeast, not *Candida*, *Cr. neoformans* or *T. glabrata*	6		6		5	
Yeast, not *C. albicans*[a]		18		25		23
Mold, no identification	17		12		70	7

[a]The identification of *Aspergillus* groups and of yeasts that are not *C. albicans* is not done in the Mycology Unit of the Dermatology Clinic.

Processing of Individual Specimens

The procedures outlined below, which are summarized in Table 4, are given for the transport and processing of different kinds of specimens for fungal isolation. These are the methods in use in our own laboratory. The choice of isolation media may vary within the guidelines that have been set out in the previous discussion. References are given with these procedures for alternative methods used by other large mycology laboratories.

BLOOD

PRINCIPLE

C. albicans, which is the fungus most commonly isolated from the blood, can be isolated on aerobic routine bacteriologic blood cultures incubated at 37°C for seven days. Other *Candida* species, *Cr. neoformans, Torulopsis glabrata*, and pathogenic molds may require four to six weeks of incubation at room temperature or 30°C before growth is observed. For this purpose, the biphasic medium developed by Roberts and Washington, described here, is more satisfactory. This medium is in general use in many large medical centers. Haley and Callaway (p. 36) recommend and describe a membrane filter technique for good and rapid isolation of fungi.

SPECIMEN

In a pilot tube containing 1.7 ml sodium polyanetholsulfonate (liquoid), collect 8.3 ml of blood.

TRANSPORTATION

By messenger: Immediate transportation to the laboratory.

By mail: Slides are prepared, as described below, and mailed in slide containers to the laboratory for staining and observation.

Fresh media is inoculated, incubated, and examined until growth appears, as described below. Under a hood, the isolate is subcultured to brain-heart infusion agar slant and mailed to the laboratory in a biohazard container.

PREPARATION OF SPECIMEN

Disinfect the rubber diaphragms of the collecting tube and two bottles of biphasic media by swabbing with alcohol and flaming. Using a sterile syringe and needle, aseptically withdraw 8 ml of blood from the collection tube.

MICROSCOPIC PREPARATIONS

1. Two slides are cleaned with alcohol, flamed, and cooled.
2. A drop of blood is placed on a slide. The second slide is pulled across the first to make a flat, even smear.
3. Preparation is fixed with methyl alcohol.
4. Giemsa stain.

MEDIA

Two biphasic blood culture bottles, each with brain-heart infusion agar slant (25 ml) and 30 ml of brain-heart infusion broth.

INOCULATION

Four milliliters of blood specimen are injected into each of the two bottles. If 4 ml or less are obtained, only one bottle is inoculated. If more than 4 ml but less than 8 ml are obtained, an equal amount of blood is injected in each of the two bottles. Place a vent (sterile-cotton-plugged needle) in each bottle.

INCUBATION

Incubate at room temperature ($22°$ to $25°C$) or in $30°C$ incubator for four weeks. Cultures are visually examined daily for growth, which may first be evident as tiny cloudy colonies in the broth on the surface of the blood layer. These colonies will usually spread rapidly to form colonies on the agar surface. When possible growth is visible, an aliquot of broth and blood is carefully removed with a sterile loop and examined microscopically by Gram stain or with lactophenol cotton blue. Following each daily examination, cultures are gently mixed to reinoculate the agar surface of the biphasic medium.

REFERENCES

1. UOHSC Department of Clinical Pathology, Clinical Microbiology Division, Procedure No. 0318, 1979, p. 3.
2. Haley and Callaway (1978), p. 36.
3. Roberts and Washington (1975).

BODY FLUIDS (PLEURAL, PERITONEAL, SYNOVIAL)

PRINCIPLE

Body fluids may be submitted for detection of systemic fungi.

SPECIMEN

Specimen is submitted in a sterile tube containing heparin or sodium polyanetholsulfonate (liquoid).

TRANSPORTATION

By messenger: Immediate transportation to the laboratory.

By mail: Two methyl-alcohol-fixed slides and fresh media inoculated, as described below, are air mailed in special biohazard containers.

PREPARATION OF SPECIMEN

If the body fluid appears purulent, it need not be centrifuged. If the body fluid appears clear, centrifuge for 10 minutes at 1,240 RPM. Remove sediment with a sterile disposable pipette using sterile technique.

MICROSCOPIC PREPARATIONS

1. KOH.
2. A circle is made on a slide with a wax pencil. A drop of sediment is placed in the center of the circle, allowed to air dry, and fixed with methyl alcohol.
   a. Gram stain.
   b. Other stains as indicated in special situations.

MEDIA

1. Sabouraud agar slant.
2. Brain-heart infusion agar slant.
3. Inhibitory mold agar slant.
4. Mycosel agar slant.

INOCULATION
About 0.1 ml of specimen is pipetted onto each slant.

INCUBATION
Incubate at room temperature (22° to 25°C) or in 30°C incubator for four weeks.

REFERENCES

1. UOHSC, Department of Clinical Pathology, Clinical Microbiology Division, Procedure No. 0318 (1979), p. 15.
2. Haley and Callaway, p. 40.
3. Wolf, Russell, and Shimoda, p. 332.

BONE MARROW

PRINCIPLE
When disseminated histoplasmosis or other disseminated fungal disease is suspected, a bone marrow aspirate may be submitted for fungal isolation.

SPECIMEN
Material is submitted in a pilot tube with polyanethosulfonate (liquoid).

TRANSPORTATION

By messenger: Immediate transportation to the laboratory.

By mail: Two methyl-alcohol-fixed slides, with fresh media inoculated as described below, are air mailed in special biohazard containers.

PREPARATION OF SPECIMEN

Spin 10 minutes at 1,240 to 3,000 RPM. Enter the pilot tube with a sterile disposable pipette and remove the thin layer of white cells (buffy coat), between the red cells and plasma, for microscopic examination. Complete specimen is used for inoculation of media.

MICROSCOPIC PREPARATION

Two slides are cleaned with alcohol, flamed, and cooled. A drop of buffy coat material is placed on one slide. The second slide is pulled across the first to make a flat, even smear. Allow to air dry. Fix with methyl alcohol.

1. Methenamine silver nitrate stain, or if this is not available
2. Giemsa stain*.
3. Other stains as indicated in special situations.

MEDIA

1. Sabouraud agar slant.
2. Brain-heart infusion agar slant.

INOCULATION

About 0.1 ml of the total specimen is pipetted onto each slant.

INCUBATION

Incubate at room temperature (22° to 25°C) or in 30°C incubator for four weeks.

REFERENCES

1. UOHSC Department of Clinical Pathology, Clinical Microbiology Division, Procedure No. 0318, 1979 p. 5.
2. Haley and Callaway (1978), p. 37.
3. Larsh and Goodman (1975), p. 515.
4. Wolf, Russell, and Shimoda, p. 338.

---

*A Giemsa stain is traditionally performed on bone marrow aspirates for detection of intracellular yeast cells of *H. capsulatum.* The following statement by Larsh and Goodman (1974, p. 515) agrees with our own observation. "*H. capsulatum* can be stained in tissue by many techniques, with the methenamine silver technique giving the highest contrast between fungal cell and host cell."

CEREBROSPINAL FLUID

PRINCIPLE

Cerebrospinal fluid (CSF) is most often submitted to a mycology laboratory for the detection of *Cr. neoformans. C. albicans,* and other systemic yeasts and molds may also be detected in these specimens. The inoculation techniques described below are generally performed in most large medical centers. Haley and Callaway (1978, p. 37) report a higher yield of fungal isolates using a membrane filter technique.

SPECIMEN

Cerebrospinal fluid (preferably 1 ml) is collected in a clean sterile tube.

TRANSPORTATION

By messenger: Immediate transportation to the laboratory.

By mail: Two heat-fixed slides and inoculated fresh media, as described below, are mailed to the laboratory in biohazard containers.

PREPARATION OF SPECIMEN

Material is spun down, at 1,240 to 3,000 RPM for 10 minutes, and the sediment is used for microscopic preparations and for inoculation of media.

MICROSCOPIC PREPARATION

This is to be read and reported immediately.

1. India ink. A drop of India ink (diluted 1 to 5) is placed on a slide. A drop of sediment is added. A cover slip is placed over the solutions, allowing them to run together.
2. A circle is made on a clean slide with a wax pencil. A drop of sediment is placed in the center of the circle, allowed to dry, and heat fixed.
   a. Gram stain.
   b. Other stains as indicated.

MEDIA

1. Sabouraud agar slant.
2. Brain-heart infusion agar slant.

INOCULATION

From 0.1 to 0.5 ml of sediment is pipetted onto each slant.

INCUBATION
Incubate at 30°C for four weeks.

REFERENCES

1. UOHSC, Department of Clinical Pathology, Clinical Microbiology Division, Procedure No. 0318, 1979, p. 6.
2. Haley and Callaway (1978), p. 37.
3. Wolf, Russell, and Shimoda (1975), p. 334.

EAR

PRINCIPLE
Fungal invasion of the ear is usually secondary to bacterial infection. Media with antibacterial antibiotics is used to suppress the bacteria. Media without the antifungal antibiotic cycloheximide is used to allow growth of common molds, particularly the *Aspergillus* species, which frequently invade the ear. In addition, a cycloheximide-containing medium is inoculated to allow growth of *C. albicans* and to suppress any common molds that may be present as colonizers.

SPECIMEN
The specimen is submitted on a swab in a sterile tube or on transport medium. A middle ear drainage specimen may be submitted in a sterile tube. When the specimen is very small 0.5 to 1.0 ml of sterile saline may be added.

TRANSPORTATION

By messenger: Transportation within 24 hours. Refrigeration is recommended.

By mail: Specimen is immediately air mailed in a biohazard container.

PREPARATION OF SPECIMEN

From a swab: Fungal preparations are made directly from swab.

From a scraping: 0.5 to 1.0 ml of sterile saline is added.

From secretion or drainage: If specimen is small, 0.5 to 1.0 sterile saline is added.

MICROSCOPIC PREPARATIONS
Material submitted on a swab is swabbed directly onto flamed glass slides.

1. Gram stain.
2. Other stains as indicated.

Scrapings, secretions, and drainage are pipetted onto two slides.

1. KOH or direct wet mount.
2. A third slide is pulled across the second slide to make a flat, even smear.
   a. Gram stain.
   b. Other stains as indicated.

MEDIA

1. Inhibitory mold agar slant.
2. Mycosel agar slant.

INOCULATION

1. From a swab: Swab material in a streak on surface of each slant.
2. From scraping in saline and secretion or drainage: About 0.1 ml of material is pipetted onto each slant.

INCUBATION
Incubate at 30°C for four weeks.

REFERENCES

1. UOHSC, Department of Clinical Pathology, Clinical Microbiology Division, Procedure No. 0318, 1979, p. 7.
2. Wolf, Russell, and Shimoda (1975), p. 336.

EYE

PRINCIPLE
Common molds, particularly *Aspergillus* species, *Fusarium solani, Acremonium* (*Cephalosporium*) species, and *Petriellidium boydii,* and yeasts, particularly *C. albicans,* may invade the eye following damage to the cornea by disease or by trauma. In addition, *Cr. neoformans, Rhizopus* species, and *Mucor* species, may disseminate to the orbit of the eye through the central nervous system. Because all of these, except *C. albicans,* are inhibited by cycloheximide, noncycloheximide media are required.

SPECIMEN

1. Specimen is taken with a platinum spatula, inoculated directly onto fresh media, and smeared on cool, alcohol-cleaned, flamed slides.
2. If direct inoculation is not possible, specimen (scraping or secretion) is sub-

mitted in a sterile tube. When the specimen is very small, 0.1 to 0.5 ml of sterile saline may be added.

3. Specimen may be submitted on a swab or in transport medium in a sterile tube.

TRANSPORTATION

By messenger: Immediate transportation to the laboratory.

By mail: Two heat-fixed slides and inoculated fresh media, as described below, are mailed in biohazard containers.

PREPARATION OF SPECIMENS

When direct inoculation and preparation of slides are not possible, specimens are handled in the following way:

From a swab: Fungal preparations are made directly from swab.

From a scraping: 0.5 to 1.0 ml sterile saline is added.

From secretions or drainage: If a specimen is small, 0.5 to 1.0 ml sterile saline is added.

MICROSCOPIC PREPARATIONS

Specimen taken directly with platinum spatula is smeared on three or more alcohol-cleaned, flamed, and cooled slides.

1. Wet mount, either with or without KOH, is made before material dries. The remaining slides are gently heat fixed.
2. Giemsa stain.
3. Gram stain.
4. Other stains as indicated.

Material submitted on a swab is smeared directly onto flamed and cooled slides. Slides are gently heat fixed.

1. Giemsa stain.
2. Gram stain.
3. Other stains as indicated.

Scrapings, secretions, and drainage are pipetted onto three or more slides.

1. Wet mount, with or without KOH, is made before material dries. The remaining slides are gently heat fixed.
2. Giemsa stain.
3. Gram stain.
4. Other stains as indicated.

MEDIA

1. Sabouraud agar slant.
2. Brain-heart infusion slant.
3. Inhibitory mold agar slant.

If routine bacteriology has not been requested,

4. Thioglycollate broth.

INOCULATION

1. From a swab: Swab material in a streak on the surface of each slant, and if thioglycollate is included, place the swab in broth.
2. From a platinum spatula: Media is inoculated directly, in order given.
3. From scrapings in saline and secretion or drainage: About 0.1 ml of material is pipetted onto each slant.

INCUBATION

Agar slants are incubated at 30°C for four weeks.

Thioglycollate broth is incubated at 37°C for one week.

REFERENCES

1. UOHSC, Department of Clinical Pathology, Clinical Microbiology Division, Procedure No. 0318, 1979, p. 8.
2. Haley and Callaway (1978), p. 40.
3. Rebell and Forster, in Lennette et al., pp. 482–486.
4. Wolff, Russell, and Shimoda (1975), p. 336.

NASAL, NASOPHARYNGEAL, MOUTH, AND THROAT

PRINCIPLE

Specimens from the nasopharyngeal area are submitted, along with specimens from other sites, as part of the diagnostic workup of possible disseminated fungal disease, particularly aspergillosis or candidosis.

Specimens submitted from the mouth or throat are primarily for the isolation of *C. albicans.*

SPECIMEN

Specimen is submitted on a swab in a sterile container or on transport medium.

TRANSPORTATION

By messenger: Transportation within eight hours. Refrigeration is recommended.
By mail: Specimen is immediately air mailed in a biohazard container.

PREPARATION OF SPECIMEN
Fungal preparations are made directly from the swab.

MICROSCOPIC PREPARATION
Swab material, evenly, onto a flamed glass slide.

1. Gram stain.
2. Other stains as indicated in special situations.

MEDIA

1. Inhibitory mold agar slant.
2. Mycosel agar slant.

INOCULATION
Material is swabbed onto the agar slants in the order given above.

INCUBATION

1. Nasal and nasopharyngeal: Incubate at 30°C for four weeks.
2. Mouth and throat: Incubate at 30°C for four weeks or until *C. albicans* is isolated.

REFERENCES

1. UOHSC, Department of Clinical Pathology, Clinical Microbiology Division, Procedure No. 0318 (1979), p. 9.
2. Haley and Callaway (1978), pp. 40 and 43.

PUS, EXUDATE, AND DRAINAGE

PRINCIPLE
Fungi isolated from these sources may have been introduced by trauma as agents of subcutaneous fungal diseases, such as mycetoma or chromomycosis, or they may be present as the disseminated form of a systemic fungal disease, such as, coccidioidomycosis, blastomycosis, histoplasmosis, cryptococcosis, aspergillosis, or other opportunistic fungal disease, including candidosis and mucormycosis. Because many of these fungi are inhibited by cycloheximide, a noncycloheximide medium is required.

SPECIMEN

Pus, exudate, or drainage is submitted in a sterile tube or syringe. When the specimen is very small, 0.5 to 1.0 ml of sterile saline may be added to assure continued moisture. When it is not possible to obtain the specimen in this manner, the specimen may be submitted on a sterile swab in a sterile tube or in transport medium.

TRANSPORTATION

By messenger: When *B. dermatitidis* or *H. capsulatum* are to be ruled out, immediate transportation is necessary. For isolation of other fungi, transportation is made within eight hours, with refrigeration recommended.

By mail: When *B. dermatitidis* or *H. capsulatum* are to be ruled out, two heat-fixed slides and inoculated fresh media, as described below, are sent in a biohazard container. For isolation of other fungi, specimen is immediately airmailed in a biohazard container.

PREPARATION OF SPECIMEN

From a swab: Fungal preparations are made directly from the swab.

From pus, exudate and drainage:

In a sterile tube: When the specimen is small, 0.5 to 1.0 ml of sterile saline may be added to assure adequate material for processing.

In a syringe: Specimen may be processed directly from the syringe. If the specimen is small, it may be transferred to a tube containing 1.0 to 2.0 ml sterile saline. Syringe is rinsed thoroughly with the saline before it is discarded.

MICROSCOPIC PREPARATIONS

Material submitted on a swab is smeared directly on flamed and cooled slides. Slides are gently heat fixed.

1. Gram stain.
2. Other stains as indicated.

Pus, exudate, or drainage is pipetted or dropped from a syringe onto three or more slides that have been flamed and cooled.

1. Wet mount or KOH is observed grossly for presence of granules (indicative of mycetoma) and microscopically for fungal elements.

The remaining slides are allowed to dry and are gently heat fixed.

2. Gram stain.
3. Other stains as indicated.

MEDIA

1. Sabouraud agar slant.
2. Brain-heart infusion agar slant.
3. Inhibitory mold agar slant.
4. Mycosel agar slant.

Most of these specimens are routinely cultured for both bacteria and fungi. The isolation of *Nocardia* and *Actinomyces* species is usually done as part of routine bacteriology. In instances when a purulent specimen is sent to the laboratory with a request for fungal culture only, the following are included for isolation of possible *Nocardia* and *Actinomyces* species.

1. Middlebrook 7 H10.
2. Thioglycollate broth.
3. Blood agar/LBA split, anaerobic.

INOCULATION

1. From a swab: Swab material onto the surface of each slant in the order given above.
2. From pus, exudate, and drainage: About 0.1 ml of material is pipetted onto each slant.

INCUBATION

1. Fungal media: Incubate at 30°C for four weeks.
2. Media to rule out *Nocardia* and *Actinomyces* species: Incubate at 37°C for 1 week.
   In CO_2: Middlebrook 7H10, Thioglycollate broth.
   Anaerobically: Blood Agar/LBA split.

REFERENCES

1. UOHSC, Department of Clinical Pathology, Clinical Microbiology Division Procedure, No. 0318 (1979), p. 10.
2. Haley and Callaway (1978), p. 40.
3. Wolf, Russell, and Shimoda (1975), p. 328.

SKIN, HAIR, AND NAILS

PRINCIPLE

These specimens are submitted primarily for the isolation of dermatophytes, that is, fungi belonging to the *Microsporum, Trichophyton,* and *Epidermophyton* genera, and for isolation of *C. albicans*. These fungi may be easily isolated on cycloheximide media (Mycosel or Dermatophyte Test Medium). Most saprophytic molds and yeasts that may be present as contaminants in these specimens will be inhibited by cycloheximide. Occasionally a nondermatophyte, such as *Scopulariopsis* sp. or *Aspergillus* sp., may be a primary invader of nails or of the skin. Because many nondermatophytes are inhibited by cycloheximide, clinical laboratories are required to inoculate both a cycloheximide and a noncycloheximide medium with these specimens. Media with antibacterial antibiotics greatly facilitate the isolation of fungi from these nonsterile specimens. *Pityrosporum orbiculare*, the causative organism of tinea versicolor, will not grow on routine cultures. It is identified by microscopic appearance.

SPECIMEN

Hair: Examine with Wood's light. If Wood's light is positive (green fluorescence) take fluorescing hairs. If Wood's light is negative, take dull gray hairs. Submit in a sterile container.

Nail: Scrape involved areas deeply or clip generous amounts and submit in a small sterile container.

Skin: Cleanse area with alcohol. Submit skin scrapings from edge of active lesion, or tops of vesicles removed with sharp blade, or material dug out from nail folds with a toothpick or a probe. Submit in a small sterile container.

From 5 to 20 pieces of skin, hair, or nail are acceptable. Specimens submitted on swabs are less satisfactory but are acceptable, particularly from babies and from moist, mucocutaneous areas.

Fluid from within a vesicle is not acceptable for isolation of dermatophytes (fungi that invade the skin, hair, or nails). The physician should be instructed to submit skin from the surface of a vesicle.

TRANSPORTATION

By messenger: Immediate transportation is preferable but not necessary. Fungi may be isolated after several weeks. Refrigeration is not necessary.

By mail: Specimens are mailed in small screw-capped jars, in well-padded mailing cartons.

PREPARATION OF SPECIMEN

A hemostat may be used for large pieces of nail or skin. Whole nails or large pieces of nail are ground in a homogenizer with a small amount of saline. A sterile loop is used for smaller pieces of skin, hair, or nails. The loop is flamed and moistened by placing it briefly on the surface of the agar. This provides a sticky surface to which the skin and hair will adhere.

MICROSCOPIC PREPARATIONS
10% KOH or KOH-DMSO.

MEDIA

1. Mycosel agar slant.
2. Inhibitory mold agar slant.

INOCULATION

Nails: Homogenized nails are pipetted evenly over slant. Up to five small pieces of nail are dug into the medium in even distribution.

Hair and skin scrapings: Up to five pieces are distributed evenly over the surface of the agar.

INCUBATION

Incubate at room temperature (22° to 25°C) or in 30°C incubator for four weeks or until a dermatophyte is isolated*.

REFERENCES

1. UOHSC, Department of Clinical Pathology, Clinical Microbiology Division, Procedure No. 0318 (1979), p. 12.
2. Haley and Callaway (1978), pp. 38–39.
3. Ray and Campbell, p. 4.
4. Wolf, Russell and Shimoda, pp. 341–347.

EXPECTORATED SPUTUM, NASOTRACHEAL ASPIRATE, AND TRACHEOSTOMY AND GASTRIC WASHINGS

PRINCIPLE

The presence of systemic pathogenic fungi in the lungs may often be demonstrated in expectorated sputum. Significant isolates are: *C. immitis, B. dermatitidis, H. capsulatum, A. fumigatus, Cr. neoformans, P. boydii, Sp. schenckii,* and any mold isolated repeatedly from specimens of the same patient. *C. albicans* is well established as part of the normal flora in the sputum of hospitalized patients and is rarely a significant isolate in these specimens. Nasotracheal aspirates and tracheostomy and gastric washings are submitted on occasion, usually when it is difficult to obtain an expectorated sputum. Because these specimens will usually

---

*When *C. albicans* is isolated from these specimens before four weeks, a dermatophyte may subsequently be isolated. It is our policy to hold all *C. albicans* primary isolates from these specimens for four weeks.

be contaminated with bacteria, it is recommended that media with antibacterial antibiotics be used for inoculation. When *Nocardia* sp. is to be ruled out, specimens are inoculated on routine bacteriology media.

SPECIMENS

Sputum deeply expectorated in the early morning is submitted in a sterile container on three separate days. Specimens that grossly and microscopically resemble saliva are not processed, unless specifically requested by the physician.

TRANSPORTATION

By messenger: When *H. capsulatum* or *B. dermatitidis* are to be ruled out, immediate transport is necessary. For isolation of other fungi and yeasts, transportation is made within four hours, with refrigeration required to avoid overgrowth of yeasts.

By mail: Two heat-fixed slides and inoculated fresh media, as described below, are air mailed in a biohazard container.

PREPARATION OF SPECIMENS

From 0.5 to 0.1 ml of saline may be added to sticky mucoid specimen to assist in breaking up clumps and in the pipetting of specimens. (A technique for digesting and concentrating sputum specimens with N-acetyl-L-cysteine or Dithiothreitol is described by Haley and Callaway. We have obtained satisfactory results without doing this.)

MICROSCOPIC PREPARATIONS

A drop of purulent (yellow, brown, or bloody) material is pipetted onto two slides. Avoid clear watery areas (saliva).

1. KOH preparation is observed before material dries (see Table 4 and Plate 1).

A third slide is pulled across the second slide to make a flat, even smear. The slides are allowed to dry and are then heat fixed.

2. Gram stain.

3. Other stains as indicated in special situations.

MEDIA

1. Inhibitory mold agar slant.

2. Mycosel agar slant.

When an overgrowth of *C. albicans* or other yeast is present, a fresh specimen may be submitted and inoculated as follows:

3. Yeast extract phosphate agar plate.

INOCULATION

Routine Media: About 0.1 ml of yellow-brown or bloody material is pipetted onto each slant in the order given above.

Yeast Extract Phosphate Media: A drop of the specimen is pipetted onto the surface of the agar. Inoculum is distributed evenly, using a bent glass rod. Immediately after inoculation a drop of concentrated ammonia is dropped slightly off the center of the plate and allowed to diffuse throughout the agar. Plate is sealed shut in four places.

INCUBATION
Incubate at 30°C for four weeks*.

REFERENCES

1. UOHSC, Department of Clinical Pathology, Clinical Microbiology Division, Procedure No. 0318 (1979), p. 14.
2. Haley and Callaway (1978), p. 41.
3. Smith and Goodman (1974), p. 276.
4. Wolf, Russell, and Shimoda, p. 328.

SPUTUM FROM BRONCHOSCOPY AND TRANSTRACHEAL ASPIRATE

PRINCIPLE

The presence of systemic pathogenic fungi and yeasts in the lungs may be demonstrated in specimens taken by the surgical procedures of bronchoscopy and transtracheal aspirate. Competing bacterial and yeast flora, which are usually present in expectorated sputum specimens, are very much reduced in these specimens. Media with and without antibiotics are inoculated. This makes it possible for *Nocardia* species to be isolated on the nonantibiotic mycologic media.

SPECIMEN

Bronchoscopy specimens and transtracheal aspirates are collected by surgical procedures and submitted in sterile containers.

TRANSPORTATION

By messenger: Immediate transport is necessary. If there is any delay, refrigeration is required.

---

*When *C. albicans* or other yeasts are isolated from these specimens before four weeks, incubation and regular observation of media for growth of molds is continued for four weeks. When *H. capsulatum* is suspected, incubation is extended to eight weeks.

By mail: Two heat-fixed slides and inoculated fresh media, as described below, are air mailed in a biohazard container.

PREPARATION OF SPECIMEN
If necessary, a small amount of sterile saline (less than 1 ml) may be added to break up a sticky specimen.

MICROSCOPIC PREPARATIONS
A drop of purulent (yellow, brown, or bloody) material is pipetted onto two slides.

1. KOH preparation, or if specimen is clear, a wet mount without KOH added (Plate 1).

A third slide is pulled across the second slide to make a flat, even smear. These two slides are allowed to air dry and are then heat fixed.

2. Gram stain.
3. Other stains as indicated in special situations.

MEDIA
1. Sabouraud agar slant.
2. Brain-heart infusion agar slant.
3. Inhibitory mold agar slant.
4. Mycosel agar slant.

INOCULATION
About 0.1 ml of material is pipetted onto each slant.

INCUBATION
Incubate at 30°C for four weeks or longer if *Histoplasma capsulatum* is strongly suspected.

REFERENCES

1. UOHSC, Department of Clinical Pathology, Clinical Microbiology Division, Procedure No. 0318 (1979), p. 15.
2. Haley and Callaway (1978), pp. 41 and 42.
3. Wolf, Russell, and Shimoda, p. 328.

STOOL OR RECTAL SWAB

PRINCIPLE
C. albicans may be part of the normal flora in stool or rectal specimens, but it is considered significant when this fungus is isolated in large numbers as the predomi-

nant organism. Other yeasts or molds isolated from these highly contaminated specimens are rarely significant.

SPECIMEN
Stool specimens are submitted in clean containers. Rectal swabs are submitted in transport medium.

TRANSPORTATION

By messenger: Immediate transport of stool specimens is recommended, with refrigeration to avoid overgrowth of yeast if there is a delay. Rectal swabs in transport medium are to be delivered within a reasonable time, no longer than eight hours.

By mail: Stool: A heat-fixed slide and inoculated fresh media, as described below, are sent in a biohazard container.

Rectal swab: The specimen in transport medium is mailed in a biohazard container.

PREPARATION OF SPECIMEN

Stool: Remove a portion of the specimen with a cotton swab, including any part that may be bloody and/or purulent.

Rectal swab: Remove the swab with a sterile, flamed hemostat.

MICROSCOPIC PREPARATION

1. Swab material evenly onto a flamed slide.
2. Gram stain.

MEDIA

1. Inhibitory mold agar slant.
2. Mycosel agar slant.

INCUBATION
Incubate at 30°C for four weeks or until *C. albicans* is isolated.

REFERENCES

1. UOHSC, Department of Clinical Pathology, Clinical Microbiology Division, Procedure No. 0318, p. 16.
2. Haley and Callaway (1978), p. 39.
3. Wolf, Russell, and Shimoda p. 331.

TISSUE (BIOPSY OR AUTOPSY SPECIMEN)

PRINCIPLE

To detect the presence of an invasive fungus it may be necessary to culture a piece of tissue taken at biopsy or as part of an autopsy procedure. Touch-slide preparations performed and stained in a microbiology laboratory may give a preliminary indication of fungal disease. These tissues are best examined microscopically in thin paraffin or frozen sections, a procedure done in an anatomical pathology laboratory. A KOH wet mount of these tissues is rarely satisfactory because the fibrous material present is not easily distinguishable from fungal hyphae.

Laboratory workers are alerted to expect any of the systemic pathogenic fungi in these tissues. Any yeast or mold isolated from these specimens is probably significant.

SPECIMEN

The specimen is submitted in a sterile container. The addition of a small amount of sterile saline or a piece of gauze moistened with saline will allow specimen to remain moist during rapid transport to the laboratory.

TRANSPORTATION

By messenger: Immediate transport is essential, with refrigeration required if there is any delay.

By mail: Two or more heat-fixed slides and inoculated fresh media, as described below, are sent in a biohazard container.

PREPARATION OF SPECIMEN

1. The specimen is placed on a flamed slide and minced with a sharp, flamed scalpel blade, or:
2. If the specimen is small (less than 3 mm square), grind in homogenizer with 0.1 to 0.5 ml of saline.

MICROSCOPIC PREPARATION

Minced or homogenized tissue is placed on a slide. A second slide is pulled across the first to flatten the tissues and to make an even smear.

1. Gram stain.
2. Methenamine silver stain.
3. Other stains as indicated in special situations.

MEDIA

1. Sabouraud agar slant.
2. Brain-heart infusion agar slant.
3. Inhibitory mold agar slant.
4. Mycosel agar slant.

INOCULATION

1. As many as 10 pieces of minced tissue are firmly placed and evenly distributed over the surface of the agar, or:
2. About 0.1 ml of homogenized specimen is pipetted onto each slant.

INCUBATION

Incubate at 30°C for four weeks, or longer if indicated.

REFERENCES

1. UOHSC, Department of Clinical Pathology, Clinical Microbiology Division, Procedure No. 0318 (1979), p. 17.
2. Haley and Callaway (1978), pp. 33 and 34.
3. Wolf, Russell, and Shimoda, p. 337.

URINE

PRINCIPLE

Urine specimens are submitted to a mycology laboratory to detect yeast infection of the kidney and also as part of the diagnostic workup for disseminated fungal disease. Disseminated histoplasmosis, coccidioidomycosis, cryptococcosis, and candidosis may be first detected in a urine specimen.

SPECIMEN

Ten milliliters of voided urine or catheterized urine is sent immediately to the laboratory in a sterile container.

TRANSPORTATION

By messenger: Immediate transport with refrigeration if there is a delay.

By mail: Heat-fixed slide and inoculated fresh media, as described below, are sent in a biohazard container.

PREPARATION OF SPECIMEN

When *B. dermatitidis* or *H. capsulatum* isolation is requested, a portion of the specimen is centrifuged for 10 minutes at 1,240 RPM. Sediment is withdrawn with a sterile pipette and used for microscopic preparations and for inoculation.

MICROSCOPIC PREPARATION

A circle is made on a slide with a wax pencil, then flamed. A drop of urine or of sediment is placed in the center of the circle, allowed to air dry, and heat fixed.

1. Gram stain.
2. Other stains as indicated.

MEDIA

1. Inhibitory mold agar slant.
2. Mycosel agar slant.

   If suprapubic or cytoscopy specimen:
3. Sabouraud agar slant.

INOCULATION

About 0.1 ml is pipetted onto each slant.

INCUBATION

Incubate at 30°C for four weeks.

REFERENCES

1. UOHSC, Department of Clinical Pathology, Clinical Microbiology Division, Procedure No. 0318 (1979), p. 18.
2. Haley and Callaway (1978), p. 43.
3. Wolf, Russell, and Shimoda (1975), p. 330.

VAGINAL AND CERVICAL SWABS

PRINCIPLE

Vaginal and cervical specimens are submitted to a mycology laboratory for the isolation of *C. albicans*. This may also be done as part of a routine bacteriology culture. When such a culture is not being done, fungal cultures are processed as described below.

SPECIMEN

The specimen is submitted on a sterile swab in a sterile tube with a drop or two of saline or on transport medium.

TRANSPORT

By messenger: Specimen is transported within four hours, with refrigeration if there is any delay.

By mail: Specimen on transport medium is immediately mailed in a biohazard container.

PREPARATION OF SPECIMEN
Swab is removed with a sterile flamed hemostat.

MICROSCOPIC PREPARATION
A flamed slide is heavily smeared with specimen from swab, air dried, and heat fixed.

1. Gram stain.

MEDIA

1. Inhibitory mold agar slant.
2. Mycosel agar slant.

INOCULATION
Material is swabbed evenly over the surface of the agar slants in the order given above.

INCUBATION
Incubate at 30°C for one week, or until *C. albicans* is isolated.

REFERENCES

1. UOHSC, Department of Clinical Pathology, Clinical Microbiology Division, Procedure No. 0318 (1979), p. 19.
2. Haley and Callaway (1978), p. 43.
3. Wolf, Russell, and Shimoda, p. 331.

Microscopic Preparations for Examination of Fungal Elements in Specimens

Fungi are recognized in these preparations by a variety of morphologic features, described in Tables 5A and 5B, which must be distinguished from other forms, such as fibrous tissue, cell walls, powder crystals, and pollen grains. Plates 1 and 2 illustrate fungal forms in some of these preparations.

GIEMSA STAIN

PRINCIPLE

This stain is used as a rapid stain for fungal elements and for the detection of intracellular *H. capsulatum* yeast cells in bone marrow smears.

MATERIALS

1. Giemsa solution (Matheson, Coleman, and Bell #257), freshly diluted, 1:10 with each use.
2. Methyl alcohol.

METHOD

1. Flood slide with methyl alcohol, one minute; pour off.
2. Flood slide with freshly diluted giemsa solution, five minutes.
3. Wash with water; air dry.

INTERPRETATION

Fungal elements are recognized by morphologic characteristics. Cellular contents appear deep blue and occasionally rose colored. Cell walls are unstained.

REFERENCE

1. Paik and Saggs (1974), p. 942.

GRAM STAIN

PRINCIPLE

Although Gram stain is not a satisfactory stain for observation of fungal elements, it is used routinely in all microbiology laboratories. *C. albicans* may often be identified in vaginal, throat, and mouth smears using this stain.

MATERIALS AND METHODS

This is the standard Gram stain performed in all microbiology laboratories.

INTERPRETATION (PLATE 2)

Fungal elements stain either gram-positive or gram-variable and are often difficult to recognize.

Decolorizing Gram Stain

When a special fungal stain is to be made and only a Gram-stained slide of the individual specimen is available, it is possible to decolorize the stain and perform whichever other staining method is required on the same slide preparation.

MATERIALS

One percent H_2SO_4, acetone, or acid alcohol.

METHOD

1. Flood slide with one of the above reagents for 30 seconds to 60 seconds.
2. Pour off.
3. Wash with running tap water.
4. Proceed with required stain.

INDIA INK PREPARATIONS FOR CAPSULES OF *CRYPTOCOCCUS NEOFORMANS*

PRINCIPLE

This is a rapid screening test used routinely for *Cr. neoformans* on all cerebrospinal fluid (CSF) specimens submitted for fungal isolation and on all yeast isolates suspected of being *Cr. neoformans*.

MATERIALS

1. India ink.
2. Slide and cover slip.

METHOD

1. Place a drop of material (if CSF or other fluid, use sediment after centrifugation) to be examined on a clean glass slide.
2. Add a drop of India ink. This may first be diluted with 5 parts distilled water to 1 part India ink.
3. Cover with cover slip.
4. Examine for budding yeast surrounded by a capsule under microscope at low power or high power, but not with oil.

INTERPRETATION (PLATE 2)

Positive: Budding yeast cells, 4-20 μm (mean 5-8 μm), surrounded by capsule, 1-20 μm (mean 3-6 μm) in width, appear brilliant white against the background.

Negative: No cells surrounded by capsules seen.

REFERENCES

1. Silva-Hutner and Cooper (1974), p. 492.
2. UOHSC, Department of Clinical Pathology, Clinical Microbiology Division, Procedure No. 0318 (1979), p. 49.

TEN PERCENT POTASSIUM HYDROXIDE (KOH)

PRINCIPLE

This is a rapid method for observing fungal elements in a temporary preparation. The KOH digests other cellular elements more rapidly than fungi, thus clearing the specimen and leaving fungal elements more clearly visible.

MATERIALS

1. 10% potassium hydroxide (glycerin may be added in equal parts for a permanent preparation).
2. Clean glass slide.
3. 22 × 30 cover slip.

METHOD

1. Place a portion of the material to be examined on a clean glass slide.
2. Add a drop of 10% KOH.
3. Place a cover slip on preparation and allow to stand at room temperature for 5 to 10 minutes. If kept for longer than 30 minutes, the slide is placed in a dish with a piece of moistened paper. Glycerine may be added. Heating is rarely necessary and may distort fungi in specimens.
4. Examine with a microscope under low power and reduced light.

INTERPRETATION (PLATE 1)

Positive: Fungal elements are seen.
Negative: Fungal elements are not seen.

REFERENCE

1. UOHSC Department of Clinical Pathology, Clinical Microbiology Division, Procedure No. 0318 (1979), p. 49.

KOH WITH DIMETHYLSULFOXIDE (DMSO)

PRINCIPLE

The dimethylsulfoxide included in this preparation is a penetrating agent that speeds the action of the KOH in digesting cellular elements and clearing the preparation so that fungal elements are clearly visible. It is used particularly for observation of thick specimens of nail and skin.

MATERIALS

1. 20% KOH–40% DMSO.
2. Slide, cover slip.

METHOD

1. Place a portion of the material to be examined on a clean glass slide.
2. Add a drop of KOH–DMSO.
3. Cover with a cover slip. The scales may be examined immediately. Thicker scales and nails are allowed to stand at room temperature for five to 15 minutes or until clearing is observed. If kept for more than 15 minutes, place slide in a Petri dish with moistened filter paper.
4. Examine under low power or high power microscopically. Do not use oil immersion.

INTERPRETATION (PLATE 1)

Positive: Fungal elements are seen.
Negative: Fungal elements are not seen.

REFERENCE

1. UOHSC, Department of Clinical Pathology, Clinical Microbiology Division, Procedure No. 0318 (1979), p. 50.

MAYER'S MUCICARMINE STAIN FOR
CRYPTOCOCCUS NEOFORMANS

PRINCIPLE

This stain is used in fungal preparations to demonstrate the capsules of *Cr. neoformans*.

MATERIALS

1. Coplin jars, each containing one of the following:
   a. Weigert's iron hematoxylin, freshly prepared.
   b. Metanil yellow solution.
   c. Dilute mucicarmine stain, freshly prepared.
2. Coplin jar for water rinse.

3. Wash bottles containing:
    a. 95% alcohol.
    b. Absolute alcohol.
4. Dropper bottle containing xylene.
5. Histoclad or Permount mounting medium.
6. Control slide of *Cr. neoformans.*

METHOD

1. Moisten slides in distilled water or tap water.
2. Weigert's hematoxylin, seven minutes.
3. Running tap water, five minutes.
4. Dilute mucicarmine solution, 30 minutes (check control slide), 60 minutes if necessary.
5. Distilled water, quick rinse.
6. Metanil yellow solution, one minute.
7. Distilled water, quick rinse.
8. 95% alcohol, quick rinse.
9. Absolute alcohol, two changes.
10. Xylene, two changes.
11. Mount in permount.

INTERPRETATION

Capsules of *Cr. neoformans* stain deep rose, with a diffuse border surrounding a clearly outlined budding or nonbudding cell.

B. dermatitidis and *H. capsulatum* stain weakly with this stain; cell borders are clearly stained.

REFERENCES

1. Emmons et al. (1977), p. 564.
2. UOHSC, Department of Clinical Pathology, Clinical Microbiology Division, Procedure No. 0318 (1979), p. 54.

MODIFIED ACID-FAST STAIN

Hank's Method

PRINCIPLE

N. asteroides, N. caviae, and *N. brasiliensis* will usually retain carbolfuchsin stain when decolorized with weak sulfuric acid. This stain can be done by the conventional Kinyoun technique, using 1% sulfuric acid in place of acid alcohol, or by Hank's method described below, with the sulfuric acid incorporated into methylene blue.

MATERIALS

1. Hank's carbolfuchsin solution.
2. Hank's methylene blue/sulfuric acid solution.
3. Positive control: *N. asteroides* culture.
4. Negative control: *Streptomyces* sp. culture.

METHOD

1. Several smears are made. Specimen is smeared onto glass slide. Positive and negative controls are smeared onto separate slides. Culture growth on agar or broth may be smeared onto the same slide as the positive and negative control. Slides are allowed to air dry.
2. Flood slides with Hank's carbolfuchsin solution and steam gently for 60 to 90 seconds. This can be done on a staining rack with flame applied from a Bunsen burner.
3. Wash slides with tap water.
4. Flood slides with Hank's methylene blue/sulfuric acid solution for two minutes. This procedure may be varied if controls are not working.
5. Wash with tap water, drain, and allow to dry.
6. Examine under oil immersion.

INTERPRETATION (PLATE 2)

Positive: Red-stained,* thin (less than 2 μm), branching filaments are seen. Because many stain "partially" acid-fast, irregular staining of the filaments frequently occurs.
Negative: Blue-stained filaments are seen.

REFERENCE

1. Haley and Callaway (1978), p. 48.

*Ascospores and bacterial spores also stain red, as do *Mycobacteria* sp., which stain as short, red bacillae.

PERIODIC ACID-SCHIFF STAIN (PAS)

PRINCIPLE

Yeast and dermatophyte hyphae are effectively demonstrated in tissues with this stain.

MATERIALS

1. Four Coplin jars, each containing one of the following reagents:
   a. Formalin-ethanol mixture.
   b. 1% periodic acid.
   c. Schiff's reagent brought to room temperature.
   d. Light green working solution.
2. One Coplin jar for water rinsing.
3. Three wash bottles, each containing one of the following:
   a. 70% alcohol.
   b. 95% alcohol.
   c. Absolute alcohol.
4. Xylol in a dropper bottle.
5. Histoclad or permount mounting medium.
6. Clean glass slide and cover slip.
7. Control slide.

METHOD

1. Prepare smear. Do not heat fix.
2. Using forceps, place slide in Coplin jars of reagents and tap water as indicated.
   a. Formalin-ethanol, 10 minutes. (This fixes the tissue.)
   b. Running tap water, 5-10 minutes.
      NOTE: Sections that have been embedded in paraffin and rehydrated are immediately placed in periodic acid.
   c. 1% periodic acid, 20 minutes.
   d. Running tap water, 10-15 minutes.
   e. Schiff's reagent, 20 minutes.
   f. Running tap water, 10-15 minutes.
   g. Light green working solution, 12 minutes.
3. Wash slide with two rinses each from wash bottles of 70%, 95%, and absolute alcohol in sequence.

4. Wash slide with two rinses each of xylol from dropper bottle.

5. Place drop of mounting medium on slide and cover with cover slip.

6. Allow to harden one hour before examining slide.

NOTE: Formalin-ethanol and periodic acid solutions may be reused as long as they are clear but for no longer than six months. Schiff's reagent is stored in the refrigerator and may be reused as long as it is clear but for no longer than six months. When it turns pink, it is no longer usable.

INTERPRETATION (PLATE 2)

1. Fungi stain a brilliant magenta.

2. Background is green.

3. Mucin also stains a brilliant magenta, making this stain unsuitable for staining undigested respiratory secretions.

REFERENCES

1. Emmons et al. (1977), p. 566.
2. UOHSC Department of Clinical Pathology, Clinical Microbiology Division, Procedure No. 0318 (1979), p. 57.

RAPID METHENAMINE SILVER NITRATE STAINING PROCEDURE

PRINCIPLE

This is the most sensitive of fungal stains. It is used in special instances when a fungus is strongly suspected to be present in a clinical specimen and has not been detected by other procedures. The method given here is a 20-minute procedure and produces the same results as the three-hour conventional Gomori methenamine silver nitrate procedure.

MATERIALS

1. Plastic Coplin jar containing freshly made methenamine silver nitrate solution:

3% methenamine	40 ml
5% silver nitrate	2 ml
5% Borax	3 ml
Distilled water	35 ml

Pour 40 ml of 3% methenamine into plastic Coplin jar. Add 2 ml of 5% silver nitrate. A white precipitate forms but will disappear with gentle shaking. Add 3 ml of 5% borax in 35 ml distilled water to methenamine silver nitrate solution.

2. Five Coplin jars containing the following solutions:
   a. 10% aqueous chromic acid.
   b. 1% sodium metabisulfite.
   c. 1% gold chloride.
   d. 5% sodium thiosulfate.
   e. Light green working solution.
3. One Coplin jar for water rinses.
4. Three wash bottles, each containing one of the following:
   a. 70% alcohol.
   b. 95% alcohol.
   c. Absolute alcohol.
5. Xylol in a dropper bottle.
6. Mounting medium (Histoclad or Permount).
7. Clean glass slide.
8. Cover slip.
9. Positive control slide.
10. Oven set at 95°C.
11. Teflon- or paraffin-coated forceps.

METHOD

1. Place plastic Coplin jar of methenamine silver nitrate solution in oven at 95°C.
2. Fix slides by heating, or with alcohol, or in paraffin sections.
3. Wet slides with water (or rehydrate paraffin-fixed slides).
4. With forceps, place control slide and test slide in Coplin jars in the following sequence for the times given:
   a. Chromic acid, 10 minutes.
   b. Running tap water, five seconds.
   c. 1% sodium metabisulfite, one minute.
   d. Hot tap water (until Coplin jar is hot), one minute.
   e. Methenamine silver nitrate solution at 95°C, 5–10 minutes. When sections become golden brown, remove control slide, wash with water and observe microscopically. When fungal elements are positive, reaction is done. Over-heating may cause silver to precipitate. Solution is discarded after use.
   f. Rinse in hot tap water and cool gradually to avoid cracking Coplin jar.
   g. Distilled water, rinse.
   h. 1% gold chloride, 10 seconds.

    i. Distilled water, rinse.

    j. 5% sodium thiosulfate, three minutes.

    k. Running tap water, 30 seconds.

    l. Light green working solution, 30 seconds.

5. Wash slide with two rinses each from wash bottles of 70%, 95%, and absolute alcohol in sequence.

6. Wash slide with two rinses of xylol from dropper bottle.

7. Place drop of mounting medium (Histoclad or Permount) on slide and cover with cover slip.

INTERPRETATION (PLATE 2)

Positive: Fungi are sharply delineated in black, with rose-lavender to gray center parts. Mucin and certain bacteria (including *Nocardia* species and the mycobacteria) will appear lavender, gray, or black. It is necessary to use morphologic criteria to rule out *Pneumocystis* sp., bacteria (including *Corynebacterium* and *Bacillus*), and tissue elements (including recticulum fibers and elastin fibers) that may take this stain.

NOTES:

1. The methenamine silver nitrate solution is used only once. The other reagents may be reused as long as they are clear, but for no longer than one month.

2. Fungi are able to grow in these reagents and can give some extremely confusing results. We have found that by adhering strictly to the following washing procedures and diligent changing of reagents every month, we have had no problems with fungal contaminants. Coplin jars are washed in hot soapy water, rinsed three times in hot tap water, and then three times in distilled water before new reagents are poured into them.

REFERENCE

1. Mahan and Sale (1978).

REHYDRATION OF PARAFFIN-EMBEDDED TISSUE

PRINCIPLE

Thin sections of paraffin-embedded tissues are often superior to routine smears for detection of fungal elements. The paraffin must be removed before staining.

MATERIAL

1. Paraffin-embedded tissue in sections fixed on a slide prepared by the pathology laboratory.

2. Three Coplin jars, each containing xylol.
3. Three wash bottles, each containing one of the following:
   a. Absolute alcohol.
   b. 95% alcohol.
   c. 70% alcohol.
4. Distilled water.

METHOD

1. Place slide in Coplin jar of xylol for 12 minutes. This removes the paraffin. Repeat, using two more jars of xylol.
2. Using forceps, rinse the xylol from the slide with two rinses each of the following, in sequence:
   a. Absolute alcohol.
   b. 95% alcohol.
   c. 70% alcohol.
3. Rinse the slide twice with distilled water.
4. Proceed immediately with appropriate stain.

REFERENCE

1. UOHSC Department of Clinical Pathology, Clinical Microbiology Division, Procedure No. 0318 (1979), p. 56.

Microscopic Preparations for Examination of Fungal Isolates

The following microscopic procedures may be useful for identifying a fungal isolate. These are arranged in alphabetical order.

COVER-SLIP CULTURE

PRINCIPLE

The cover-slip culture is used to observe the morphologic characteristics of a fungal isolate without disturbing the arrangement of spores on hyphal structures. It is easier and quicker to do than a slide culture and has the advantage that if the first preparation fails to demonstrate adequate sporulation, there are still three left to be examined at weekly intervals.

MATERIALS

1. Two tubes (18 ml) of agar (Sabouraud, corn meal, or potato dextrose as indicated).
2. Sterile Petri dish.
3. Sharp #11 blade on #7 Bard-Parker handle.
4. 22 × 22 mm cover slips.
5. 70% alcohol.
6. Lactophenol cotton blue.

METHOD

1. Agar is melted, poured into a Petri dish, and allowed to harden.
2. With a sharp blade, sterilized by flaming, a square (about 5 mm on all sides) is cut out of the agar and placed on the surface of the agar. Several of these squares (usually four) may be cut and lifted onto the surface of the agar, taking care to allow enough room between squares for the subsequent placement of cover slips.
3. A small piece of the fungus is inoculated onto one corner of the top of each square.
4. A cover slip, held with forceps, if flamed, briefly cooled, and placed on top of each inoculated square.
5. Plates are incubated, right side up, at room temperature for one week. If preparation is not satisfactory at this time, plates are reincubated and reexamined every week for four weeks before they are discarded.
6. A drop of lactophenol cotton blue is put on a clean glass slide. When corn meal agar is used, glycerine is used in place of lactophenol cotton blue.
7. The cover slip on which the fungus is growing is lifted gently from the surface of the agar block with forceps.
8. A drop of 70% alcohol may be put on the fungus side of the cover slip and allowed to drain off into a discard container. This fixes the preparation and prevents air bubbles.
9. Cover slip is placed on the drop of lactophenol cotton blue, fungus side down.

   NOTE: If the fungus has grown over the top of the cover slip as well as on the under surface, a second drop of lactophenol cotton blue may be placed on top of the first cover slip and a second cover slip (22 × 30 mm) added.

REFERENCES

1. Ray and Campbell, p. 6.
2. UOHSC Department of Clinical Pathology, Clinical Microbiology Division, Procedure No. 0318 (1979), p. 43.

LACTOPHENOL COTTON BLUE OR ANILINE BLUE: (TEASED PREPARATION)

PRINCIPLE

This is a time-honored mounting medium, routinely used for making microscopic preparations of mold isolates. It contains phenol, which serves as a fungicide; glycerine, which gives a semipermanent preparation; cotton blue* or aniline blue, which stains the outer wall of the fungus; and lactic acid, which acts as a clearing agent. A permanent preparation may be made by incorporating polyvinyl alcohol into the medium in place of glycerine, following a method described by Wolf, Russell, and Shimoda, p. 351.

MATERIALS

1. Lactophenol cotton blue* or aniline blue in a dropper bottle.
2. Glass slide and cover slip.

METHOD

1. A drop of lactophenol cotton blue or aniline blue is placed on a clean glass slide.
2. Using a flamed firm needle or blade (such as #11 blade on a Bard-Parker handle) a small amount of colony is cut from the culture, preferably from the most granular area. It may be advantageous to take a small amount of agar with the piece of mold colony.
3. This piece of mold is placed in the drop of lactophenol cotton blue or aniline blue.
4. The material is gently teased with the aid of a flamed dissecting needle.
5. A cover glass is pressed gently over the preparation, which may be gently heated if agar has been included in the specimen. This helps to spread the fungus evenly throughout the preparation and to remove bubbles.
6. Examine under the microscope with lowered light, at low power or high power.
7. A semipermanent preparation may be made as follows:
   a. All air bubbles are removed from preparation by pressure, gentle heating, or the addition of more lactophenol blue.
   b. Excess lactophenol blue is removed from around cover slip with 70% alcohol on a cotton swab.
   c. Cover slip is rimmed with clear nail polish and allowed to dry overnight. It is rimmed again with a second coat of nail polish.

*Cotton blue has been reported to be carcinogenic. The carcinogenic potential of aniline blue is not known.

NOTE: When it is necessary to use the oil immersion lens for observing these preparations, great care is to be taken in removing the oil from the cover slip.

REFERENCES

1. UOHSC, Department of Clinical Pathology, Clinical Microbiology Division, Procedure No. 0318 (1979), p. 52.
2. Wolf, Russell, and Shimoda, p. 351.

SCOTCH TAPE PREPARATION

PRINCIPLE

This is a rapid method for preparing a temporary microscopic mount of a mold without disturbing the arrangement of spores and hyphae.

MATERIALS

1. 10 cm strip of clear Scotch tape (No. 800, No. 600, or equivalent).
2. Microscope slide.
3. Lactophenol cotton blue or aniline blue.
4. Mold colony on agar plate.

METHOD

1. A drop of lactophenol cotton blue or aniline blue is placed on a microscope slide.
2. The Scotch tape is held between the thumb and forefinger of each hand with the sticky side down.
3. The center of the sticky side is pressed firmly onto the surface of the mold colony.
4. Tape is pulled gently away from the colony and placed on drop of lactophenol cotton blue or aniline blue.
5. Ends of tape will extend beyond the end of the slides. These are folded over the ends of the slide.
6. Preparation is observed through the microscope and then discarded.

REFERENCE

1. Koneman, Roberts, and Wright (1978), pp. 19 and 20.

SLIDE CULTURE

PRINCIPLE

A slide culture is made to observe the morphologic characteristics of a fungal isolate without disturbing the arrangement of spores and hyphae. The advantage of this relatively complicated procedure over the more simple cover-slip procedure is that it is possible to follow the morphologic development of spores and hyphae over a period of time in a given area of the preparation.

MATERIALS

1. 18 ml of agar poured and cooled in 100 X 15 mm Petri dish.
2. Sterile Petri dish, one for each culture.
3. Glass microscope slide.
4. Cover slip, 22 X 30 mm.
5. Sterile applicator sticks, 7 cm long.
6. Filter paper (Whatman #2 qualitative).
7. Clean dissecting needle.
8. Forceps.
9. Fresh Bard-Parker #11 blade on #7 handle.
10. Sterile distilled water.
11. 95% alcohol.

METHOD

1. Place one or two pieces of filter paper in bottom of sterile Petri dish and moisten with sterile water.
2. With flamed forceps, place two applicator sticks across filter paper.
3. With forceps, sterilize slide by flaming and place across applicator sticks.
4. With flamed Bard-Parker blade, cut a 10-mm square agar block and place gently on center of slide in Petri dish.
5. Inoculate a very small portion of fungal colony onto each of the four corners of the agar block.
6. With forceps, flame the cover slip and place gently but firmly on surface of agar block. Replace top of Petri dish.
7. Incubate, right side up, at room temperature.
8. Examine daily for growth and moisten filter paper when it becomes dry.
9. Remove slide from Petri dish at intervals, up to one month, and examine microscopically for sporulation.

10. Two semipermanent mounts may be made as follows:
   a. From cover slip:
      1. With forceps, cover slip is lifted gently from the surface of the agar.
      2. A drop of 95% alcohol is put on fungus side of cover slip and allowed to drain into discard container.
      3. Cover slip is placed in drop of lactophenol cotton blue or aniline blue on clean slide.
   b. From slide:
      1. With a clean blade, agar block is gently removed from slide and placed in discard container with disinfectant solution.
      2. A drop of 95% alcohol is put on fungal growth on slide and allowed to drain into discard container.
      3. A drop of lactophenol cotton blue or aniline blue is placed on fungal growth and covered with a clean cover slip.

REFERENCES

1. Koneman, Roberts, and Wright (1978), p. 21.
2. Wolf, Russell, and Shimoda, p. 373.

Differential Tests

A battery of differential tests is available to aid in identifying fungal isolates. The procedure for each of these tests in alphabetical order follows. They are listed by use in Table 6 (yeast, dermatophyte, dimorphic fungus, and mold identification).

ANIMAL INOCULATION

PRINCIPLE

On occasion it is necessary to use animal inoculation for the demonstration of the tissue phase of a dimorphic fungus. The following procedure is based primarily on the instructions given by Emmons et al. (1977). Immunodiffusion techniques that are now described for the identification of *C. immitis, B. dermatitidis,* and *H. capsulatum* will give a rapid identification and, it is hoped, eliminate the need for animal inoculation. References to these tests are given in Chapter 5 under individual descriptions of each of these organisms.

MATERIALS

1. Fungal isolate in pure culture on agar slant.
2. Sterile saline.
3. 5% hog gastric mucin.
4. Sterile screw-capped tube.
5. Two sterile 5 ml syringes.
6. Sterile needle #18.
7. Two sterile needles #21.
8. 70% alcohol.
9. Cotton balls.
10. Four mice.

METHOD
Inoculation of animals is performed in an isolation room in the animal quarters.

1. 5 ml sterile saline is added with a syringe and #18 needle to suspected fungal isolate, *under the hood,* and suspension is drawn back into the syringe. Suspension is added to 5 ml of gastric mucin in sterile tube.
2. The abdominal area of each mouse is cleaned with 70% alcohol.
3. With a #21 needle, each of the three mice is inoculated intraperitoneally with 1 ml of equal parts of the saline fungus suspension and 5% hog gastric mucin.
4. A control mouse is inoculated with sterile saline in the same manner.
5. Animal cages are cleaned thoroughly, bedding material is discarded, and fresh bedding material is used at least every three days.
   NOTE: Extreme caution is to be used in the handling of animals and animal cages in which animals infected with pathogenic fungi are held. Inoculated animals should be kept in isolation, away from other animals or people. According to Emmons, "Infectious forms of *Cryptococcus neoformans* and *Histoplasma capsulatum* are discharged in the exudate from ulcerated and crusted lesions about the eyes and nose of animals experimentally infected with these fungi." It is possible for the fungus to be passed into the sawdust or other bedding in the cage through the excrement or exudate of infected animals. *C. immitis,* in particular, can thus be converted from the noninfectious tissue form to the highly infectious filamentous form. Regular cleaning of the cages is recommended.
6. The three experimental mice are killed, one at four days and two at two weeks.
7. Impression smears and histologic sections of tissue are examined using H&E stain, PAS stain, and silver stain.

8. Cultures and microscopic preparations are made according to procedure for culture of tissue (biopsy and autopsy specimens) for fungal isolation.

INTERPRETATION

Positive: Fungal elements are observed.

Negative: Fungal elements are not observed.

REFERENCES

1. Beneke and Rogers (1971), p. 49.
2. UOHSC, Department of Clinical Pathology, Clinical Microbiology Division, Procedure No. 0318 (1979), p. 60.
3. Emmons, et al. (1977), p. 545.

ASCOSPORE PRODUCTION

PRINCIPLE

The perfect form of many yeasts, particularly the *Saccharomyces* species, may be demonstrated by production of ascospores on ascospore agar.

MATERIALS

1. Two ascospore agar slants.
2. Modified acid-fast stain reagents.
3. Positive control: *Saccharomyces cerevisiae.*

METHOD

1. Yeast isolate is streaked onto one slant of ascospore agar.
2. A control colony of *S. cerevisiae* is streaked onto the other slant of ascospore agar.
3. Incubate at room temperature for three days. Examine microscopically with a modified acid-fast stain. If the test is negative (regardless of the control test), reincubate and reexamine weekly for three weeks. At this time if the control is positive and the test isolate is negative, the test is negative.

INTERPRETATION

Positive: Red ascospores are seen among counterstained yeast cells.

Negative: No red ascospores are seen.

REFERENCES

1. Vera and Dumoff, in Lennette, et al. (1974), p. 925.
2. UOHSC, Department of Clinical Pathology, Clinical Microbiology Division, Procedure No. 0318 (1979), p. 62.

BROMCRESOL GREEN (BCG) AGAR WITH NEOMYCIN FOR DIFFERENTIATING SPECIES OF YEAST

PRINCIPLE

Various species of *Candida* and other yeasts produce colonies of specific color patterns and texture on bromcresol green (BCG) agar. This observation is useful in determining the purity of a yeast isolate and, with experience, in the early presumptive identification of some yeasts. Neomycin is added to the agar to reduce bacterial contaminants.

MATERIALS

Bromcresol green (BCG) agar plate.

METHOD

1. Plate may be divided into two sections for two isolates.
2. Each yeast isolate is streaked for purity on one section.
3. Incubate three days at room temperature. If growth is minimal, incubate until growth is easily observed.
4. Observe and record gross morphologic characteristics of isolated colonies; color and texture of surface, color pattern of reverse.
5. If culture appears to be mixed, the test is repeated from isolated colony types until a pure culture is obtained.

INTERPRETATION (PLATE 3)

Pure culture: Isolated colonies are similar in color and texture.

Mixed culture: Isolated colonies are varied in color and texture.

NOTE: Occasional strains of yeast, particularly some strains of *C. tropicalis,* will consistently produce more than one colony type. This phenomenon is apparently a kind of mutation. When it is observed repeatedly, it may be assumed that the culture is pure.

Presumptive identification of yeast isolate: See Table 9 and Plate 3.

REFERENCES

1. Harold and Snyder (1969), p. 8.
2. Haley and Callaway, p. 113.
3. UOHSC, Department of Clinical Pathology, Clinical Microbiology Division, Procedure No. 0318 (1979), p. 64.

CARBOHYDRATE ASSIMILATION TESTS

Wickerham Tube Method

PRINCIPLE

This test provides a definite biochemical basis for determining species of yeasts. The Wickerham tube method, given here, provides easy-to-read, clear-cut results. The API 20C system is a modification of the Wickerham tube method and provides a large battery of carbohydrates.

MATERIALS

1. Yeast nitrogen base control — liquid in screw-top tube.
2. Yeast nitrogen base (liquid in screw-top tube) with the following carbohydrates added:

Sucrose	Maltose	Cellobiose	Xylose
Dextrose	Lactose	Inositol	Other carbohy-
Galactose	Raffinose	Trehalose	drates as
			needed

3. Sterile distilled water in screw-top tube.
4. Sterile Pasteur pipette and bulb.

METHOD

1. A suspension of a pure colony of the yeast from a three-day-old culture is made in sterile distilled water (about #1 McFarlane density).
2. Two drops of this suspension are pipetted into each of the tubes containing carbohydrates and into the yeast nitrogen base control tube.
3. Tubes are loosely closed and incubated at 37°C for three days.
4. Observe turbidity of solution.

INTERPRETATION (SEE TABLE 9)

Positive: Solution is turbid (turbidity greater than negative control).

Negative: Solution is clear (turbidity equal to negative control).

NOTE: Solutions will usually be equally turbid. Occasionally, one of the tests will be less turbid than the others but more turbid than the control. Result is recorded as positive, and a note is made that the turbidity of this solution was less than the others. *Cr. neoformans* may assimilate galactose weakly. A weak false-positive maltose assimilation may occur because of impurities in the maltose.

REFERENCES

1. UOHSC, Department of Clinical Pathology, Clinical Microbiology Division, Procedure No. 0318 (1979), p. 65.
2. Silva-Hutner and Cooper, in Lennette, et al. (1974), p. 500.

Auxanographic Plate

PRINCIPLE

In this test the yeast is inoculated onto an agar plate. Carbohydrates are provided, usually in discs, at even intervals on the surface of the agar. Growth or absence of growth is observed. A nitrogen source may be provided either in the agar or in the carbohydrate discs. The method given here is based on the one described by Silva-Hutner and Cooper. Several others are in general use. Haley and Callaway suspend the yeast in the agar before the plate is poured and claim highly accurate results with their system. Huppert et al. incorporate bromothymol blue into the basal agar. A color change indicating growth may be observed before growth is visually apparent. The Corning Uni-yeast-Tek system is based on this method.

MATERIALS

1. Six tubes, each containing 20 ml of 2% Noble agar with yeast nitrogen base.
2. Two sterile Petri dishes, 150 × 15 mm.
3. Carbohydrate discs* as needed.

Sucrose	Maltose	Cellobiose	Others as required
Dextrose	Lactose	Inositol	
Galactose	Raffinose	Trehalose	

4. Heavy suspension of yeast from three-day-old colony in sterile distilled water.
5. Sterile cotton swab.
6. Two diagrams, one for each Petri dish, indicating placement of discs at even

*Mini-tek discs available from BBL.

intervals over the surface of the agar. Not more than six discs are placed on each dish.

METHOD

1. Three tubes of agar are melted and poured into each of the two Petri dishes. These are allowed to cool and harden.
2. With the sterile cotton swab, yeast suspension is distributed evenly over the surface of the agar.
3. Petri dish is placed over the diagram. Using flamed forceps, carbohydrate discs are placed in indicated places.
4. Plates are incubated at 30°C for 48 hours.
5. Plates are observed, against a dark background, for growth around each disc.

INTERPRETATION (SEE TABLE 9)

Positive: Growth
Negative: No growth.

REFERENCES

1. Silva-Hutner and Cooper, in Lennette et al., p. 500.
2. Haley and Callaway (1978), p. 116.
3. Huppert, Harper, Sun, et al. p. 22.

CARBOHYDRATE FERMENTATION TESTS

Durham Tube

PRINCIPLE

Fermentation tests aid in the identification of yeasts, but they are less reliable than assimilation tests. This method uses carbohydrate in a liquid broth with a Durham tube.

MATERIALS

1. Four tubes of fermentation broth with four Durham tubes, each containing one of the following carbohydrates:
    Sucrose   Dextrose   Maltose   Lactose
2. Yeast suspension in sterile distilled water. (Inoculation is the same as that used in assimilation tests.)

METHOD

1. Two drops of the yeast suspension are pipetted into each of the tubes containing carbohydrate.
2. Tubes are *tightly* capped and incubated at 37°C for three days. If results are indefinite at this time, tubes are reincubated and reexamined at regular intervals for up to three weeks.
3. Tubes are examined grossly for yellow color and for a bubble in the Durham tube. If there is no bubble in the Durham tube, the tube is gently shaken and observed for rising bubbles in the broth.

INTERPRETATION

1. Positive fermentation:
   a. Acid-Gas (AG): Solution turns yellow and bubbles are seen.
   b. Acid (A): Solution turns yellow. No bubbles are seen.
2. Negative fermentation: Solution is purple. Bubbles are not seen.

REFERENCES

1. UOHSC, Department of Clinical Pathology, Clinical Microbiology Division, Procedure No. 0318 (1979), p. 66.
2. Silva-Hutner and Cooper in Lennette et al. (1974), p. 501.

Rapid Method with Fermentation Tablets

PRINCIPLE

This is a rapid test using fermentation tablets and Vaspar to demonstrate the ability of certain yeasts to ferment carbohydrates under anaerobic conditions.

MATERIALS

1. Fermentation tablets*: glucose, maltose, sucrose, and lactose.
2. Heavy suspension of yeasts from three-day-old colonies in sterile distilled water. (Black lines on Wickerham card are completely obscured.)
3. Four 11-mm-diameter clean test tubes.
4. Melted Vaspar at 50°C.

METHOD

1. Approximately 1 ml of yeast suspension is placed in each of the four test tubes.

*Available from Key Scientific Products, Los Angeles, California.

2. Fermentation tablets are added, one to each tube.
3. With a Pasteur pipette, 1 ml of melted Vaspar, cooled to 50°C, is added carefully to avoid trapping any air bubbles.
4. Tubes are incubated at 35° to 37°C for 24 hours.

INTERPRETATION

Positive: Vaspar plug rises and is completely separate from liquid suspension.
Negative: Vaspar plug does not separate from liquid suspension.

REFERENCE

1. Huppert, Harper, Sun et al. (1975), p. 21.

CONVERSION OF ARTHROCONIDIUM FORM TO SPHERULE FORM OF *COCCIDIOIDES IMMITIS*

PRINCIPLE

It is reported by Sun et al (1976) that the arthroconidium form of *C. immitis* may be converted to the spherule form on defined media at 40°C in 20% CO_2, using a slide culture procedure. The conversion may also be accomplished on the same defined media according to the following procedure.

MATERIALS

1. Four glucose yeast extract agar slants.
2. One tube Converse liquid medium, modified.
3. Four tubes 1% ionagar slants.
4. Incubator set at 40°C with 15% to 20% CO_2.

METHOD

All work is done under the hood.
1. Production and suspension of arthroconidia.
   a. Four glucose yeast extract agar slants, numbered 1, 2, 3, and 4, are inoculated with the test culture and incubated at room temperature for 10 days to 2 weeks.
   b. For safety of workers, formalin may be added to Tube #1. Tube #1 with formalin is incubated at room temperature for 24 hours. The fixed culture is observed in lactophenol cotton blue preparation for the presence of arthroconidia.
   c. If arthroconidia are present, proceed to next step. If arthroconidia are

absent, incubate the remaining cultures and examine at intervals until arthro-conidia are observed.

 d. Using a Pasteur pipette and working under the hood, prepare a conidium suspension by adding several drops of Converse liquid medium modified to surface of viable glucose yeast extract culture.

2. Inoculation and incubation.

 a. Suspension is flooded over surface of four ionagar slants.

 b. Incubate at 40°C in 15% to 20% CO_2 for one to four weeks.

3. Observation of spherules.

NOTE: It is reported that only the noninfectious spherules are produced at 40°C. The following precautions, using formalin killed cultures, are given to guard against any accidental infection due to incomplete conversion of the highly infectious arthroconidia.

 a. After one week, **under the hood**, add 0.5 ml. formalin to one of the ionagar slants. Incubate at 37°C for 24 hours.

 b. With a Pasteur pipette, withdraw several colonies of mold in the liquid suspension.

 c. Place these colonies on a slide and observe in lactophenol cotton blue prep-aration.

 d. If test is negative, continue incubation of remaining cultures at 40°C in 15% to 20% CO_2 and repeat steps a, b, and c at intervals until test is positive or until all are negative at four weeks.

INTERPRETATION

Positive: Spherules containing endospores are observed.

Negative: No spherules are observed.

REFERENCES

1. UOHSC, Department of Clinical Pathology, Clinical Microbiology Division, Procedure No. 0318 (1979), pp. 68–69.
2. Sun, Huppert, and Vukovich (1976), p. 186.
3. Sun, Personal Communication (1980).

CONVERSION OF MOLD FORM TO YEAST FORM FOR IDENTIFICATION OF DIMORPHIC FUNGI

PRINCIPLE

 The dimorphic pathogenic fungi, *H. capsulatum, P. brasiliensis, B. dermatitidis,* and *Sp. schenckii,* may be converted from a mold (hyphal) form at room tempera-ture to a yeast form at 35°C.

MATERIALS

1. One of the following enriched agars as indicated.
   a. Brain-heart infusion agar or Eugonagar slant with 1% sheep blood.
   b. Brain-heart infusion agar slant.
   c. Pharmamedia slant, when *B. dermatitidis* is strongly suspected.
2. Sabouraud agar slant for control culture.

METHOD

1. A small amount of the fungus is inoculated onto enriched agar and onto Sabouraud agar.
2. Enriched agar is incubated at 35°C in 10% CO_2.
3. Sabouraud control culture is incubated at room temperature.
4. Enriched agar cultures are examined grossly and microscopically for the presence of budding cells at weekly intervals for four weeks.
5. Control (room temperature) cultures are examined for continued hyphal growth.
6. When yeast forms are present, dimorphism is confirmed by reconverting the colony to the filamentous form (see next procedure).
7. When hyphal forms only are observed, isolate is subcultured three successive times to enriched agar before dimorphism is ruled out.

INTERPRETATION

Budding cells, characteristic of each species, are recognized. (See Table 13.) NOTE: It may be extremely difficult to convert a filamentous form to a yeast form. Animal inoculation may be necessary.

REFERENCE

1. UOHSC, Department of Clinical Pathology, Clinical Microbiology Division, Procedure No. 0318 (1979), p. 69.

CONVERSION OF YEAST FORM TO MOLD FORM
FOR CONFIRMATION OF IDENTIFICATION
OF DIMORPHIC FUNGI

PRINCIPLE

C. albicans or other yeasts are often found in specimens submitted for fungal isolation, along with filamentous fungi. These yeasts have on occasion been misinterpreted as the dimorphic form of a filamentous fungus. Dimorphism of *H. capsulatum*, *B. dermatitidis*, *P. brasiliensis*, and *Sp. schenckii* is confirmed by demonstrating conversion of yeast phase to mold phase.

MATERIAL

Sabouraud agar slant.

METHOD

1. Yeast colony to be tested is inoculated onto a Sabouraud agar slant.

2. Incubate at room temperature for one week, or until growth is observed.

INTERPRETATION

Dimorphism is confirmed: Mold grows.

Dimorphism is not confirmed: A yeast colony continues to grow.

REFERENCE

1. UOHSC, Department of Clinical Pathology, Clinical Microbiology Division, Procedure No. 0318 (1979), p. 70.

CORN MEAL AGAR SLANT WITH 0.2% DEXTROSE FOR PRODUCTION OF RED COLOR BY *TRICHOPHYTON RUBRUM*

PRINCIPLE

   T. rubrum is characterized by development of a deep red pigment on the reverse of the colony. Many isolates do not produce this pigment on the routine Sabouraud or cycloheximide agar used for primary isolation from clinical specimens. On corn meal agar with 0.2% dextrose *T. rubrum* isolates will usually develop a deep red colony color. Other common dermatophytes do not produce this color on corn meal agar. (The nonpathogenic *T. terrestre* may also produce a deep red pigment. The nonpathogenic *T. fishcheri,* which is similar to *T. rubrum* in colony and microscopic characteristics, will not produce a red color.)

MATERIAL

Corn meal Tween-80 with 0.2% dextrose agar slant.*

METHOD

1. Inoculate a small piece of fungal isolate to be tested on corn meal Tween-80 agar slant.

*We have found that pigment is consistently produced by *T. rubrum* on prepared corn meal agar with 0.2% dextrose supplied by Difco. This pigment was not consistently produced by *T. rubrum* isolates on other prepared corn meal agar mixes.

2. Incubate at room temperature for one week and if test is negative, reincubate and observe weekly thereafter for four weeks.

INTERPRETATION

Positive: Colony develops a deep red pigment.

Negative: Colony remains colorless, pale yellow to brown.

Preliminary tests with five *T. rubrum* isolates using the erythritol albumen agar described by Kane have been extremely satisfactory. A deep ruby-red color developed in three weeks on the reverse of each isolate. Flourishing white cottony or velvety surface growth occurs, in contrast to the slow, flat, waxy growth that is seen on Difco corn meal agar with 0.2% dextrose.

REFERENCES

1. Kane, p. 238.
2. UOHSC, Department of Clinical Pathology, Clinical Microbiology Division, Procedure No. 0318 (1979), p. 71.

CORN MEAL AGAR WITH TWEEN-80 FOR HYPHAE AND BUDDING CELLS OF *CANDIDA* SPECIES

PRINCIPLE

Candida species are differentiated from *Cryptococcus* species, *Torulopsis* species, and *Saccharomyces* species by the development of hyphae as well as budding cells on corn meal agar with Tween-80. A rice extract agar (Haley and Callaway, p. 195) is also used for this purpose.

MATERIAL

Corn meal Tween-80 agar plate, freshly poured with 18 ml agar.

METHOD

1. Plate may be divided into quarters for four isolates.
2. A short streak (about 20 mm) is made with a loop carrying the inoculation across a quarter section.
3. Four stabs are cut crossways through the streak, using the side of a loop.
4. A cover slip is flamed, briefly cooled, and placed over the inoculum.
5. After inoculations are complete, the plate is sealed all around with tape.
6. Incubate at room temperature for three days.
7. Examine through the reverse side of the plate with the low-power objective.

If test is negative, plates are reincubated for another three to four days and examined again.

INTERPRETATION (PLATE 5)

Positive: Hyphae and budding cells are seen.

C. albicans: Hyphae, budding cells, and chlamydoconidia are seen.

Negative: Budding cells only are seen.

NOTE: An early presumptive identification of different *Candida* species may often be made by workers who have developed a skill in morphologic recognition.

REFERENCES

1. Dolan and Roberts in Washington (1974), pp. 155–156.
2. UOHSC, Department of Clinical Pathology, Clinical Microbiology Division, Procedure No. 0318 (1979), p. 72.

CORN MEAL AGAR WITH TWEEN-80
FOR SPORE PRODUCTION

PRINCIPLE

Sporulation of molds may be enhanced by growth on corn meal agar with Tween-80. This is particularly true of the dematiaceous (dark-colored) fungi.

MATERIAL

Follow procedure for cover-slip culture. Cover slip is mounted in glycerine instead of in lactophenol cotton blue.

REFERENCES

1. UOHSC, Department of Clinical Pathology, Clinical Microbiology Division, Procedure No. 0318 (1979), p. 73.
2. Koneman, Roberts, and Wright (1978), pp. 125–126.

CYCLOHEXIMIDE SENSITIVITY
FOR RULING OUT SOME
CANDIDA SPECIES

PRINCIPLE

Some *Candida* species are sensitive to cycloheximide. Susceptibility to cycloheximide may be used as a test in identification procedure.

MATERIALS

1. Mycosel agar slant.
2. Sabouraud agar slant.
3. Sterile distilled water in screw-top tube.

METHOD

1. A suspension of pure colony of *Candida* species is made in sterile distilled water (about No. 1 McFarlane density).
2. A loopful of suspension is streaked onto the agar slants in the following sequence to avoid transfer of cycloheximide to control slant.
   a. Sabouraud agar slant.
   b. Mycosel agar slant.
3. Incubate at room temperature for three days.
4. Observe both cultures for growth and record as (=) or (+ to ++++).

INTERPRETATION

Positive: Growth on the mycosel equal to growth on the Sabouraud agar slant.

Negative: No growth on the mycosel, or less growth on mycosel than on the Sabouraud.

NOTE: After three days, the sensitive strains may begin to grow on mycosel, and the test is read as negative when there is less growth on mycosel than on the Sabouraud agar control slant.

The following *Candida* species usually grow well on mycosel:

C. albicans (1% are sensitive to cycloheximide and will not grow);

C. pseudotropicalis;

C. guillermondii;

C. stellatoidea.

The following *Candida* species are inhibited on (sensitive to) mycosel.

C. parapsilosis

C. tropicalis;

C. krusei.

REFERENCE

1. UOHSC, Department of Clinical Pathology, Clinical Microbiology Division, Procedure No. 0318 (1979), p. 80.

CYCLOHEXIMIDE TOLERANCE FOR IDENTIFYING A POSSIBLE MAJOR PATHOGENIC FUNGUS

PRINCIPLE

This is a useful test to determine whether a mold isolate could be one of the major pathogenic fungi that is able to grow in the presence of cycloheximide.

MATERIAL

1. Mycosel agar slant.
2. Sabouraud agar slant for control.

METHOD

1. An equal amount of fungus is inoculated onto each slant.
2. Incubate at room temperature until Sabouraud control shows growth, up to four weeks.
3. Examine both slants for growth and record as a (=) or (+ to ++++).

INTERPRETATION

Fungi that are tolerant of cycloheximide will grow as well on mycosel as on Sabouraud. Those that are sensitive will grow less well or not at all on mycosel.

Pathogenic fungi that are able to grow on mycosel:

Microsporum species

Trichophyton species

Epidermophyton floccosum

H. capsulatum at room temperature (inhibited by cycloheximide at 37°C)

B. dermatitidis at room temperature (inhibited by cycloheximide at 37°C)

C. immitis

F. pedrosoi

Sp. schenckii

C. albicans

Pathogenic fungi that are inhibited by cycloheximide:

P. boydii

A. fumigatus

A. flavus

Aspergillus species

Cr. neoformans

T. glabrata

Many common molds and yeasts that may be opportunists:

Most agents of mycetoma

Most agents of keratomycosis

Also *Nocardia, Actinomadura,* and *Streptomyces* species

REFERENCES

1. UOHSC, Department of Clinical Pathology, Clinical Microbiology Division, Procedure No. 0318 (1979), pp. 81–82.
2. Wolf, Russell, and Shimoda (1975), pp. 359–360.

DERMATOPHYTE TEST MEDIUM (DTM) FOR THE PRESUMPTIVE IDENTIFICATION OF DERMATOPHYTES

PRINCIPLE

DTM is a selective medium containing cycloheximide, which inhibits the growth of many common molds (see cycloheximide tolerance and sensitivity tests), and gentamicin and tetracycline, which inhibit most bacterial contaminants. The phenol red indicator detects the production of alkali by the dermatophytes and related fungi. This test is more useful as a general screening test than as an identification test. Occasional dermatophytes will be slow to give a color reaction, and several molds that are not dermatophytes *will* give a color reaction. For example, the fungi listed below have been observed to produce a positive (red) color reaction on DTM within one week.

Dermatophytes	*Nondermatophytes*
E. floccosum	*Acremonium* sp.
Microsporum sp.	*B. dermatitidis*
Trichophyton sp.	*Chrysosporium* sp.
	E. jeanselmei
	F. pedrosoi
	H. capsulatum
	P. boydii
	Ph. verrucosa
	Scopulariopsis sp.
	S. schenckii
	Verticillium sp.

MATERIALS

1. DTM agar slant.
2. Sabouraud agar slant for control.

METHOD

1. A small amount of fungus is placed on the surface of the DTM slant.
2. A small amount of fungus is placed on the surface of the Sabouraud agar slant.
3. Incubate both cultures at room temperature for one week, or until growth is observed on the control slant after one week.

INTERPRETATION

Positive: Red color is observed around fungal growth on DTM agar within one week*.

Probably not a dermatophyte: Growth is observed on both slants. There is no color change on the DTM.

Not a dermatophyte: Growth is observed on Sabouraud but not on DTM.

REFERENCES

1. UOHSC, Department of Clinical Pathology, Clinical Microbiology Division, Procedure No. 0318 (1979), p. 74.
2. Salkin (1973), p. 135.
3. Taplin et al. (1969), p. 203.

EOSIN METHYLENE BLUE (EMB) AGAR WITH TETRACYCLINE FOR *CANDIDA ALBICANS* IDENTIFICATION

PRINCIPLE

C. albicans is differentiated from other *Candida* species, from *Cryptococcus* species, and from *Torulopsis glabrata* by the ability to produce germ tubes at three hours, and hyphae and budding cells at 24 hours when grown at 35° to 37°C on EMB agar in 10% CO_2. *Trichosporon* species also produce germ tubes and hyphae in these conditions, but the microscopic characteristics are easily distinguished from *C. albicans*.

*It is important that this test be read at one week, or when the first growth is observed after that time. Most nondermatophyte fungi that are able to grow on this medium will eventually produce the red alkaline reaction.

MATERIALS

Eosin methylene blue plate with tetracycline.
Positive control: *C. albicans,* fresh isolate.
Negative control: *C. tropicalis.*

METHOD

1. For performing several tests, the plate may be divided into as many as eight sections. A positive and a negative control are inoculated on each plate.
2. A light inoculum of yeast is streaked for isolation onto one section of the plate.
3. Within 10 minutes of inoculation, incubate in 5% to 10% CO_2 at 35° to 37°C. After three hours, plates may be examined. If test is negative, plates are incubated overnight.
4. Plates are observed microscopically on the reverse side through the low-power objective.

INTERPRETATION (PLATE 4)

1. Positive:
   a. At three hours: Germ tubes (tubelike projections with parallel walls and no constriction at point of production from parent cells)
   b. At 24 hours: True hyphae and groups of budding cells (feathering)
2. Negative: Only budding cells, or pseudohyphae and budding cells at 24 hours

REFERENCES

1. UOHSC, Department of Clinical Pathology, Clinical Microbiology Division, Procedure No. 0318 (1979), p. 75.
2. Walker and Huppert (1959), p. 551.

0.4% GELATIN FOR ACTINOMYCETE IDENTIFICATION

PRINCIPLE

   This test is used in differentiating aerobic actinomycetes (*Nocardia* sp., *Actinomadura* sp., and *Streptomyces* sp.).

MATERIALS

1. 0.4% gelatin in tube, one tube for control and one for each test.
2. Positive control: *N. brasiliensis.*

METHOD

1. A positive control is inoculated each time the test is done.
2. A fragment of the colony is inoculated just below the surface of the medium.
3. Incubate at 35° to 37°C for 10 days.
4. Examine for growth.

INTERPRETATION (TABLE 17)

Positive: Growth occurs.
Negative: No growth occurs.

REFERENCE

1. Wolf, Russell, and Shimoda (1975), p. 359.

**GERM-TUBE TEST FOR
IDENTIFICATION OF
*CANDIDA ALBICANS***

PRINCIPLE

   On incubation in human serum or fetal bovine serum, *C. albicans* produces characteristic projecting tubes (germ tubes) that distinguish it from other yeasts.

MATERIALS

1. Straight-sided glass test tubes (one for each test).
2. Human serum or fetal bovine serum.
3. One-ml pipette.
4. Pasteur pipettes (one for each test).
5. Glass slides.
6. Glass cover slips.
7. Positive control: *C. albicans*, fresh isolate.
8. Negative control: *C. tropicalis.*

METHOD

1. 0.5 ml serum is pipetted into each tube.
2. A light inoculum of yeast is emulsified in serum so as to make a barely cloudy suspension (McFarland #1 or less).
3. Tubes are placed in 35°C incubator for two to three hours.

4. One drop of suspension is placed on a microscope slide, covered with a cover slip, and examined under high-power lens.

INTERPRETATION (PLATE 4)

Positive: Germ tubes (tubelike projections with parallel walls and no constriction at point of production from parent cell).

Negative: Budding cells or pseudohyphae only are seen.

REFERENCES

1. UOHSC, Department of Clinical Pathology, Clinical Microbiology Division, Procedure No. 0318 (1979), p. 76.
2. Silva-Hutner and Cooper, in Lennette et al. (1974), pp. 496 and 498.

GROWTH AT 35° TO 37°C

PRINCIPLE

For some species of yeasts and fungi, the ability or failure to grow at 35° to 37°C is an identifying characteristic. For example, *A. fumigatus* grows well at 35°C. *A. glaucus* grows poorly or not at all at 35°C. A common mold that grows well at 35°C is more likely to be an opportunistic invader than one that does not grow well at 35°C.

MATERIALS

Two Sabouraud agar slants.

METHOD

1. Slants are inoculated with equal amounts of the yeast or fungal isolate.
2. Incubate one slant at 35°C. Incubate one slant at room temperature as a control.
3. Examine 35°C cultures grossly for growth at three days, comparing with growth of room-temperature control. If there is no growth on either culture, slants are reincubated and examined for growth at regular intervals for four weeks, or until growth is observed on control culture.

INTERPRETATION

Positive: Good growth at 35°C, growth at room temperature.

Negative: No growth at 35°C, growth at room temperature.

REFERENCE

1. UOHSC, Department of Clinical Pathology, Clinical Microbiology Division, Procedure No. 0318 (1979), p. 77.

HAIR PENETRATION TEST FOR THE IDENTIFICATION OF *TRICHOPHYTON MENTAGROPHYTES*

PRINCIPLE

T. mentagrophytes and some of the uncommon *Microsporum* species produce an enzyme which penetrates and makes holes in human hair in vitro. This test is helpful in distinguishing *T. mentagrophytes* from *T. rubrum.*

MATERIALS

1. 10% yeast extract, sterile.
2. Sterilized human hair (hair of a child under 5 years old).
3. Two screw-capped tubes, each containing 10 ml of sterile distilled water.
4. Sterile Pasteur pipette.
5. *T. mentagrophytes* control culture.

METHOD

1. With a pipette, one drop of yeast extract is placed in each tube of sterile distilled water.
2. With flamed and cooled forceps, several pieces (10 to 30) of sterile human hair are dropped into each tube of water and yeast extract.
3. A small amount of unknown fungal isolate is placed in one tube. A small amount of *T. mentagrophytes* is placed in the other tube as a control.
4. Incubate both tubes at room temperature for two weeks. If test is negative, (even if control is positive) reincubate and examine weekly for a total of four weeks. If both the control and the test isolate are still negative the test is repeated, using a different strain of *T. mentagrophytes* for a control.
5. Hairs are removed from water with a flamed loop and placed on a slide in a drop of lactophenol cotton blue. Cover with a cover slip.
6. Examine hairs microscopically in this preparation for splitting and pitting, indicative of penetration. (See drawing in Rebell and Taplin, p. 5 and illustration in Chapter 5 of *T. mentagrophytes*.)

INTERPRETATION

Positive: Splitting, pitting, and holes are seen.

Negative: Splitting, pitting, and holes not seen in test isolate.

REFERENCES

1. UOHSC, Department of Clinical Pathology, Clinical Microbiology Division, Procedure No. 0318 (1979), p. 78.
2. Rebell and Taplin (1974), p. 5.

HYDROLYSIS TESTS FOR NOCARDIA, ACTINOMADURA, AND STREPTOMYCES SPECIES

PRINCIPLE

A presumptive identification of *Nocardia* species, *Actinomadura* species, and *Streptomyces* species may be made by observing the pattern of hydrolysis on casein, xanthine, and tyrosine agars.

MATERIALS

1. Casein agar plate, freshly poured and cooled.
2. Xanthine agar plate, freshly poured with crystals distributed evenly and cooled.
3. Tryosine agar plate, freshly poured with crystals distributed evenly and cooled.
4. Control strains.
    a. Casein positive control: *N. brasiliensis*.
    b. Xanthine positive control: *N. caviae*.
    c. Tyrosine positive control: *N. brasiliensis*.

METHOD

1. A positive control is set up for each kind of agar.
2. Plate may be divided in quarters for three isolates and positive control.
3. Using a sharp blade, a generous amount of inoculum is transferred to the agar.
4. After inoculation, plate is sealed around with tape.
5. Incubate plates at room temperature for one week, or until control is positive (up to three weeks).

INTERPRETATION

Positive: Clearing is observed around inoculum.

Negative: No clearing is observed around inoculum.

REFERENCE

1. Haley and Callaway (1978), p. 143.

NITRATE-ZEPHIRAN SWAB TEST

PRINCIPLE

Cotton swabs impregnated with KNO_3-Zephiran are used to test yeasts for the ability to form nitrite from nitrate (presence of nitrate reductase). The formation of nitrite is detected by the addition of a color reagent. The reaction (color changes) occurs on the cotton swab.

MATERIALS

1. Three swabs treated with buffered nitrate-Zephiran solution.
2. Six straight-sided, clean test tubes (10 cm × 1 cm).
3. Control cultures.
   Positive: *Cr. albidus*, var. *albidus*.
   Negative: *Cr. neoformans*.
4. Solution A: 0.5% α-naphthylamine in 5N acetic acid.
   Solution B: 0.8% sulfanilic acid in 5N acetic acid.

PROCEDURE

1. A positive and negative control are run each time the test is done.
2. Coat swabs with yeasts from several colonies to be tested.*
3. Swirl against the bottom of a clean, empty test tube to assure adequate contact between organism and substrate within the swab.
4. Incubate tube with swab for 10 minutes at 45°C.
5. Remove swab from tube and insert in a second tube containing two drops each of Solution A and Solution B.

INTERPRETATION

Controls must work before test is valid.

Positive: Bright red color develops in cotton swab.

Negative: Swab retains only the color of the test organism.

REFERENCES

1. UOHSC, Department of Clinical Pathology, Clinical Microbiology Division, Procedure No. 0318 (1979), p. 83.
2. Hopkins and Land (1977), pp. 497–500.

POTATO DEXTROSE AGAR FOR SPORE PRODUCTION

PRINCIPLE

Sporulation of fungi is enhanced by growth on potato dextrose agar, made from fresh ingredients. This medium does not work effectively when made from a commercially prepared mixture.

---

*When testing a red yeast (*Rhodotorula* sp.), confine the organism solely to the tip of the swab. This is most easily done by touching colonies grown on a Petri-dish culture. Use *R. rubra* for a negative control and *R. glutinis* for a positive control.

MATERIAL

1. Potato dextrose agar plate poured with 36 ml of agar, or
2. Potato dextrose agar slant.

METHOD

1. Follow procedure for cover slip culture, or
2. Inoculate slant with culture and, when good growth is established, follow procedure for lactophenol cotton blue mount.

REFERENCES

1. Haley and Callaway (1978), p. 59.
2. UOHSC, Department of Clinical Pathology, Clinical Microbiology Division, Procedure No. 0318 (1979), p. 84.

PROTEOLYTIC ACTION DEMONSTRATED ON LÖEFFLER'S SERUM SLANT OR ON 12% GELATIN DEEP FOR IDENTIFICATION OF NONPATHOGENIC *CLADOSPORIUM* SPECIES

PRINCIPLE

The nonpathogenic species of *Cladosporium* are proteolytic and liquefy gelatin or Löeffler's serum slants. The pathogenic *Cladosporium* species do not digest serum or liquefy gelatin.

MATERIALS

1. Three Löeffler's serum slants or three 12% gelatin slants.
2. Three Sabouraud agar slants.
3. Control strains: Positive control: *Cladosporium* sp.
                        Negative control: *Fonsecaea pedrosoi*

METHOD

1. A positive and negative control is set up each time this test is done.
2. A small amount of fungus to be tested is placed on the surface of the gelatin deep or on the Löeffler's and on the Sabouraud agar slant.
3. Cultures are incubated at room temperature and examined weekly until test is positive or for four weeks.
4. Gelatin or Löeffler's serum slant is observed for liquefaction. Sabouraud slant is observed for growth.

INTERPRETATION

Positive: Liquefaction of serum slant or gelatin, growth on control culture.

Negative: No liquefaction of serum slant or gelatin, growth on control culture.

REFERENCES

1. UOHSC, Department of Clinical Pathology, Clinical Microbiology Division, Procedure No. 0318 (1979), p. 79.
2. Nielsen in Lennette et al. (1974), p. 543.

RICE (BOILED) FOR THE IDENTIFICATION OF *MICROSPORUM AUDOUINI*

PRINCIPLE

M. audouini is the only dermatophyte that does not grow well on boiled rice. This test is a comparison of the growth of the unknown on boiled rice with the growth of *M. audouini,* which grows poorly or not at all, and with another dermatophyte (e.g., *M. canis*) that grows well.

MATERIALS

1. Three tubes of boiled rice medium.
2. One tube of Sabouraud agar slant.

METHOD

1. A small amount of the fungal isolate is inoculated onto the surface of the boiled rice.
2. An equal amount of *M. canis* and *M. audouini* control cultures are each inoculated onto one of the other tubes of boiled rice medium.
3. A Sabouraud agar slant is inoculated with the unknown. This is a control for viability for fungal isolates.
4. Incubate at room temperature. Examine grossly at one week and, if necessary, weekly thereafter for four weeks.

INTERPRETATION

If the unknown is *M. audouini,* it will show poor growth equal to that of the *M. audouini* control. If the growth is equal to that of the *M. canis* control, the unknown is not *M. audouini.*

NOTE: Excess water covering the boiled rice is poured off before rice is inoculated. This medium is also useful for production of macroconidia by *M. canis.*

REFERENCE

1. UOHSC, Department of Clinical Pathology, Clinical Microbiology Division, Procedure No. 0318 (1979), p. 63.

SABOURAUD BROTH FOR SURFACE FILM PRODUCTION BY SOME *CANDIDA* SPECIES

PRINCIPLE

Some *Candida* species consistently produce a characteristic film and gas on Sabouraud broth. Others are variable and some never produce film. The primary use of this test is to differentiate *C. krusei* and *C. tropicalis* from the common *Candida* species.

MATERIAL

Sabouraud broth in tube with loose top.

METHOD

1. A loopful of yeast colony from a three-day-old culture is inoculated into a tube of Sabouraud broth.
2. Incubate at room temperature for three days. If results are inconclusive, culture may be held for as long as three weeks.
3. Observe broth for production of film on the surface. Tube is shaken gently, held to the light, and examined for rising bubbles, indicating production of gas.

INTERPRETATION

The following *Candida* species will always produce a surface film and gas on this media:

C. tropicalis (narrow film)

C. krusei (wide film)

Many other yeasts may, on occasion, produce a surface film and/or gas on this medium, including

C. parapsilosis

Candida species (other than those listed above and below)

Torulopsis glabrata

The yeasts that will produce a surface film but no gas on this medium, include

Trichosporon species

The following yeasts do not produce a surface film on this medium and may not produce gas:

C. albicans

C. stellatoidea

C. guillermondii

Cr. neoformans

Cryptococcus species

REFERENCES

1. UOHSC, Department of Clinical Pathology, Clinical Microbiology Division, Procedure No. 0318 (1979), p. 85.
2. Conant, Smith, Baker, et al. (1963), p. 183.

SEED AGAR (STAIB'S MEDIUM) OR CAFFEIC ACID AGAR FOR IDENTIFICATION OF *CRYPTOCOCCUS NEOFORMANS*

PRINCIPLE

Cr. neoformans produces a brown color on seed agar at room temperature. This effect has been shown on caffeic acid to be due to phenoloxidase activity located within the cell wall. Other *Cryptococcus* sp., *Candida* sp., *Torulopsis* sp., and *Saccharomyces* sp. do not produce a brown color on seed agar.

MATERIAL

1. Seed or caffeic acid agar plate.
2. *Cr. neoformans* culture for positive control.
3. Sabouraud agar slant for test-culture control.

METHOD

1. Divide plate into two sections with one of the following:
   a. Test isolate.
   b. *Cr. neoformans.*
3. Incubate Sabouraud agar slant with test isolate.
4. Incubate all cultures at room temperature for three days or until *Cr. neoformans* control is brown.
5. Observe plate grossly for brown colonies, similar to the color of the positive control and darker than the color of the test yeast growing on Sabouraud agar.

INTERPRETATION (PLATE 3)

Positive: Brown colonies on seed agar, light-colored colonies on Sabouraud control.

Negative: Colonies same color as Sabouraud agar control.

NOTE: *Aureobasidium, Sporothrix, Wangiella,* and *Phialophora* species may grow in a yeast form in early cultures and develop dark brown colonies on Sabouraud and other agar as the cultures mature. Careful observation of the Sabouraud control culture and the microscopic characteristics will assure that these and any other dark brown fungi are not recorded as positive.

REFERENCES

1. UOHSC, Department of Clinical Pathology, Clinical Microbiology Division, Procedure No. 0318 (1979), p. 86.
2. Healey, Dillavou, and Taylor (1977), p. 387.
3. Rippon (1974), p. 548.

TRICHOPHYTON AGARS FOR DIFFERENTIATION
OF SOME *TRICHOPHYTON* SPECIES

PRINCIPLE

Some of the *Trichophyton* species have a definite and unique pattern of nutritional requirements. Chemically defined media are used for demonstrating the vitamin requirements of these fungi.

NOTE: Media used for these tests are prepared and numbered by Difco.

MATERIALS

1. Control agar slant, containing no vitamins; either #1, with casamino acids as a base, or #6, with ammonium nitrate as a base (see below).
2. One or more of the following slants with vitamins added, as indicated.
    a. Those with casamino acid as a base.
        1. #2 inositol.
        2. #3 inositol and thiamine.
        3. #4 thiamine.
        4. #5 nicotinic acid.
    b. Those with ammonium nitrate as a base.
        1. #7 histidine.
3. Sabouraud agar slant for a control.

METHOD

1. A small and equal (about 1 mm) amount of the test fungus is placed on the surface of each of the test media; be careful not to transfer agar from the media on which the test isolate is growing.
2. A small amount of the test fungus is placed on the surface of a Sabouraud agar slant.

3. Incubate all cultures at room temperature for two weeks and if results are not conclusive at this time, reincubate cultures for two more weeks or until the Sabouraud control shows good growth after this time, for a total of six weeks.

4. Cultures are examined grossly and quantitation is made in comparison with No. 3 or No. 7 tube and recorded as + to ++++.

INTERPRETATION
See Table 12.

REFERENCES

1. Difco (1972), pp. 76-77.
2. Georg and Camp (1957), p. 74.
3. UOHSC, Department of Clinical Pathology, Clinical Microbiology Division, Procedure No. 0318 (1979), p. 88.

UREASE PRODUCTION BY *CRYPTOCOCCUS* SPECIES

PRINCIPLE

Cr. neoformans, other *Cryptococcus* species, and some other yeasts produce urease. Many other yeasts do not, including most of the *Candida* species and *Torulopsis glabrata.* This characteristic provides a useful screening test to determine if a yeast isolate could be *Cr. neoformans.* The urea agar used in this test contains phenol red, which serves as an indicator of the alkaline reaction that results when the urea is split and ammonia is produced.

MATERIALS
Urea agar slant.

METHOD

1. Yeast isolate is streaked onto a slant.
2. Incubate at room temperature for three days. Observe color.

INTERPRETATION

Positive: Deep magenta color is produced, indicating production of urease.

Negative: Agar remains the same color or becomes yellow, indicating an acid reaction.

NOTE: False-positive results will occur when a urease positive bacterial contaminant is present.

REFERENCES

1. UOHSC, Department of Clinical Pathology, Clinical Microbiology Division, Procedure No. 0318 (1979), p. 90.
2. Difco (1972), p. 427.

UREA DEXTROSE AGAR SLANT FOR DIFFERENTIATING *TRICHOPHYTON MENTAGROPHYTES* FROM *TRICHOPHYTON RUBRUM*

PRINCIPLE

T. mentagrophytes splits urea (in urea agar with dextrose added) more rapidly than do other dermatophytes. *T. rubrum* (except for some granular strains) gives a negative or a weak positive reaction.

MATERIALS

1. Urea dextrose agar slant.
2. Sabouraud agar control slant.

METHOD

1. A small amount of fungus is placed on the surface of each slant.
2. Incubate at room temperature for four days.
3. Observe for production of color in urea agar and for growth in Sabouraud agar.

INTERPRETATION

Strong positive: Deep magenta color throughout media, growth on control slant.

Weak positive: Pale pink color in media, growth on control slant.

Negative: No color change on urease slant, growth on control slant.

NOTE: A positive test *after* four days is not significant.

NOTE: False positive results will occur when a urease positive bacterial contaminant is present.

REFERENCES

1. Philpot (1967), p. 189.
2. UOHSC, Department of Clinical Pathology, Clinical Microbiology Division, Procedure No. 0318 (1979), p. 91.

BIBLIOGRAPHY

Ajello L, Padhye AA: Dermatophytes and the agents of superficial mycoses, in Lennette EH, Spaulding EH, Truant JP (eds): *Manual of Clinical Microbiology,* ed 2. Washington DC: American Society for Microbiology, 1974, p. 469.

Beneke ES, Rogers AL: *Medical Mycology Manual,* ed 3. Minneapolis: Burgess Publishing Co, 1970.

Campbell MC: Mycology Procedure, University of Oregon Health Sciences Center, Department of Clinical Pathology, Clinical Microbiology Division Procedure No. 0318. Portland: Oregon, 1979.

Conant NF, Smith DT, Baker RD, Callaway JL: *Manual of Clinical Mycology,* ed 3. Philadelphia: W.B. Saunders Co, 1971.

Difco Supplementary Literature. Detroit: Difco Laboratories, 1972.

Dolan CT, Roberts GD: "Mycology" Section II, in Washington JA (ed): *Laboratory Procedures in Clinical Microbiology,* Boston: Little Brown Co, 1974.

Ellis MB: *Dematiaceous Hyphomycetes.* Kew, Surrey, Commonwealth Mycological Institute, 1971.

Ellis MB: *More Dematiaceous Hyphomycetes.* Kew, Surrey, Commonwealth Mycological Institute, 1976.

Emmons CW, Binford CH, Utz JP, Kwon-Chung KJ: *Medical Mycology,* ed 3. Philadelphia: Lea and Febiger, 1977.

Georg LK, Camp LB: Routine nutritional tests for the identification of dermatophytes. *J Bacteriol* 74:113, 1957.

Gordon MA: Aerobic Pathogenic Actinomycetaceae in Lennette EH, Spaulding EH, Truant JP (eds): *Manual of Clinical Microbiology,* Washington DC: American Society for Microbiology, 1974, p 175.

Haley LD, Callaway CS: *Laboratory Methods in Medical Mycology,* ed 4. US Department of Health Education and Welfare. HEW Publication No. (CDC) 78-8361. 1978.

Harold W, Snyder M: Scheme for cultural identification of *Candida* species of medical importance. *Difco Technical Information Bulletin No. 0615,* 1969.

Healey ME, Dillavou CL, Taylor GE: Diagnostic medium containing inositol, urea and caffeic acid for selective growth of *Cryptococcus neoformans. J Clin Microbiol* 6:387, 1977.

Hopkins JM, Land GA: Rapid method for determining nitrate utilization by yeasts. *J Clin Pathol* 5:497, 1977.

Huppert M, Harper G, Sun HS, et al: Rapid methods for identification of yeasts. *J Clin Microbiol* 2:21, 1975.

Huppert M, Sun SH, Rice EH: Specificity of exoantigens for identifying cultures of *Coccidioides immitis. J Clin Microbiol* 8:346, 1978.

Kane J: *Trichophyton fischeri* sp. Nov. A saprophyte resembling *Trichophyton rubrum. Sabouraudia* 15:231, 1977.

Koneman EW, Roberts GD, Wright SF: *Practical Laboratory Mycology,* ed 2. Baltimore: The Williams and Wilkins Co, 1978.

Larsh HW, Goodman NL: Fungi of the systemic mycoses, in Lennette EH, Spaulding EH, Truant JP (eds): *Manual of Clinical Microbiology,* ed 2. Washington DC: American Society for Microbiology, 1974, p 508.

Mahan CT, Sale GE: Rapid methenamine silver stain for *Pneumocystis* and fungi. *Arch Pathol Lab Med* 102:352, 1978.

Nielsen HS Jr: Dematiaceous fungi, in Lennette EH, Spaulding EH, Truant JP (eds): *Manual of Clinical Microbiology,* ed 2. Washington DC: American Society for Microbiology, 1974, p 528.

Paik G, Suggs MT: Reagents stains and miscellaneous procedures, in Lennette EH, Spaulding EH, Truant JP (eds): *Manual of Clinical Microbiology,* ed 2. Washington DC: American Society for Microbiology, 1974, p 930.

Philpot C: The differentiation of *Trichophyton mentagrophytes* from *Trichophyton rubrum* by a simple urease test. *Sabouraudia* 5:189, 1967.

Ray, LF, Campbell MC: A *Syllabus on Fungi for Dermatologists.* University of Oregon Medical School, 1973.

Rebell CG, Forster RK: Fungi of keratomycosis, in Lennette EH, Spaulding EH, Truant JP (eds): *Manual of Clinical Microbiology,* ed 2. Washington DC: American Society for Microbiology, 1974, p 482.

Rebell G, Taplin D: *Dermatophytes, Their Recognition and Identification.* Coral Gables: University of Miami Press, 1974.

Rippon JW: *Medical Mycology.* Philadelphia: W.B. Saunders Co, 1974.

Roberts GD, Washington JA: Detection of fungi in blood cultures. *J Clin Microbiol* 1:309, 1975.

Schneidau JD: Fungi of maduromycosis, in Lennette EH, Spaulding EH, Truant JP (eds): *Manual of Clinical Microbiology,* ed 2. Washington DC: American Society for Microbiology, 1974, p 522.

Salkin IF: Dermatophyte test medium: Evaluation of nondermatophyte pathogens. *Appl Microbiol* 26:134, 1973.

Silva-Hutner M, Cooper BH: Medically important yeasts, in Lennette EH, Spaulding EH, Truant JB (eds): *Manual of Clinical Microbiology,* ed 2. Washington DC: American Society for Microbiology, 1974, p 491.

Smith CD, Goodman NL: Improved culture methods for the isolation of *Histoplasma capsulatum* and *Blastomyces dermatitidis* from contaminated specimens. *Am J Clin Pathol* 63:276, 1974.

Sun SH, Huppert M, Vukovich KR: Rapid in vitro conversion and identification of *Coccidioides immitis. J Clin Microbiol* 3:186, 1976.

Taplin D, Zaias N, Rebell G, et al: Isolation and recognition of dermatophytes on a new medium (DTM). *Arch Dermatol* 99:203, 1969.

University of Oregon Health Sciences Center, Department of Clinical Pathology Clinical Microbiology Procedure No. 0318, 1979, Campbell MC (author), Kim KSW (ed).

Vera HD, Dumoff M: Media, reagents and stains, in Lennette EH, Spaulding EH, Truant JP (eds): *Manual of Clinical Microbiology,* ed 2. Washington DC: American Society for Clinical Microbiology, 1974, p 881.

Walker I, Huppert M: A rapid reliable technique for the identification of *Candida albicans*. *Am J Clin Pathol* 31:551, 1959, p 551.

Wolf PL, Russell B, Shimoda A: *Practical Clinical Microbiology and Mycology: Techniques and Interpretations*. New York: John Wiley and Sons, Inc, 1975.

5. Indentification of Individual Fungal Isolates

The identification of the fungi is still an exercise in contemplative observation.

Rippon, page 3

Individual isolates may be identified, starting at this point, by observing the gross color and texture and by observing the microscopic characteristics. Table 20 is a rudimentary color guide to gross colony appearance, designed to help a beginning worker screen out some groups of molds and to seek an identification among those remaining. The color given refers to the surface of the colony unless otherwise indicated, as when the color refers to the reverse of the colony. An example of this is *T. rubrum,* which is almost always white on the surface, but which may be red on the reverse. It is, therefore, listed in the white group and again in the red group as red (reverse). Different strains of many molds are extremely variable in the color of the gross colony. Also, the color of a given isolate will often change as the culture matures. For example, *A. fumigatus* may be white at one to two days, blue-green in five to 10 days, gray-brown at 14 days, and almost black in a month. This species and others that are variable in this way are listed in all of the appropriate color groups.

The microscopic guide shown in Table 21 has been designed to be used as a practical key to the identification of fungi described in this chapter. A review of Chapter 2 (*Taxonomy*) will be helpful in following this key, which is a guide only. It is not to be used for final identification of fungal isolates.

Identification of all yeasts and molds is ultimately confirmed by comparing each given isolate with written descriptions, drawings, and, when available, photo-

Table 20

**A RUDIMENTARY COLOR AND TEXTURE GUIDE TO THE
GROSS DIFFERENTIATION OF MEDICALLY SIGNIFICANT FUNGI[a]**

Color	Pathogenic Fungi	Common Molds or Opportunistic Fungi
	Granular, Velvety, or Cottony Colonies	
White to cream-color	*Blastomyces dermatitidis*	*Acremonium (Cephalosporium)* sp.
	Coccidioides immitis	*Aspergillus* sp.
	Histoplasma capsulatum	*Chrysosporium* sp.
	Microsporum audouini	*Fusarium* sp.
	Microsporum canis	*Geotrichum* sp.
	Microsporum distortum	*Mucor* sp.
	Microsporum gypseum	*Neurospora* sp.
	Microsporum nanum	*Paecilomyces* sp. (early)
	Paracoccidioides brasiliensis	*Penicillium* sp. (early)
	Trichophyton ajelloi	*Rhizopus* sp.
	Trichophyton concentricum	*Scopulariopsis* sp. (early)
	Trichophyton mentagrophytes	*Sepedonium* sp.
	Trichophyton rubrum	*Streptomyces* sp.
	Trichophyton schoenleinii	*Trichothecium* sp. (early)
	Trichophyton soudanense	*Verticillium* sp.
	Trichophyton tonsurans	
	Trichophyton verrucosum	
	Trichophyton yaoundei	
Tan to light brown	*Blastomyces dermatitidis*	*Alternaria* sp.
	Coccidioides immitis	*Aspergillus terreus*
	Epidermophyton floccosum	*Chrysosporium* sp.
	Histoplasma capsulatum	*Cladosporium* sp.
	Microsporum audouini	*Curvularia* sp.

Table 20 (continued)

Color	Pathogenic Fungi	Common Molds or Opportunistic Fungi
Tan to light brown	*Microsporum canis* *Microsporum cookei* *Microsporum gypseum* *Microsporum nanum* *Paracoccidioides brasiliensis* *Trichophyton ajelloi* *Trichophyton equinum* *Trichophyton mentagrophytes* *Trichophyton rubrum* (reverse) *Trichophyton terrestre* *Trichophyton tonsurans*	*Epicoccum* sp. *Mucor* sp. *Paecilomyces* sp. *Penicillium* sp. *Rhizopus* sp. *Scopulariopsis* sp. *Sepedonium* sp. *Streptomyces* sp. *Verticillium* sp.
Yellow to orange	*Coccidioides immitis* *Epidermophyton floccosum* *Microsporum audouini* *Microsporum canis* (reverse) *Microsporum cookei* (reverse) *Microsporum ferrugineum* *Microsporum nanum* *Trichophyton rubrum* (reverse) *Trichophyton tonsurans* *Trichophyton verrucosum* *Trichophyton soudanense* *Trichophyton yaoundei*	*Aspergillus* sp. *Chaetomium* sp. *Epicoccum* sp. *Neurospora* sp. *Phoma* sp. *Trichoderma* sp. (early) *Trichothecium* sp. *Verticillium* sp.
Rose-red to lavender	*Actinomadura (Streptomyces) pelleterei* *Coccidioides immitis* *Microsporum audouini* (reverse)	*Acremonium (Cephalosporium)* sp. *Aspergillus* sp. (reverse) *Chrysosporium* sp. (reverse, may diffuse)

	Microsporum cookei (reverse) *Microsporum gallinae* (reverse, diffusible) *Microsporum gypseum* (reverse) *Microsporum nanum* (reverse) *Trichophyton ajelloi* (reverse) *Trichophyton equinum* (reverse) *Trichophyton megninii* *Trichophyton mentagrophytes* (reverse) *Trichophyton rubrum* (reverse) *Trichophyton terrestre* (reverse) *Trichophyton tonsurans* (reverse) *Trichophyton violaceum*	*Epicoccum* sp. *Fusarium* sp. *Penicillium* sp. (reverse or surface) *Phoma* sp. *Streptomyces* sp.
Dark brown to black	*Cladosporium carrionii* *Cladosporium trichoides* *Coccidioides immitis* (reverse, may be diffuse) *Exophiala* (*Phialophora*) *jeanselmei* *Exophiala* (*Cladosporium*) *werneckii* *Fonsecaea pedrosoi* *Madurella grisea* *Madurella mycetomi* *Phialophora verrucosa* *Piedraia hortai* *Sporothrix schenckii* *Trichophyton tonsurans* *Wangiella* (*Phialophora*) *dermatitidis*	*Alternaria* sp. *Aspergillus niger* *Aspergillus* sp. *Aureobasidium pullulans* *Chaetomium* sp. *Cladosporium* sp. *Curvularia* sp. *Drechslera* sp. *Epicoccum* sp. (reverse) *Helminthosporium* sp. (reverse) *Humicola* sp. *Nigrospora* sp. (reverse) *Phoma* sp. (reverse)
Gray	*Coccidioides immitis* *Madurella grisea* *Madurella mycetomi*	*Absidia* sp. *Alternaria* sp. *Botrytis* sp.

Table 20 (continued)

Color	Pathogenic Fungi	Common Molds or Opportunistic Fungi
Gray	*Petriellidium (Allescheria) boydii*	*Chaetomium* sp. *Cladosporium* sp. *Drechslera* sp. *Fusarium* sp. *Helminthosporium* sp. *Mucor* sp. *Nigrospora* sp. *Paecilomyces* sp. *Phoma* sp. *Streptomyces* sp. *Syncephelastrum* sp. *Rhizopus* sp.
Green	*Aspergillus fumigatus* *Cladosporium carrionii* *Cladosporium trichoides* *Epidermophyton floccosum* *Exophiala (Phialophora) jeanselmei* *Fonsecaea pedrosoi* *Petriellidium (Allescheria) boydii* *Phialophora verrucosa*	*Aspergillus* sp. *Cladosporium* sp. *Gliocladium* sp. *Paecilomyces* sp. *Penicillium* sp. *Sepedonium* sp. *Trichoderma* sp.

Waxy to Moist Colonies (White to cream-color unless otherwise indicated)

	Pathogenic Fungi	Common Molds or Opportunistic Fungi
	Actinomadura sp. (tan to cream-color) *Blastomyces dermatitidis* (hard, waxy, tufts) *Blastomyces dermatitidis* (37°C)	*Acremonium (Cephalosporium)* sp. *Aureobasidium pullulans* (cream-color to black) *Candida* sp. *Chrysosporium* sp.

214

Candida albicans
Coccidioides immitis
Cryptococcus neoformans
Nocardia asteroides (white to orange)
Nocardia brasiliensis (white, tan, brown)
Paracoccidioides brasiliensis (37°C)
Exophiala (*Phialophora*) *jeanselmei* (early, black)
Sporothrix schenckii (leathery, cream-color to black)
Sporothrix schenckii (37°C)
Trichophyton rubrum (early)
Trichophyton violaceum (cream-color to violet)
Trichophyton yaoundei
Trichosporon cutaneum/beigelii
Wangiella (*Phialophora*) *dermititidis* (black)

Cryptococcus sp.
Geotrichum sp.
Phialophora sp. (early, black)
Rhodotorula sp. (pink, orange)
Saccharomyces sp.
Scopulariopsis sp. (early)
Sepedonium sp.
Streptomyces sp.
Torulopsis sp.
Trichosporon sp.
Ustilago sp.

[a]Different isolates of any given species of fungus may vary considerably in color and texture. Cultures are incubated at room temperature unless otherwise indicated. Colors given describe surface of colony unless otherwise indicated.

Reference:

Adapted from Ray LF, Campbell MC: *A Syllabus on Fungi for Dermatologists.* Portland, University of Oregon Medical School, 1973.

TABLE 21
MICROSCOPIC GUIDE

Microscopic Appearance	Fungus	Illustration
Predominantly wide hyphae >8 μm		
Many cross walls		
1. Conidia borne on pegs on swollen cells	*Botrytis*	
2. Waxy colony, thick-walled zygospores with beak, also sporangia and chlamydospores	*Basidiobolus*	
Cross walls absent or rarely present, increasing in number as colony ages		
1. Sporangiospores in fingerlike projections (merosporangia)	*Syncephalastrum*	
2. Sporangiospores in round sacks (sporangia)		
a. Columellae present		
• Rhizoids not present		
Sporangiophore with lateral curved branches bearing small sporangia	*Circinella*	
Sporangiophore with long, straight branches	*Mucor*	
Rhizoids present		
Sporangiophores originating just above rhizoids	*Rhizopus*	
Sporangiophores originating on stolon connecting rhizoids	*Absidia*	
b. No columellae, zygospores enveloped in dense hyphal covering, hyphae start broad and then thin out, stylospores also present	*Mortierella*	
Hyphae predominantly thinner than 5 μ		
Hyphae form into arthroconidia		
1. Hyphae branch in Y shape, colonies orange	*Neurospora*	
2. Every other section matures into arthroconidia	*Coccidioides*	
3. Arthroconidia germinate at corner into hyphae	*Geotrichum*	
4. Yeast, budding cells (blastoconidia), pseudo-hyphae present	*Trichosporon*	
5. Short hyaline hyphae with aseptate terminal extensions; pigmented hyphae form arthroconidia, some curled forms, some swollen areas divided	*Hendersonula*	

216

Table 21 (continued)

Microscopic Appearance	Fungus	Illustration
Conidia formed within very large structures		
1. Large structure (perithecia) with spike appendages	*Chaetomium*	
2. Besides perithecia, large oval conidia, growth occurs at 37° C	*Petriellidium*	
3. Pycnidia containing small, hyaline pycnidiospores	*Phoma*	
4. Colony blackish, dark closely septate hyphae, swollen, irregular cells, asci, ascospores rarely seen	*Piedraia*	
Conidia multicelled		
1. Macroconidia with brown pigment		
a. Cross walls transverse only		
• Thick-walled macroconidia usually originate from round conidiogenous cell that has a tough, thick bottom and thin collapsible top	*Torula*	
• Macroconidia originate through tiny pores of conidiogenous cell (tretic conidia)		
Conidiogenous cell sympodial		
Central cell of macroconidium is larger and darker than other cells; conidium is curved or bent	*Curvularia*	
Cells are equally dark, conidium is not curved or bent	*Drechslera*	
Conidiogenous cell is smooth (not sympodial); macroconidia are attached at right angles	*Helminthosporium*	
b. Cross walls at various angles		
• Conidia round with rough wall, arising from short special hyphae in clumps	*Epicoccum*	
• Conidium-bearing (conidiogenous) structure sympodial; conidia also in chains resembling hand grenades; conidia are tretic	*Alternaria*	
2. No brown pigment		
a. Conidia club-shaped in branches	*Epidermophyton floccosum*	

Table 21 (continued)

Microscopic Appearance	Fungus	Illustration
b. Conidia shaped like canoes	*Fusarium*	
c. Conidia one to three celled, attached at right angles (except first one) like a golf club	*Trichothecium*	
d. Conidia long, thin, smooth-walled	*Trichophyton*	
e. Conidia wider, thick outer wall, rough walls (may not always be evident)	*Microsporum*	
• Spores spindle-shaped	*Microsporum canis*	
• Spores one to three cells	*Microsporum nanum*	
• Spores three to six cells, one end cut off, other end rounded	*Microsporum gypseum*	
• Spores distorted	*Microsporum distortum*	
Conidia produced endogenously from phialides or annellides		
1. Phialides produced on swollen structure	*Aspergillus*	
2. Phialides and annellides hyaline (light-colored) a. Conidia held in clumps by sticky substance, not always evident • Phialides long slender delicate, in verticils	*Verticillium*	
• Phialides robust, point toward tip of hyphae, conidia in chains	*Gliocladium*	
• Phialides short, fat, irregular, colony bright green	*Trichoderma*	

Table 21 (continued)

Microscopic Appearance	Fungus	Illustration
b. Conidia not held in clumps • Conidia rough walled, in chains Conidia lemon-shaped, phialides with long slender tip, divergent	*Paecilomyces*	
Annellides fat, corase, conidia with one flat side	*Scopulariopsis*	
Conidia round, phialides not slender, not coarse, colony usually bluish green	*Penicillium*	
• Conidia not rough-walled, not in chains Phialides long, slender, at right angles to hyphae, conidia may clump	*Acremonium*	
Small phialides, small spores, sclerotia in old colonies	*Madurella*	
3. Phialides, conidia, and hyphae brown pigmented a. Three types of sporulation: (1) phialides; (2) conidia in chains (Cladosporium-type); (3) sympodial	*Fonsecaea pedrosoi*	
b. Phialides have a flared tip; no other type of sporulation	*Phialophora verrucosa*	
c. Long, slender phialides, conidia tend to clump along side of phialide, enlarged yeast cells, colony begins as yeast	*Wangiella*	
d. Annellides long, slender or short and chunky rings around tip, conidia clump, early growth yeastlike	*Exophiala*	
e. Annellides on bundles of long hyphae produce chains of brown conidia	*Doratomyces*	

219

Table 21 (continued)

Microscopic Appearance	Fungus	Illustration

Single-celled conidia

1. Conidia contain brown pigment
   a. Conidia in chains with youngest at the tip
      (acropetal); black spot where conidia are
      attached — *Cladosporium*

   b. Conidia not in chains
      • Conidia with hyaline ring around center — *Arthrinium*

      • Large round conidia borne on swollen
        tip — *Nigrospora*

2. Colonies are yeast at 37° C, pathogenic
   a. Yeast small, conidia large with projections
      through cell wall — *Histoplasma capsulatum*

   b. Yeast larger, broad-based budding, conidia
      not distinctive — *Blastomyces dermatitidis*

   c. Yeast all with multiple budding, mold
      form rarely produces conidia — *Paracoccidioides brasiliensis*

3. Conidia and colonies not as above
   a. Small conidia borne on thin zigzag
      (sympodial) tip of conidiophore, which
      form rosettes — *Beauveria*

   b. Conidiogenous structures resemble phialides
      but are sympodial cells with thin branches
      in daisy form at end, yeast phase at 37° C — *Sporothrix schenckii*

   c. Conidia borne directly on hyphae or short
      stalk, separate by fragmentation often
      leaving a "frill" on conidium (aleurioconidia)

      • Broad-based conidia, knobby hyphae, no
        macroconidia; in most species conidia
        are large (5–8 μm) — *Chrysosporium*

      • Small conidia predominate, macroconidia
        produced sometimes, hyphae not
        knobby, conidia usually not broad based — *Trichophyton*

      • Macroconidia predominate in most species,
        microconidia not distinctive — *Microsporum*

   d. Large elliptical conidia with rough walls,
      no growth at 37° C — *Sepedonium*

220

Table 21 (continued)

Microscopic Appearance	Fungus	Illustration
e. Large round to elliptical conidia with smooth walls, borne on simple conidiophore, perfect stage produced	*Monosporium*	

Colonies are yeasts predominantly
Hyphae present at some stage
1. Two sizes of hyphae, thin and wide, blastoconidia produced on sides, colony becomes black with age — *Aureobasidium pullulans*

2. Colony cream-color, blastoconidia produced on hyphae — *Candida*

3. Yeast with very irregular long shapes, black chlamydospores may develop — *Ustilago*

No true hyphae present
1. Yeast produces ascospores — *Saccharomyces*

2. Yeast colony normally red or orange — *Rhodotorula*

3. Yeast requires olive oil to grow on artificial media; budding cell leaves a collar on mother cell — *Pityrosporum*

4. Inositol assimilated, yeast produces capsule in most species — *Cryptococcus*

5. Inositol not assimilated, small yeast, acid and gas produced on dextrose and trehalose — *Torulopsis glabrata*

6. Alga, no growth on cycloheximide, cells 8–24 × 10–27 μm, spores 9–11 μm — *Prototheca*

No growth on artificial media
Chains of oval budding cells in tissue, may bud at more than one point — *Loboa loboi*
Tissue form has sporangia 100–350 μm, contains endospores, 6–7 μm at discharge — *Rhinosporidium seeberi*

Branching filaments <2 μm
Strict anaerobe — *Actinomyces*
Aerobic colonies
1. Positive on modified acid-fast stain — *Nocardia*
2. Negative acid fast stain, chains of spores <2 μm — *Streptomyces*

graphs of individual fungi. The following descriptions are arranged alphabetically. While it is hoped that these descriptions will be useful by themselves, additional references are given that we have found helpful in these identifications. These references are cited by author and page number. A complete bibliography is given at the end of the chapter.

There is no reason to expect that each fungal isolate will absolutely match the handful of descriptions given here. Rare and unusual isolates are not as rare and unusual as one would hope. It is helpful to have several books available for the identification of odd fungal isolates. Those marked with an asterisk in the bibliography have been proven indispensable for this purpose.

FUNGI INCLUDED IN CHAPTER 5

Absidia sp.
Acremonium (Cephalosporium) sp.
Actinomadura madurae
Actinomyces bovis
Actinomyces israelii
Alternaria sp.
Arthrinium sp. (Papularia sp.)
Aspergillus sp.
Aspergillus (clavatus group)
Aspergillus (flavus group)
Aspergillus (fumigatus group)
Aspergillus (glaucus group)
Aspergillus (nidulans group)
Aspergillus (niger group)
Aspergillus (terreus group)
Aspergillus (versicolor group)
Other *Aspergillus* groups
Aureobasidium (Pullularia)
  pullulans

Basidiobolus haptosporus
Beauveria sp.

Blastomyces dermatitidis
Botrytis sp.

Candida sp.
Candida albicans
Candida guillermondii
Candida krusei
Candida parapsilosis
Candida pseudotropicalis
Candida stellatoidea
Candida tropicalis
Cephalosporium sp.
  (See *Acremonium* sp.)
Chaetomium sp.
Chrysosporium sp.
Chrysosporium keratinophilum
Chrysosporium pannorum
Chrysosporium parvum
Chrysosporium parvum, var. *crescens*
Chrysosporium pruinosum
Chrysosporium tropicum
Cladosporium sp.

Cladosporium carrionii
Cladosporium trichoides
Circinella sp.
Coccidioides immitis
Cryptococcus sp.
Cryptococcus neoformans
Curvularia sp.

Doratomyces (Stysanus) stemonitis
Drechslera sp.

Epicoccum sp.
Epidermophyton floccosum
Exophiala jeanselmei
Exophiala salmonis
Exophiala spinifera
Exophiala werneckii

Fonsecaea pedrosoi
Fusarium sp.

Geotrichum candidum
Gliocladium sp.

Helminthosporium sp.
Hendersonula toruloidea (See
  Scytalidium sp.)
Histoplasma capsulatum
Histoplasma capsulatum, var.
  duboisii

Loboa loboi

Madurella mycetomi
Madurella grisea
Microsporum audouini
Microsporum canis
Microsporum cookei
Microsporum distortum
Microsporum ferrugineum
Microsporum fulvum
Microsporum gallinae
Microsporum gypseum
Microsporum nanum
Microsporum persicolor
Microsporum vanbreuseghemii

Monilia sp. (See *Neurospora* sp.)
Monosporium apiospermum (See
  Petriellidium boydii)
Mortierella sp.
Mucor sp.

Neurospora sitophila
Nigrospora sp.
Nocardia asteroides
Nocardia brasiliensis
Nocardia caviae

Paracoccidioides brasiliensis
Paecilomyces sp.
Penicillium sp.
Petriellidium boydii
Phialophora sp.
Phoma sp.
Piedraia hortai
Pityrosporum furfur
Prototheca sp.

Rhinosporidium seeberi
Rhizopus sp.
Rhizopus arrhizus
Rhizopus nigricans
Rhizopus rhizopodiformis
Rhodotorula sp.

Saccharomyces sp.
Scopulariopsis sp.
Scytalidium sp.
Sepedonium sp.
Sporothrix schenckii
Streptomyces sp.
Syncephalastrum sp.

Torula sp.
Torulopsis glabrata
Trichoderma sp.
Trichophyton ajelloi
Trichophyton concentricum
Trichophyton equinum
Trichophyton fischeri
Trichophyton megninii
Trichophyton mentagrophytes

continued

Trichophyton rubrum
Trichophyton schoenleinii
Trichophyton soudanense
Trichophyton terrestre
Trichophyton tonsurans
Trichophyton verrucosum
Trichophyton violaceum
Trichophyton yaoundei

Trichosporon beigelii
Trichosporon cutaneum
Trichothecium sp.

Ustilago sp.

Verticillium sp.

Wangiella dermatitidis

INDIVIDUAL DESCRIPTIONS

***Absidia* sp. (Class, Zygomycete; Order, Mucorales)**

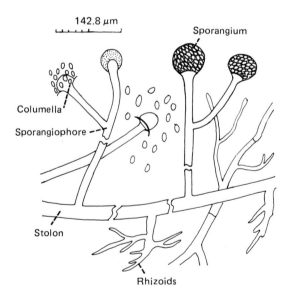

GROSS: Rapidly growing mold, fills tube or plate in one week; coarse, gray or brown, and woolly.

MICRO: Sporangiophores usually occur in groups of two to five, rising from stolons at points away from rhizoid formation. Sporangia are pyriform (pear-shaped). Spores are usually smooth walled and round or oval.

Sporangiophores: 10–15 X 25–70 μm
Spores: 5–6 μm

For more descriptions see

Emmons et al., p. 273
Gillman, pp. 15–19
Rippon, p. 445
Wilson and Plunkett, p. 323

PATHOGENICITY: Agent of mucormycosis (see Chap. 3); also a common mold.

TISSUE FORM: Aseptate hyphae, 10 to 20 μm in diameter, best seen with H & E stain.

SERODIAGNOSIS: Immunodiffusion test has given promising preliminary results (Jones and Kaufman, 1978).

Acremonium **(***Cephalosporium***) sp. (hyphomycete)**

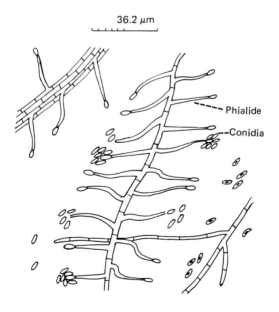

GROSS: Growth rate moderate; at first may be smooth and waxy or velvety, becoming velvety to cottony, white, cream-yellow to rose. *A. falciforme* is described as gray-violet at maturity, with a violet-purple pigment on the reverse (Halde et al., 1976). Most species are colorless on the reverse.

MICRO: Conidiophores are slender phialides. Phialoconidia are elongate, sometimes slightly curved with one septation and often remaining in a slimy ball at the tip of the phialide.

Conidiophores: 15–30 X 3 μm

Conidia: 2–3 X 4–8 μm

For more descriptions see

Chapter 4, Table 18A

Barnett and Hunter, pp. 90–91

Emmons et al., p. 528

Gillman, pp. 210–212, 293

Kendrick and Carmichael, Plate 3c, p. 438

Wilson and Plunkett, pp. 348 and 355

PATHOGENICITY: Agent of mycetoma (see Chap. 3 and Halde et al., 1976). Common mold.

TISSUE FORM: Soft white to yellow granules, 0.2 to 0.5 mm, hyphal forms in tissue.

Actinomadura madurae: **See Chapter 4, Table 18B.**

PATHOGENICITY: Mycetoma.

Actinomyces israelii **(anaerobic to microaerophilic actinomycete)**

GROSS: On anaerobic blood agar plates, colonies appear in five to seven days. They are rough, nodular, and sometimes adherent to the agar. These are described as "molar tooth" in appearance. In thioglycollate broth, colonies appear as small, white flocculent balls throughout the deep part of the media in four to six days. These colonies are catalase negative, do not liquefy gelatin, and do not peptonize milk.

MICRO: Gram's stain shows short, gram-positive bacillary forms.

Gas-liquid chromatography for the detection of volatile fatty acids is the usual method of *Actinomyces* identification.
For more descriptions see

Dowell and Sonnenwirth (in Lennette et al.), pp. 396–401
Rippon, pp. 25–29

PATHOGENICITY: Agent of actinomycosis (see Chap. 3).

TISSUE FORM: Small, yellow to light tan gritty flecks called "sulfur granules" are seen in sputum and draining sinuses. On being crushed between a slide and cover glass and stained by Gram's stain, these granules are shown to consist of delicate, branching, intertwined gram-positive filaments, 1 μm in diameter. The ends of the radial hyphae are frequently sheathed with a gelatinous mass, giving the appearance of club-shaped structures, which has led to the term *actino* or *ray* fungus.

SERODIAGNOSIS: Fluorescent antibody conjugates are used routinely at the Center for Disease Control as an aid in the identification of cultures of *Actinomyces* species (Dowell and Sonnenwirth, pp. 399–400, Rippon, p. 24).

Actinomyces bovis (anaerobic actinomycete)
Similar to *Actinomyces israelii,* with the following exceptions:

GROSS: Colonies on anaerobic blood agar plates are smooth, moist, and glistening. In thioglycollate broth, colonies produce a soft, diffuse growth with downward streamers.

PATHOGENICITY: Usual cause of actinomycosis in cattle.

Alternaria sp. (hyphomycete)

GROSS: Rapid woolly growth, surface varies from white to gray to brown to dark green, reverse is brown or black.

MICRO: Macroconidia are longitudinally and transversely septate, dark yellow or brown. The macroconidia are produced in chains, acropetally, or directly on the sides of the hyphal conidiophores. Detached macroconidia may produce hyphae directly from the septations. Conidiogenous (conidium-producing) cells are sympodial (enlarging and becoming knobby with the production of each conidium), and

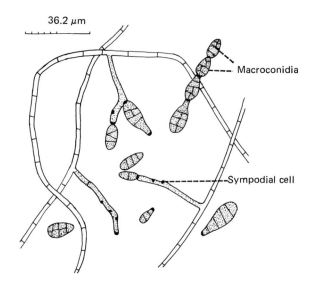

may be monotretic or polytretic. The word *tretic* indicates that the conidium is produced from the inner wall of the conidiogenous cell.

Macroconidia: 6-16 × 16-90 μm (average 14 × 36 μm)

For more descriptions see

Barnett and Hunter, pp. 128–129

Barron, p. 88

Ellis, 1971, pp. 464–497

Emmons et al., p. 528

Gillman, pp. 346–348

Kendrick and Carmichael, Plate 36h, p. 471

Wilson and Plunkett, p. 382

PATHOGENICITY: Commonly implicated in allergies, rarely seen as a cause of cutaneous mycoses (see Chap. 3). Frequently occurs as a common mold.

TISSUE FORM: Dark, highly septate hyphae are seen (see Plate II).

Arthrinium sp. (*Papularia* sp.) (hyphomycete)

GROSS: Early growth is dirty white, woolly, becoming gray to black with age.

MICRO: Lens-shaped, flattened conidia are black and often have a characteristic

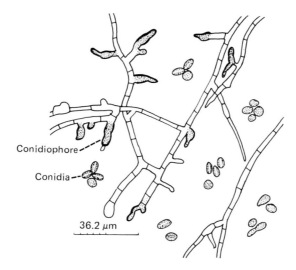

Conidiophore

Conidia

36.2 μm

light slit and a light rim. These conidia are produced from oval, round, or barrel-shaped cells that are borne laterally on chunky conidiophores. These conidiophores are "basauxic," which means that, as the conidia are produced, the conidiogenous cell grows at the base.

For more descriptions see

Barnett and Hunter, p. 78
Barron, p. 90
Ellis, 1971, pp. 567–575
Gillman, p. 316

PATHOGENICITY: Not known as a pathogen.

Aspergillus sp. (hyphomycete)

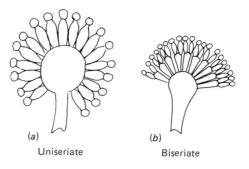

(a)
Uniseriate

(b)
Biseriate

GROSS: Textures are fine velvety to coarse, rough, woolly or cottony, varying in color from white to pink, orange, yellow, green, blue-green, gray, brown, sometimes with deep red or lavender reverse. Descriptions given are based on colonies grown on Czapek Dox agar.

MICRO: This genus is characterized by the presence of a swollen vesicle at the tip of a conidiophore, to which phialides (formerly called "sterigmata") are attached. Phialoconidia are produced basipetally from the phialides. The phialides may be borne directly on the vesicle (uniseriate) or they may be borne on prophialides that arise from the vesicle (biseriate).

The *Aspergillus* species have been divided into 18 groups by Raper and Fennell (1973). The characteristics of the groups in which species commonly isolated are placed are given below. The report of an *Aspergillus* isolate identified by the criteria given here would correctly state the group, not the species, identification. For instance, the report would be written "*Aspergillus (fumigatus* group)," not "*Aspergillus fumigatus.*" For species descriptions the book by Raper and Fennell is consulted.

PATHOGENICITY: *Aspergillus* species have been implicated in systemic subcutaneous, cutaneous, and nail infections. These species are also toxin producers and are frequently a cause of allergic reactions. They occur commonly in the environment. Animals and birds are frequently infected.

TISSUE FORM: *Aspergillus* forms are seen in tissue or respiratory secretions as hyphae, 2.5 to 8 μm wide, usually septate, and dichotomously (divided in two equal parts) branched, at a 45° angle. *Aspergillus* hyphae may be seen in KOH preparations and are most easily seen in the methenamine silver nitrate stain. They are not easily seen in a Gram stain, where they are usually stained gram-negative or not at all. *Aspergillus* fruiting heads may occasionally be seen in tissues from lung cavities and also in exudates from ear infections, where aerobic conditions may exist.

SERODIAGNOSIS: Because of the ubiquitousness of the *Aspergillus* species, nearly all people, animals, and birds have circulating antibodies to the aspergilli. Skin tests, immunodiffusion, complement fixation, and radio immunoassay tests are found to correlate with clinical types of aspergillosis, often with specific species isolated.

For further information about serodiagnosis see

Bardana et al. (three papers cited)

Gerber et al.

Rippon, pp. 423–424; (preparation of antigen, p. 552)

Aspergillus (*clavatus* **group**)

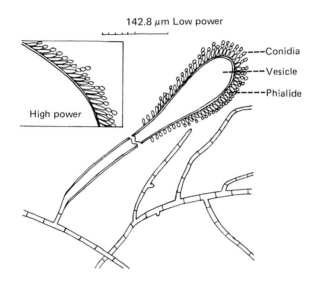

GROSS: Texture is coarse and fluffy. These organisms are rapid growers. The early growth is white, rapidly developing blue-green spore heads that are easily seen on gross examination. Alkaline conditions are preferred.

MICRO: Vesicles are elongate (clavate), from 300 μm to 400 μm when mature. Phialides are uniseriate, conidiophores are smooth and colorless.

PATHOGENICITY: A toxin, called patulin, is produced on grains. (Patulin is also an antibiotic with fungistatic properties.) It is toxic to mice and there is evidence that it is toxic to cattle fed with grain infected with *A. clavatus*. Tissue invasion is rare. One case of nail invasion has been reported.

For more information see

Raper and Fennell, pp. 137–146

Aspergillus (flavus group)

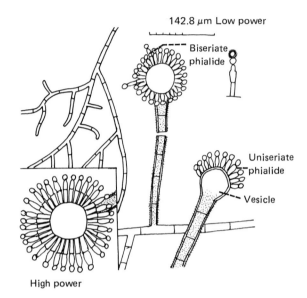

GROSS: Surface is bright yellow-green to deep yellow-green, rough and woolly. Dark red-brown to purple-red sclerotia may produce a variegated color pattern. Reverse ranges from colorless to deep red-brown. Many isolates grow better at 37°C than at 25°C.

MICRO: Radiate heads are predominant, but some are columnar and similar to the aspergilli of the *fumigatus* group. Phialides may be uniseriate or borne on prophialides (biseriate). Both forms occur simultaneously. Conidiophores are colorless and distinctly roughened. Young vesicles may be flask shaped and morphologically indistinguishable from those of the *A. fumigatus* group. At maturity the vesicles are globose (round) or subglobose (almost round).

Vesicle: young, 10–20 µm; mature, 10–65 µm
Phialide: 6–10 µm
Prophialide: 6–10 X 4–5 µm
Conidiophore: 10–20 X 300 µm

The rough, woolly texture and greenish yellow color of the colony and the development of rough-walled conidiophores aid in separating the *A. flavus* group from the *A. fumigatus* group (Raper and Fennell, pp. 357–388).

PATHOGENICITY: Major toxin producer, bronchial and pulmonary lesions and skin lesions are seen. Animals are frequently infected.

For more information, see

Raper and Fennell, pp. 388–404

Aspergillus (*fumigatus* group)

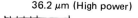

36.2 μm (High power)

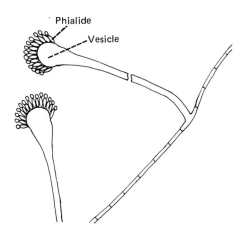

GROSS: Early growth is white, becoming blue-green to gray. Old cultures become dark brown to brown-gray. Texture is velvety and flat or folded. Isolates grow well at 37° to 45°C, some at even higher temperatures, up to 65°C.

MICRO: Heads are columnar. Vesicle is flask shaped and usually fertile over the upper half to one-third. Phialides are uniseriate and crowded evenly together. In the Fischerii series, which are less often seen in a medical lab, white to yellow cleistothecia are present.

Vesicle: 20–30 μm wide
Phialides: 6–8 × 2–3 μm
Conidia: 2.5–3 μm
Conidiophore: up to 300 μm

PATHOGENICITY: Major systemic pathogen, and most frequent cause of pulmonary aspergillosis. Often seen in ear infections. Not often a cause of cutaneous or nail infections. Endotoxins are produced by growth on grain.

For more information, see

Raper and Fennell, pp. 242–268

Aspergillus (glaucus **group)**

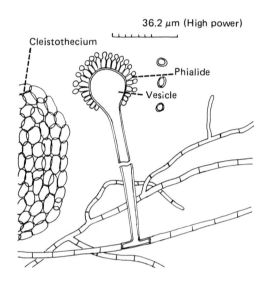

36.2 μm (High power)

Cleistothecium

Phialide

Vesicle

GROSS: Colonies are green to green-gray, with yellow, red, or orange aerial growth, due to cleistothecia, which can be seen grossly. Texture is coarse, uneven, and woolly. Growth at room temperature is good. At 37°C growth is inhibited or poor.

MICRO: Heads are radiate or columnar, with uniseriate and coarse phialides. Yellow, red, or orange cleistothecia are present.

Vesicle: 25–40 μm (average)
Phialides: 7–10 × 3–4 μm
Conidia: 4–7 μm
Cleistothecia: 75–100 μm

PATHOGENICITY: Infrequently reported as a pathogen. Skin, eye, and ear infections are reported, and a toxin that causes death in calves has been extracted.

For more information, see

Raper and Fennell, pp. 152–196

Aspergillus (*nidulans* group)

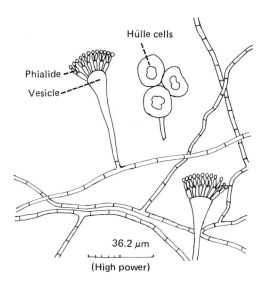

GROSS: Texture is flat and velvety, with irregular margins. Color varies from creamy buff to honey yellow to dark green. The reverse is purplish red.

MICRO: Conidiophores are distinctly brown and usually smooth. They may be slightly roughened. Vesicles are small and hemispherical, fertile at the top, which is distinctly flattened. Phialides and prophialides are present (biseriate). Both cleistothecia and Hülle cells are also seen.

Vesicle: 8–10 μm
Phialide: 6–10 × 3–5 μm
Prophialide: 5–6 × 2–3 μm
Conidiophore: 60–130 × 2.5–5 μm
Cleistothecia: 100–200 μm
Hülle cells: 25 μm

PATHOGENICITY: Rarely a pathogen. Has been reported from appendicitis, pulmonary infections, mycetoma, ear, nails, and skin infections.

For more information, see

Raper and Fennell, pp. 495–542

Aspergillus (*niger* **group**)

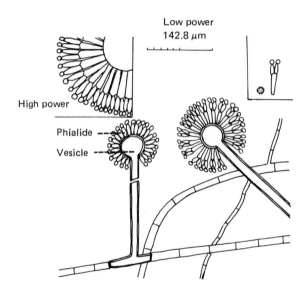

GROSS: Surface is charcoal black, granular, flat. Growth may be white at first. Reverse is colorless to white.

MICRO: These heads may be uniseriate or biseriate. Vesicle is large and round. Radiate heads with numerous black conidia make it difficult to see phialides and prophialides if they are present.

Vesicle: 60–80 μm (average)
Phialide: 2–3 $\times$ 7–11 μm
Prophialide: 3–5 $\times$ 8–11 μm

PATHOGENICITY: Ear infections, lung invader, mycetoma. Oxalic acid is produced in animal feed and associated with oxalic-acid poisoning.

For more information, see

Raper and Fennell, pp. 293-344

Aspergillus (*terreus* group)

36.2 μm (High power)

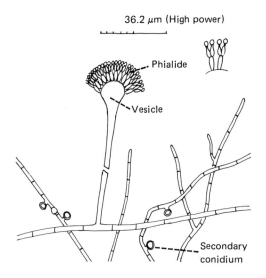

GROSS: Colony is pale buff to dark brown, velvety folded.

MICRO: Vesicle is small and hemispherical with phialides borne on prophialides (biseriate). Phialoconidia are small. A secondary type of conidium is seen, uniquely in the *A. terreus* group, which is larger then the phialoconidia and borne directly on the side of the hypha or on a small hyphal projection.

Vesicle: 10-15 μm
Phialide: 5-7 X 1-2 μm
Prophialide: 5-7 X 2-5 μm
Phialoconidia: 1-8 X 2-4 μm
Secondary conidia: 6-7 μm

PATHOGENICITY: Skin, nails, and ear are infected. Incidence of pulmonary invasion is debated. Secondary spores, 6 to 7 μm are seen in tissue sections.

For more information, see

Raper and Fennell, pp. 567-577

Aspergillus (versicolor **group)**

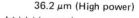

36.2 μm (High power)

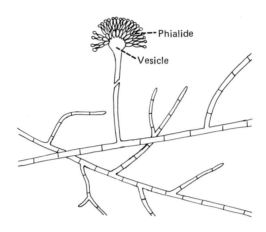

GROSS: Folded, velvety colonies that occur in shades of white and green, become darker with age.

MICRO: Heads are radiate or loosely columnar, biseriate. Vesicle is small, hemispherical and fertile over the upper half. Conidiophores are smooth and hyaline (light-color).

Vesicle: 12–16 μm
Phialide: 5–7 × 2 μm
Prophialide: 5–8 × 3 μm

PATHOGENICITY: Rarely isolated as a pathogen.

For more information, see

Raper and Fennell, pp. 442–490

Other *Aspergillus* groups, not usually implicated as pathogens, are described by Raper and Fennell as follows:

Aspergillus (ornatus group): Uniseriate, grayish yellow to olive-brown, white to purplish cleistothecia (p. 199).
Aspergillus (cervinus group): Uniseriate, pinkish fawn (p. 213).

Aspergillus (restrictus group): Uniseriate, requires 20 to 40% sucrose (p. 222).

Aspergillus (sparsus group): Uniseriate and biseriate, constriction below vesicle head (p. 431).

Aspergillus (ochraceus group): Uniseriate and biseriate, yellow-orange or buff (p. 269).

Aspergillus (candidus group): Uniseriate and biseriate, white to yellow-cream (p. 345).

Aspergillus (wentii group): Uniseriate and biseriate, large (up to 500 μm) heads, yellow to light brown (p. 407).

Aspergillus (cremeus group): Uniseriate and biseriate, requires 20 to 40% sucrose (p. 418).

Aspergillus (ustus group): Biseriate, phialides longer then prophialides. Hülle cells elongated, curved, or twisted (p. 545).

Aspergillus (flavipes group): Biseriate, white, flesh color or buff (p. 559).

As Raper and Fennell (p. 130) have said, "It should be emphasized that we are dealing with living and variable organisms and that species and group concepts must be reasonably elastic."

Aureobasidium (Pullularia) pullulans (hyphomycete)

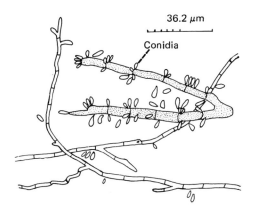

GROSS: Growth is shiny, moist, yeastlike. Early cultures are white to cream and become brown to black with age. Sometimes a white fringe is seen. Colonies may become folded and wrinkled with age.

MICRO: Thick-walled, black, large hyphal cells and delicate thin-walled hyphae produce conidia that continue to multiply by budding.

For more descriptions see

Chapter 4, Table 17
Barnett and Hunter, pp. 64–65
Barron, p. 96
Ellis, 1971, p. 515
Gillman, p. 316
Wilson and Plunkett, p. 372

PATHOGENICITY: Rarely seen as a pathogen. (See Chap. 3: Aureobasidio-mycosis.) Commonly isolated as a contaminant mold.

Basidiobolus haptosporus (zygomycete)

GROSS: Colonies are buff to gray, turning brown when older, thin, flat, glabrous radial folds. Surface becomes covered with a "bloom" of sporangia, chlamydo-spores, and zygospores.

MICRO: Wide, occasionally septate hyphae. "Sporangiospores are produced by cleavage of the sporangial cytoplasm. Zygospores are spherical and thick walled, formed following the conjugation of adjacent hyphal cells." (Emmons et al., pp. 281–282.) Chlamydospores may replace zygospores in laboratory cultures.

Hyphae: 8 to 20 μm wide
Zygospores: 30 to 50 μm

PATHOGENICITY: Cause of entomophthoromycosis.

TISSUE FORM: Aseptate hyphae, 10 to 20 μm in diameter, stain best with H & E stain.

Beauveria sp. (hyphomycete)

GROSS: Surface is white, velvety to powdery to fluffy.

MICRO: Conidiophores are sympodial, developing a zigzag effect as conidia are produced on small projections.

For more descriptions see

Barnett and Hunter, pp. 96 and 97

36.2 μm

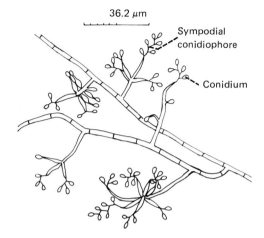

Sympodial
conidiophore

Conidium

Barron, p. 99
Kendrick and Carmichael, p. 459, Plate 24E

PATHOGENICITY: Rarely seen as a pathogen. (See Chap. 3: Beauveriosis.)

Blastomyces dermatitidis (hyphomycete),
Ajellomyces dermatitidis (Ascomycotina)

36.2 μm

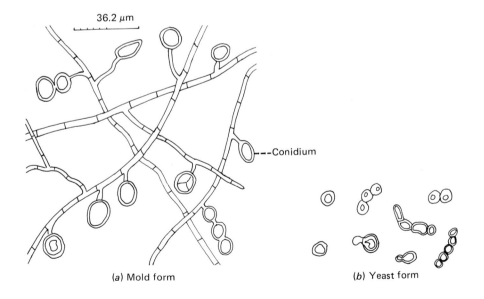

Conidium

(a) Mold form   (b) Yeast form

GROSS: Dimorphic fungus.

Mold form: Optimal growth is seen on enriched agar, such as brain-heart infusion agar at 22°-30°C. Energetic growth occurs on all routine isolation media at 22°-30°C, including media with cycloheximide. Colonies are waxy at first, and may develop a prickly appearance. The entire surface may become covered with a white woolly mat. Cultures are white at first and may become tan with age.

Yeast form: Slow-growing, wrinkled pasty colonies appear on enriched agar at 37°C. Growth at 37°C is inhibited by cycloheximide.

MICRO:

Mold form: Many spherical to pyriform conidia are borne on short hyphal branches or on slender conidiophores.
Conidia: 2 to 10 μm.

Yeast form: Broad-based budding cells (multinucleate) are seen.
Budding cells: 8 to 15 μm.
Broad base: 4 to 5 μm.

Special Tests: Conversion of mold form to yeast form on enriched agar is necessary to establish the identification of *B. dermatitidis*. It may be necessary to make several sequential subcultures at 37°C for complete conversion. See Chapter 4, flow chart Table 13C.

For more descriptions see

Chapter 4, Tables 13C and 14

Carmichael, p. 1154

Emmons et al., pp. 359–363

McGinnis and Katz, 1979

Rippon, pp. 315–318

Wilson and Plunkett, pp. 357–358

PATHOGENICITY: Causative organism of blastomycosis (see Chap. 3).

TISSUE FORM: 8 to 15 μm multinucleate budding cells, broad-based budding (4 to 5 μm), are seen in KOH and methenamine silver nitrate stains, and by fluorescent staining methods.

SERODIAGNOSIS: An antigen prepared from cell sap has been reported as a specific immunodiffusion technique (Rippon, pp. 312 and 353, and Rippon,

Anderson, et al.). Kaufman, McLaughlin and others (p. 559) have also reported a specific immunodiffusion technique using reference sera containing A and B precipitins that have been recognized in sera of patients with blastomycosis. Less than 50% of patients with proven blastomycosis give a positive reaction in a routine complement fixation test. Commercially prepared antigens show cross-reactions with histoplasmin and coccidiodin. A fluorescent antibody technique has been developed by Kaplan and Kaufman (1963) which is useful in recognizing the yeast form of *B. dermatitidis* in tissue sections.

Discussions of the serology of blastomycosis are found in

Kaufman (in Lennette et al.), p. 559
Rippon, pp. 312-313, 353 (Preparation of Cell Sap Antigen)

Botrytis sp. (hyphomycete)

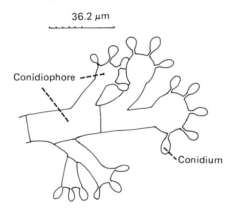

36.2 μm

Conidiophore

Conidium

GROSS: Gray to brown, woolly.

MICRO: Conidiophores are long, often pigmented, branched apical cells that are enlarged or rounded. These bear clusters of conidia on short denticles. These conidia are hyaline or ash colored, one celled, and ovoid. Black irregular sclerotia (hard masses of hyphae) are frequently produced.

For more descriptions see

Barnett and Hunter, pp. 70 and 71
Barron, pp. 105-107

Gillman, pp. 298–300
Wilson and Plunkett, p. 356

PATHOGENICITY: None reported.

Candida species (blastomycete)

The *Candida* species described on the following pages are those most commonly isolated in a medical laboratory. Occasionally there will be other *Candida* species that do not fit these criteria. These may be more completely identified with reference to the work of Lodder, or by use of the API 20C system, or they may be reported as *Candida* species if they fit the following simple criteria.

GROSS: White to cream color, moist or pasty.

MICRO: Budding cells on routine media and on EMB agar test and in serum. On corn meal Tween-80 agar or rice agar, hyphae, pseudohyphae, and budding cells are seen.

For more descriptions see

Lodder and Kreger-Van Rij (ed 2), 1970.
Kreger-Van Rij NJW (ed): *The Yeasts, A Taxonomic Study,* ed 3 is currently in preparation, with a chapter by Sally A. Meyer on *Candida* species.)

Candida albicans (blastomycete)

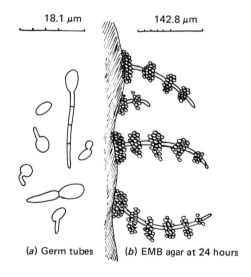

(a) Germ tubes   (b) EMB agar at 24 hours

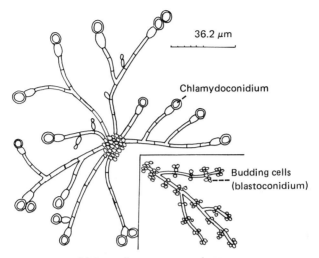

36.2 μm

Chlamydoconidium

Budding cells
(blastoconidium)

(c) Seven days on corn meal agar.

GROSS: Growth at three days is moist and white, with a satinlike sheen. At one week, reverse of colony may show mycelium extending into the medium. Older cultures often become heaped and rough. On eosin–methylene blue agar, incubated in 5 to 10% CO_2 at 35°C to 37°C (EMB agar test), feathering may be seen. On bromcresol green agar, at room temperature, colonies are white to pale green or pale yellow.

MICRO: Budding cells are seen on routine isolation media. In serum within two hours, or on EMB agar test in two to three hours, germ tubes, pseudohyphae and budding cells are seen. On EMB agar test at 24 hours, hyphae, pseudohyphae and clusters of budding cells are seen. On corn meal or rice agar in three to seven days chlamydoconidia are usually seen. These are diagnostic. Budding cells occurring in tight clusters along the hyphae are also seen.

Budding cells (blastoconidia): 3 to 8 μm

For more descriptions see

Chapter 4, Table 9
Plates 3, 4, and 5
Haley and Callaway, p. 125
Silva-Hutner and Cooper in Lennette et al., Table I, pp. 497 and 502
All mycology texts

246   Doing It

PATHOGENICITY: *C. albicans* is an opportunistic fungus that invades all areas of the body, causing cutaneous, mucocutaneous and opportunistic systemic infections (see Chap. 3 and Bakerspigel, Proc. 4th Int. Conf. Mycoses, Part II, pp. 141–175).

TISSUE FORM: Hyphae, pseudohyphae, and budding cells are seen in tissue, by all microscopic techniques.

SERODIAGNOSIS: Satisfactory *C. albicans* antigen can be purchased from Hollister-Stier Laboratories in Spokane, Washington, or can be prepared according to methods described (see Rippon, p. 553). The latex agglutination test and the immunodiffusion test are helpful in the diagnosis and monitoring of systemic *Candida* disease.

Further discussions on the serodiagnosis of *C. albicans* are found in

Kaufman (in Lennette et al.), p. 559
Rippon, pp. 195–196

Candida guillermondii (blastomycete),
Pichia guillermondii (Ascomycotina)

36.2 μm

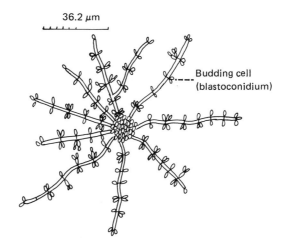

Budding cell
(blastoconidium)

GROSS: Growth is moist and creamy. Early cultures, grown in three to seven days, are white. After two to three weeks, a pale pink color may develop. On brom-cresol green agar, colonies develop more slowly then *C. albicans* and at seven days are blue to blue-green and glossy.

MICRO: Small budding cells (blastoconidia) are seen on routine media, in serum, and on EMB agar test. On corn meal Tween-80 or rice agar, short hyphae and compact clusters of small budding cells are seen. Hyphae are often slow to develop. Chlamydoconidia are absent.

For more descriptions see

Chapter 4, Table 9
Plates 3 and 5
Dolan and Roberts, p. 156
Haley and Callaway, p. 132
Harold and Snyder, pp. 8-9

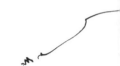

PATHOGENICITY: This may be an opportunistic yeast. (See Bakerspigel, Proc. 4th Int. Conf. Mycoses, p. 143).

Candida krusei (blastomycete),
Pichia kudriavezii (Ascomycotina)

36.2 μm

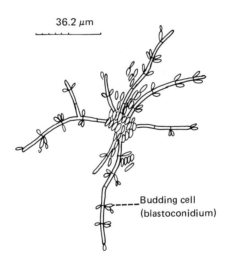

Budding cell
(blastoconidium)

GROSS: Growth is white, flat, and dry. On bromcresol green agar, colonies are yellow or pale green and usually flat and dry. Occasional strains are raised and a pasty dull yellow.

MICRO: Elongated budding cells (blastoconidia) and occasional pseudohyphae are seen on routine media, in serum, and on EMB agar test. On corn meal Tween-80 or on rice agar, hyphae and elongated budding cells in parallel formation are seen.

For more descriptions see

Chapter 4, Table 9
Plates 3 and 4
Dolan and Roberts, p. 156
Haley and Callaway, p. 129
Harold and Snyder, pp. 8–9
Rippon, p. 198

PATHOGENICITY: May invade the skin of burn patients and other compromised hosts. Also associated with infant diarrhea. (See Chap. 3 and Bakerspigel, Proc. 4th Int. Conf. Mycoses, 1978, p. 144.)

Candida parapsilosis (blastomycete), *Lodderomyces elongisporus* (Ascomycotina)

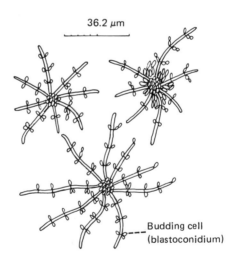

36.2 μm

Budding cell
(blastoconidium)

GROSS: Growth is moist and creamy, occasionally becoming brown on the border and dry and wrinkled with age. On bromcresol green agar, colonies are pale yellow to pale green, moist and pasty. At seven days, on the reverse, a sharp yellow border with a dark green center is seen.

MICRO: Budding cells (blastoconidia) are seen on routine media, in serum at 37°C, and on EMB agar test. On corn meal Tween-80 agar, or rice agar, hyphae are seen, with short branches, pseudohyphae and slender budding cells, making up compact colonies and giving a splattered starry effect. Occasionally giant hyphae are seen.

For more descriptions see

Chapter 4, Table 9
Plates 3 and 5
Dolan and Roberts, p. 155
Haley and Callaway, p. 128
Harold and Snyder, p. 819

PATHOGENICITY: This organism may be an opportunistic fungus and is seen in endocarditis and in nail disease. It is frequently isolated as a saprophytic yeast on the skin. (See Bakerspigel, Proc. 4th Int. Conf. Mycoses, 1978, p. 143.)

Candida pseudotropicalis (blastomycete),
Kluyveromyces fragilis (Ascomycotina)

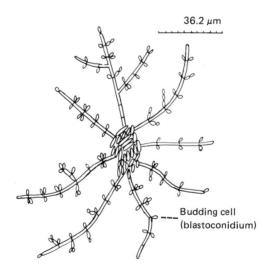

36.2 μm

Budding cell
(blastoconidium)

GROSS: Growth is moist and creamy. On EMB agar a metallic sheen is seen, indicating lactose fermentation. On bromcresol green agar, at three to seven days, colonies are an intense glossy green to yellow-green, with a thin yellow border.

MICRO: Budding cells (blastoconidia) are seen on routine media and on EMB agar test and on serum at 37°C. On corn meal Tween-80 or rice agar, hyphae and elongated budding cells (similar to those of *C. krusei*) are often seen in parallel formation.

For more descriptions see

Chapter 4, Table 9
Plates 3 and 5
Dolan and Roberts, p. 156
Haley and Callaway, p. 128
Harold and Snyder, p. 8

PATHOGENICITY: May be an opportunistic fungus, seen in lung and nail infections.

Candida stellatoidea (blastomycete)

GROSS: Colonies are white to cream colored, moist and pasty. Cultures may become heaped and rough with extending fringes of mycelium submerged into the medium. On bromcresol green agar, colonies are light yellow to yellow-green, with feathery growth penetrating into the medium.

MICRO: *C. stellatoidea* is similar to *C. albicans* in microscopic forms seen on all media. Budding cells (blastoconidia) are seen on routine media. Germ tubes are formed on serum at 37°C within two hours and on EMB agar test in three hours. Hyphae and chlamydoconidia are produced on corn meal Tween-80 agar or on rice agar. This species is distinguished from *C. albicans* by its inability to assimilate sucrose. The descriptions given by Harold and Snyder describe some of the morphologic differences between these species.

For more descriptions see

Harold and Snyder, p. 8

PATHOGENICITY: *C. stellatoidea* is rarely a pathogen.

Candida tropicalis (blastomycete)

GROSS: Growth is typically rough, heaped, and waxy. It may also be moist and smooth. Both forms may be present in isolates from the same specimen. On brom-

36.2 μm

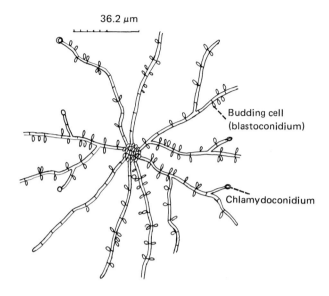

Budding cell
(blastoconidium)

Chlamydoconidium

cresol green agar, the surface is pale green to pale yellow, often with a gray sheen. Texture may be smooth to rough, with irregular borders. More than one colony type may be present.

MICRO: Budding cells (blastoconidia) and occasionally pseudohyphae are seen on routine media. In serum at 37°C in two to three hours, and on EMB agar test in three hours, budding cells in chains of three and short pseudohyphae may be present. At two hours on EMB agar test, budding cells only may be seen, or pseudohyphae and budding cells, borne singly, may be seen. These are distinguished from the hyphae and budding cells of *C. albicans* by the constrictions at the points of pseudohyphal growth and by the singly borne conidia. On corn meal agar, blastoconidia are typically borne singly along the hyphae, often not at the septations. The long filamentous hyphae are seen to extend from a central group of large refractile budding cells. Small chlamydoconidia may be seen.

For more descriptions see

Chapter 4, Table 9
Plates 3, 4 and 5
Dolan and Roberts, p. 155
Haley and Callaway, p. 127
Harold and Snyder, p. 8

PATHOGENICITY: *C. tropicalis* is frequently implicated as a pathogen, particularly in endocarditis and in compromised patients. *C. tropicalis* and *C. albicans* will often be seen in succession or, occasionally, together in seriously ill patients. (See Bakerspigel, Proc. 4th Int. Conf. Mycoses, 1978, pp. 142–165.)

Cephalosporium sp. (see *Acremonium* sp.)

Chaetomium sp. (Ascomycotina)

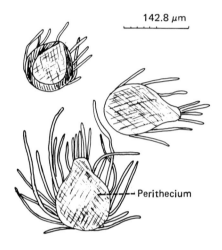

142.8 μm

Perithecium

GROSS: Growth is scant and olivaceous, later brown, or black and fluffy.

MICRO: Perithecia vary in size, depending on the species. The asci are clavate and are quickly destroyed when the perithecium erupts, leaving only the ascospores to be observed. The ascospores are lemon shaped, single-celled, and light brown.

Perithecia: 110–225 × 100–150 μm

For more descriptions see

Gillman, pp. 175–182
Wilson and Plunkett, p. 336

PATHOGENICITY: Rarely isolated as a skin invader.

Chrysosporium sp. (hyphomycete)
See also *Blastomyces dermatitidis, Epidermophyton floccosum, Histoplasma*

capsulatum, Microsporum sps., *Monosporium apiospermum, Paracoccidioides brasiliensis, Sepedonium* sp., and *Trichophyton* sps.

GROSS: Colonies are extremely varied, from waxy to velvety to powdery, and predominantly white to tan, but also pink, orange, yellow, tan, brown, gray-green, gray, lavender, or violet. The reverse is most often colorless to tan, but may range from brown to red, orange, yellow, gray-green, blue-green to deep violet, and may diffuse into the medium. Most isolates are positive on Dermatophyte Test Medium.

MICRO: Conidiophores are not easily differentiated from hyphae and may be irregularly branched. Conidia are aleurioconidia, globose to clavate, borne singly or in short chains, terminally, sessile, or intercalary. Conidial size varies from an average of 2-10 μm, with larger multiseptate macroconidia, or chlamydoconidium-like conidia occurring in some species. A broad basal scar may be seen when aleurio-conidium is released from the aleuriophore. Arthroconidia and phialoconidia may also be observed in some species.*

For further descriptions see

Carmichael, pp. 1137-1174
Emmons et al., p 524
Wilson and Plunkett, p. 357

PATHOGENICITY: The imperfect forms of several pathogenic species are in-cluded in this genus by Carmichael. These forms are agents of dermatomycoses (*E. floccosum, Microsporum* species and *Trichophyton* species), of blastomycosis (*B. dermatitidis*), histoplasmosis (*H. capsulatum*), and mycetoma (*M. apiosper-mum*), and of paracoccidiomycosis (*P. brasiliensis*).

Chrysosporium keratinophilum (hyphomycete)

GROSS: Colonies are velvety to granular, white to pale cream to sulphur yellow or brown. Reverse is colorless to tan. Grows poorly at 37°C. Digests but does not penetrate hair in vitro.

MICRO: Pyriform conidia may be borne on the tips of hyphae, on short or long pedicels, or may be intercalary. They may be smooth to slightly roughened.

---

*Species of fungi are placed in the genus *Chrysosporium* primarily on the basis of aleruio-conidium production.

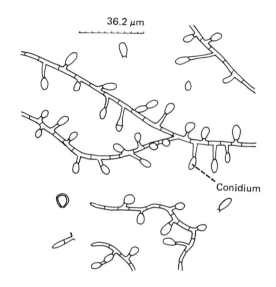

Conidia: 6-9 × 9-15 μm, average: 7-8 × 10-12 μm.

For more descriptions see

Carmichael, pp. 1157-1158
Rebell and Taplin, p. 71

PATHOGENICITY: Not known as a pathogen.

Chrysosporium pannorum (hyphomycete)

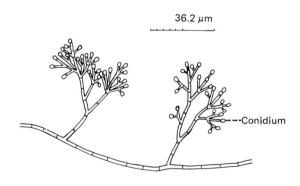

GROSS: Surface is waxy to fine chalky, powdered, flat or heaped and wrinkled, white to yellow or pale brown, or gray, pink, or lavender. Reverse color may diffuse into the medium, and may vary in subculture. There is no growth at 37°C and hair is not digested.

MICRO: Conidia are typically borne on the ends of conidiophores that are verticillately branched. The conidia may also be borne on the sides of the conidiophores or in an intercalary position, giving the appearance of arthroconidia, or, when broken loose, giving a budding appearance.

Conidia: 2–4 X 2–5 μm, average: 2 X 3 μm.

For more descriptions see

Carmichael, pp. 1163–1164
Rebell and Taplin, p. 71

PATHOGENICITY: Not known as a pathogen.

Chrysosporium (Haplosporangium) parvum,
Emmonsia parva (hyphomycete)

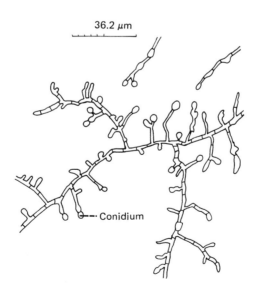

36.2 μm

Conidium

GROSS: Colorless, waxy colony may become completely velvety, or may develop tufts of hyphae, or may have alternate zones of waxy and velvety growth. Growth is inhibited at 37°C. Color varies from white to cream to tan or pale brown. Reverse is white or yellow or brown.

MICRO: At 25° to 30°C, conidia may be flattened at the tip and smooth or slightly roughened and are borne at the tips of hyphae or on narrow short pedicels. Pedicel may inflate and produce more conidia, often giving a budding appearance. At 37°C, hyphae are contorted and at 40°C, chlamydoconidia (adiaspores) are produced. These adiaspores are uninucleate.

Conidia: 2.5-5 × 3-5 μm
Adiaspores: 10-25 μm

For more descriptions see

Carmichael, pp. 1164-1166
Emmons et al., p. 500

PATHOGENICITY: Adiaspiromycosis, adiasporosis.

TISSUE FORM: In the mouse, uninucleate adiaspores, 40 μm in diameter with walls 4 μm are seen.

Chrysosporium parvum, var. crescens
(Emmonsia crescens) (hyphomycete)

GROSS: See *Chrysosporium parvum*

MICRO: Structures are similar to *C. parvum* at 25° to 30°C. At 37°C, hyphae disappear and large, thick-walled multinucleate chlamydoconidia (adiaspores) appear.

Adiaspores: 200-700 μm
Adiaspore walls: 70 μm

For more descriptions see

Carmichael, pp. 1164-1166
Emmons et al., p 502

PATHOGENICITY: Adiaspiromycosis, adiasporosis.

Chrysosporium pruinosum (hyphomycete)

36.2 μm

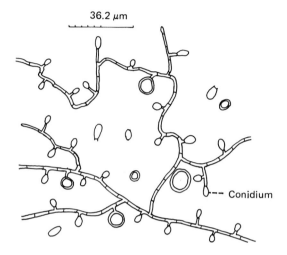

-- Conidium

GROSS: Colony is velvety to granular, white to cream colored, becoming tan with age. Grows well at 37° to 40°C and does not digest hair.

MICRO: Conidia are smooth walled, subglobose to pyriform to clavate, borne at the tips of hyphae or directly on the sides, on short or long side branches, or are intercalary. At 37°C large globose chlamydoconidia are formed.

Conidia: 3-15 X 4-20 μm

Chlamydoconidia: up to 65 μm

For more descriptions see

Carmichael, pp. 1166-1168

Rebell and Taplin, p. 72

PATHOGENICITY: Not reported as a pathogen.

Chrysosporium tropicum (hyphomycete)

GROSS: Flat, velvety to granular, white to cream. Grows well at 37°C and penetrates hair in vitro.

MICRO: At both 25° and 37°C, conidia are borne on the tips of hyphae, on the sides or on lateral branches, varying in length. Some are intercalary. The conidia

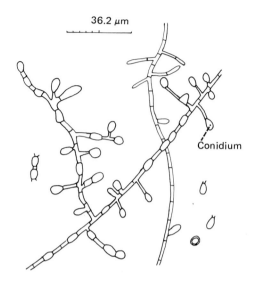

36.2 μm

Conidium

are smooth or slightly roughened and pyriform to clavate. Arthroconidia may be present.

Conidia: 3-5 X 4-9 μm, average: 3-5 X 6-7 μm.

For more descriptions see

Carmichael, pp. 1170-1171
Rebell and Taplin, p. 71

PATHOGENICITY: Not known as a pathogen.

Circinella sp. (zygomycete)

GROSS: Rapid, woolly, tan to gray.

MICRO: Many branched hyphae, with divisions. Sporangiophores carry lateral whorled branches on which are borne spherical sporangia. Walls of sporangia are encrusted with calcium oxalate crystals. Columellae are large. Spores are spherical.

Sporangia: 60 to 150 μm (depending on species)
Columella: up to 30 μm wide
Spores: 3 to 5 μm

For more descriptions see

Gillman, p. 24
Wilson and Plunkett, p. 327

PATHOGENICITY: Not known to be a pathogen.

Cladosporium (*Hormodendrum*) sp. (hyphomycete)

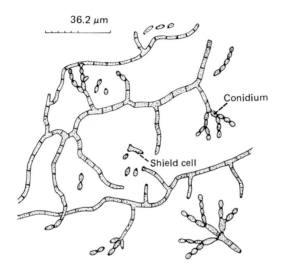

36.2 μm

Conidium

Shield cell

GROSS: Growth is rapid to moderate, velvety, folded, dark olive-green, gray-green, black or brown. Reverse of colony is black. Majority of isolates are laboratory contaminants and are proteolytic (liquefy 12% gelatin or Löeffler's serum slant). Those that are currently recognized as pathogenic are not proteolytic. Ellis (p. 308) states that over 500 species have been described.

MICRO: Hyphae are dark and segmented. Early hyphae may be hyaline (light). Conidiophores are pigmented and either branched or unbranched. Conidiogenous cells produce conidia from two or more points (polyblastic), and these are generally called *shield cells*. Conidia are produced acropetally in chains and, depending on the species, may vary in size. These may be rough (echinulate) or smooth, and they may be single celled or with septations. Scars at the attachment point, known as disjunctors, are usually prominent on both the conidia and the conidiogenous cells. These scars serve as an identification criterion for this species.

Conidia: 3-6 to 40-50 X 12-15 μm

For more descriptions see

Chapter 4, Table 17
Barnett, pp. 102–103
Barron, p. 128
Ellis, 1971, pp. 308–319
Emmons et al., pp. 528–529
Kendrick and Carmichael, p. 64
Wilson and Plunkett, pp. 377–378

PATHOGENICITY: Pathogenic species with *Cladosporium*-type of sporulation include *Cl. carrionii, Cl. trichoides,* and *Fonsecaea pedrosoi.*

Cladosporium carrionii (hyphomycete)

GROSS: Colonies are slow growing (3 to 4 cm at one month), dull gray to lavender-gray. These do not liquefy gelatin or Löeffler's serum. They grow well at room temperature and sometimes at 37°C, will not grow at 42°C and they hydrolize casein within one month.

MICRO: Conidia are produced in long chains (as described for *Cladosporium* sp.) and are 4-5 X 2-3 μm.

For more descriptions see

Emmons et al., p. 403
Nielsen (in Lennette et al.), p. 534
Wilson and Plunkett, p. 378

PATHOGENICITY: Agent of chromomycosis, particularly in Australia.

TISSUE FORM: Sclerotic bodies (round, deeply pigmented bodies), septate or unicellular (4-12 μm) and dark segmented hyphae.

SERODIAGNOSIS: Complement-fixing antibodies and precipitins have been demonstrated. (Buckely and Murray, 1966; Martin et al., 1936).

Cladosporium trichoides (*Cladosporium bantianum*) (hyphomycete)

GROSS: ·Colony is slow-growing, 3-4-cm colony at one month, olive-gray to black, with jet-black reverse. It does not liquefy 12% gelatin or Löeffler's serum and does not hydrolize casein. It grows well at 42° to 43°C.

MICRO: Long chains of small conidia (2–2.5 × 4–7 μm) are produced, as described for *Cladosporium* sp.

For more descriptions see

Emmons et al., pp. 476–482

Neilsen (in Lennette, et al.), p. 535

Wilson and Plunkett, p. 379

PATHOGENICITY: Agent of cerebral chromomycosis, pulmonary lesions, dermal and ulcerative lesions, cerebral abscesses, and meningitis are described by Emmons et al. (p. 472).

TISSUE FORM: Narrow brown hyphae (1 × 2 to 3 μm) and larger cells (up to 20 μm) are seen.

SERODIAGNOSIS: Fluorescent antibody procedures have been described by Al Doory and Gordon (1963). Antigen differences have been observed between this and other similar molds by Nielsen and Conant (1968).

Coccidioides immitis (hyphomycete)

GROSS: Dimorphic fungus

Mold form: 22°–37°C. Characteristically, a moist, flat, membranous colony is produced in three to five days. At about seven days, a central tuft of white mycelium forms. By the tenth day, the central tuft is surrounded by a zone of sparse growth, which, in turn, is surrounded by a wider zone of cottony mycelium. At two weeks, the entire culture may be white and completely cottony, becoming tan or brown with increasing age. Good growth is generally observed at temperatures ranging from 22° to 37°C and on all routinely used mycologic media. Growth is not inhibited by cycloheximide. Considerable variation of this colonial morphology in 70 out of 301 isolates is described by Huppert et al. (1967), with some strains showing only waxy growth and some strains with colors ranging from gray to pale lavender, pink, buff, cinnamon, yellow, and brown. CULTURES WILL BE FILLED WITH HIGHLY INFECTIOUS ARTHROCONIDIA. SAFETY PRECAUTIONS ARE TO BE OBSERVED (See methods section).

Spherule form: 40°C. This form may be produced by in vitro conversion. (See page 184).

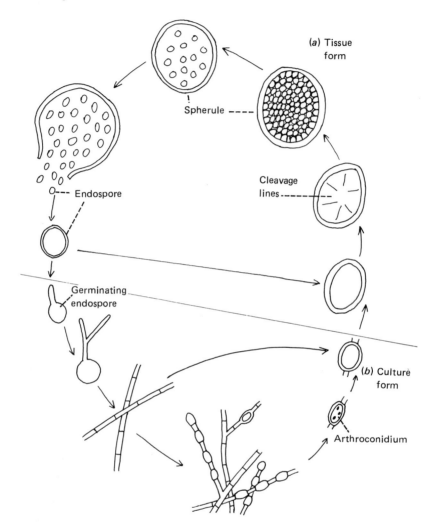

MICRO:

Mold form: At 7 to 10 days, arthroconidia, which are typically barrel shaped, are produced by septation in hyphal branches. These arthroconidia are usually thick walled and are connected by thin-walled segments. Remmants of connecting segments are observed in loose arthroconidia. Variations in size and shape of arthroconidia are described by Huppert et al. (1967). Arthroconidia may be thin walled and may be either long or oval.

36.2 μm

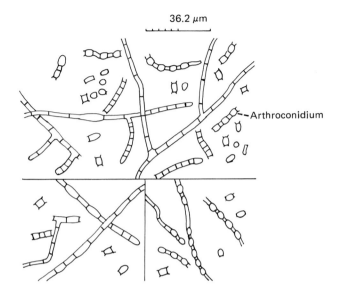

Arthroconidia: average 2.5–4 × 6 μm; may range 1.5–2.3 × 1.5–15 μm

Spherule form: See Tissue Form.

SPECIAL TESTS: *C. immitis* is differentiated from other arthroconidium-producing fungi (see Sigler and Carmichael) by demonstrating the conversion of
arthroconidia to spherules containing endospores (in vitro or by animal inoculation)
and by immunodiffusion techniques described below.

For more descriptions see

Chapter 4, Table 14
Emmons et al., pp. 250–252
Huppert, Sun and Bailey, pp. 323–328
Larsh and Goodman (in Lennette et al.), pp. 517–518
Rippon, pp. 384–386
Wilson and Plunkett, pp. 346–347

PATHOGENICITY: Causative agent of coccioidomycosis.

Tissue form: The parasitic form of *C. immitis* occurs as spherules (round cells)
            with highly refractile walls that develop into sporangia that contain
            endospores. These endospores are produced by a process known as

cleavage, in which the protoplasm of the inner sperule wall divides into multinucleate masses (protospores), which are further divided into uninucleate endospores. (Sporangia produced in animal tissue or by in vitro conversion may be quite large.) These are demonstrated in tissue in KOH (wet-mount) preparations, methenamine silver nitrate stain, periodic acid-Schiff stain, Papanicolaou stain, and the H & E stain. Gram stains are not satisfactory. The spherules of *C. immitis* may have the same appearance as nonbudding *Blastomyces dermatitidis* cells and the endospores, when seen free of the sporangium, are similar to *Histoplasma capsulatum* cells seen in tissue.

Sporangia: 30–60 μm in humans; 30–200 μm in animals, or by in vitro conversion. Endospores: 2–5 μm.

SERODIAGNOSIS: Coccidioidin is an antigen prepared from broth filtrate of *C. immitis.* Several different strains are usually used. Spherulin is an antigen made from the spherule form of *C. immitis* and will sometimes produce a positive-complement fixation test when other tests are negative to coccidioidin. Anticoccidioidin is serum containing antibodies to *C. immitis,* produced by rabbits that have been inoculated with a concentrated supernatant of broth cultures of *C. immitis.*

Skin tests: Individuals who have or have had coccidioidomycosis will have a positive skin test to Spherulin or Coccidioidin. As the disease progresses and disseminates, a subsequent negative skin test is a poor prognostic sign.

Testing of serum, spinal fluid, plasma, pleural, and joint fluids:

1. The latex particle agglutination test, available from Hyland Laboratories, Los Angeles, California, detects precipitins and gives a positive result within four minutes. It is useful in detecting early disease in 70% of proven cases of coccidioidomycosis.

2. The immunodiffusion test detects complement fixing antibodies and is 80% accurate. Together, these two tests are 93% accurate.

3. The complement fixation test is done at intervals throughout the course of the disease. A rising titer is indicative of progressive disease. A declining titer may indicate that the patient is improving or it may be a poor prognostic sign indicating energy.

Seroidentification of cultures of *C. immitis:* Anticoccidioidin is used in an immunodiffusion test for the early identification of cultures of *C. immitis.* A technique that is 100% successful in producing identifying bands for over 100 *C. immitis* isolates, including variant strains, and that does not produce identifying bands with other arthroconidium-producing molds, is described by Huppert et al. (1978). This test gives a presumptive identification of *C. immitis,* usually within five days after the initial isolation of the mold. A more rapid technique is described by Kaufman and Standard (1978).

For more information about serodiagnosis of coccidioidomycosis see

Emmons et al., pp. 236-237

Huppert, Sun, and Rice, pp. 346-348

Kaufman, L. (in Lennette, et al.), pp. 559-560

Kaufman and Standard, pp. 42-45

Rippon, p. 379; preparation of antigen, p. 554

Cryptococcus sp. (blastomycete)

GROSS: Cream to tan, moist, glassy, mucoid; urea positive, inositol positive.

MICRO: Single budding cells. Hyphae are rarely seen. In most species a polysaccharide capsule is produced, which can be seen in India ink preparations.

For species differentiation, see:

Chapter 4, Table 9.

PATHOGENICITY: The species *Cr. neoformans,* described below, is a major pathogen. Other species are generally isolated as saprophytic fungi.

Cryptococcus neoformans (blastomycete); *Filobasidiella neoformans* (subdivision, Basidiomycotina; Class, Teliomycete).

GROSS: Growth is cream colored to tan, moist, glassy, mucoid. Urea and inositol are positive. Brown colonies are produced in six hours on seed agar or on caffeic acid medium with ferric citrate added (Hopfer and Gröschel, 1975). Good growth occurs at room temperature and at 37°C. Growth is inhibited by cycloheximide. Lactose is not assimilated.

MICRO: Budding cells are produced from the parent cell, through a narrow pore. The cell is surrounded by a mucopolysaccharide capsule, which is generally narrow

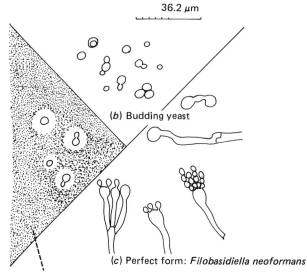

36.2 μm

(b) Budding yeast

(c) Perfect form: *Filobasidiella neoformans*

(a) India ink preparation, showing capsule

in culture. The size of the capsule in culture may be increased by repeated subcultures on brain-heart infusion agar at 37°C. Hyphae are occasionally produced.

Budding cells: 4 to 20 μm

Capsule: 1 to 2 μm, in culture may vary up to 4 μm

The perfect form, *F. neoformans,* has been demonstrated by Kwon-Chung, by the mating of two compatible isolates and the production of basidia, basidiopspores, and clamp connections in the fertilized hyphae.
Special tests:

Urea: positive

Capsule on India ink

Brown colonies on seed agar, or caffeic acid medium.

For other tests see Table 9.

For more descriptions see

Chapter 4, Table 9
Emmons et al., pp. 223–228
Kwon-Chung, 1975 and 1976

Larsh and Goodman (in Lennette et al.), p. 519

Rippon, p. 221

Silva-Hutner and Cooper (in Lennette et al.), pp. 492, 493, 497, and 503

Proceedings of the fourth International Conference on Mycoses, Part II, pp. 176–217

PATHOGENICITY: Causative agent of cryptococcosis.

Tissue form: Budding and single cells, 4 to 20 μm, are seen. These cells are surrounded by a capsule that, in tissue, may be twice the radius of the cell. Capsules are demonstrated in India ink preparation by negative staining as the particles of India ink are dispersed. Capsules also may be stained a diffuse rose color by Mayer's mucicarmine method. Budding cells, but not capsules, stain well with the methenamine silver nitrate stain and the periodic acid-Schiff stain. Capsules may often be seen in these preparations as clear, white areas surrounding the cells. KOH (wet mounts) and Gram-stained preparations are less satisfactory, but cells may be seen. Small *Cryptococcus* cells may occur intracellularly, making it difficult to distinguish them from *H. capsulatum* cells.

Budding cells: 4 to 20 μm

Capsule: varies, may be twice the radius of the cell

SERODIAGNOSIS: The latex slide agglutination test detects cryptococcal antigen in sera and CSF and may also be used to give a rapid presumptive identification of *Cr. neoformans* in culture form (Muchmore, et al., 1978). A commercial Crypto-La kit may be obtained from International Biological Laboratories, Inc., Rockville, Maryland.

An indirect fluorescent antibody (IFA) technique is described by Kaufman as a valuable and sensitive tool, but not entirely specific. Tube agglutination tests are specific, but Rippon cites a high incidence (40%) of negative results.

For more information and further references about cryptococcal serodiagnosis see:

Kaufman, L. (in Lennette et al.), pp. 560–561

Muchmore, et al., pp. 166–170

Rippon, p. 219

Curvularia sp. (hyphomycete)

36.2 μm

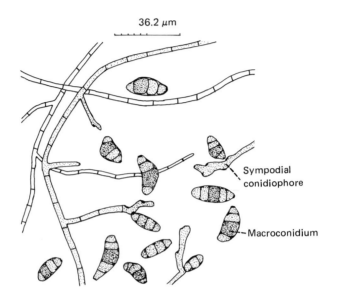

Sympodial conidiophore

—Macroconidium

GROSS: Colony is black or black-brown velvety with black reverse.

MICRO: Spindle-shaped (fusiform) macroconidia have three septations. Central cell or cells are larger and darker than the end cells and may be bent, giving a curved (geniculate) appearance. Conidiogenous cells are polytretic and may be sympodial, similar to conidiophores of *Drechslera* sp.

Macroconidia: 7–45 × 19–60 μm

For more descriptions see

Barnett, p. 118
Barron, p. 137
Ellis, 1971, pp. 452–459
Emmons et al., pp. 529–530
Gillman, p. 336
Rebell and Forster (in Lennette et al.), pp. 487–488

PATHOGENICITY: *C. lunata* is verified as causative agent in keratomycosis (eye

invasion) (Rippon, p. 480, Rebell and Forster, p. 487). *C. geniculata* has been reported in endocarditis (Rippon, p. 472; Emmons et al., p. 461) and as an agent of
phaeohyphomycosis.

TISSUE FORM: Septate hyphae are seen.

Doratomyces (Stysanus) stemonitis (hyphomycete)

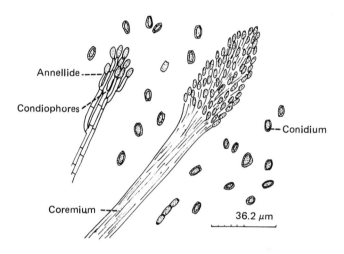

GROSS: Surface is gray-brown to black, velvety; moderate rate of growth. Reverse
is black.

MICRO: Tightly packed strands of conidiophores are formed in a bundle called a
coremium. These are graduated in length. Each one terminates in an annellide that
produces lemon-shaped conidia.

For more descriptions see

Barnett and Hunter, p. 156
Barron, p. 157
Ellis, 1971, p. 328
Gillman, p. 352

PATHOGENICITY: Not known as a pathogen.

Drechslera sp. (hyphomycete)

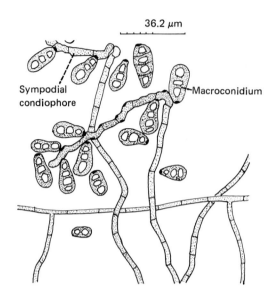

GROSS: Surface is gray, brown or blackish brown, hairy or velvety. Mycelial growth is immersed. Reverse is black or dark brown-black.

MICRO: Conidia are pale to dark brown, multiseptate, and varied in size and shape. Conidia (tretoconidia) are blown out from conidiogenous cells through tiny pores (polytretic) and are distinguished by the nubby conidiophores that enlarge with the production of each new conidium and are marked by scars at the point of attachment of loose conidia (sympodial growth).

For more descriptions see

Ellis, 1971, pp. 303–452

Emmons et al., pp. 531–532

Kendrick and Carmichael (in Ainsworth IVA), pp. 433 and 485

PATHOGENICITY: Rare pathogen. Agent of meningoencephalitis (Rippon, p. 473); also reported in a case of primary cutaneous phaeohyphomycosis (Estes, cited in Chapter III).

Epicoccum sp. (hyphomycete)

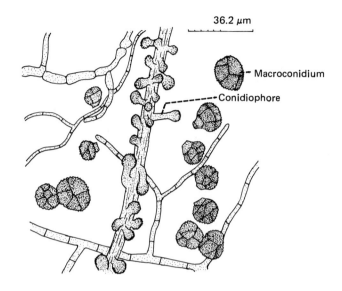

GROSS: Growth is moderately fast. Colony is white, yellow, orange, red, brown, and black with rough irregular velvety surface, which becomes dark brown or black with age. Young cultures appear to be several species due to varying colors and surfaces.

MICRO: Thick, round, or pear-shaped conidia are at first clear and nonseptate, becoming rough, septate and black with age. These are borne on short, thick conidiogenous cells that are formed from cells in intertwined strands of septate hyphae or from short septate conidiophores that rise from these hyphal septations.

Conidia: 16 to 25 µm.

For more descriptions see

Barnett, p. 152
Barron, p. 163
Ellis, 1971, pp. 72–73
Emmons et al., pp. 532–533
Gillman, p. 398 and Plate 13

Kendrick and Carmichael (in Ainsworth IVA), pp. 419 and 470
Wilson and Plunkett, p. 384

PATHOGENCITY: Not known as a human pathogen.

Epidermophyton floccosum (hyphomycete)

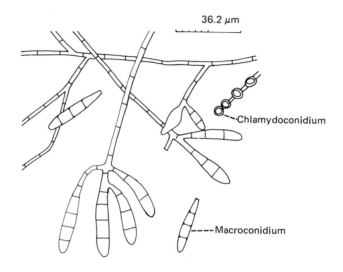

There is only one species in this genus.

GROSS: Initial growth may be golden tan with spreading border, similar to, but more intensly colored than *M. canis*. Good growth in two weeks, greenish-yellow, mustard-yellow, or golden tan. Reverse is dark orange. Surface of colony becomes heaped and folded. White cottony tufts of sterile mutants appear on surface of colony, which usually completely mutates on repeated subculture to become white and velvety.

MICRO: Paddle-shaped macroconidia with rounded ends and smooth walls and up to four or five cross walls occur singly or in bunches on the same conidiophore. Microconidia are absent. Chlamydoconidia may become abundant as culture matures.

Macroconidia: 6-12 X 20-40 μm.

For more descriptions see

Chapter 4, Table 11
Emmons et al., pp. 160 and 163
Kendrick and Carmichael (in Ainsworth IVA), pp. 432 and 486
Rebell and Taplin, p. 62
Rippon, p. 169
Wilson and Plunkett, p. 363

PATHOGENICITY: Dermatophyte invades skin and nails, causing tinea cruris, tinea corporis, tinea pedis, tinea manuum, and onychomycosis. (It does not produce tinea capitis.)

TISSUE FORM: Septate hyphae are observed.

Exophiala jeanselmei, Phialophora jeanselmei, Phialophora gougerotii
(hyphomycete)

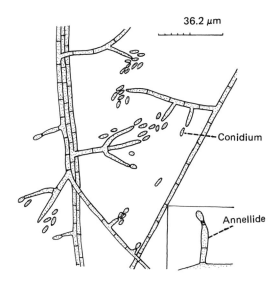

GROSS: Initial colony is moist and black, becoming gray to black or brown and velvety. Good growth is observed at 37°C on potato dextrose agar.

MICRO: Conidiogenous cells occur as either (1) annellides, or (2) thick-walled budding cells of varied sizes and shapes. Annelloconidia are formed outside the annellide (exogenously). As these are formed and freed, they will often slip down the side of the conidiophore, giving the appearance, superficially, of being attached.*

Annellides: 1.0–3.1 × 5.0–1.9 μm; average: 1.7 × 12.5 μm.
Annelloconidia: 0.9–2.9 × 1.0–5.0 μm; average: 1.5 × 2.5 μm.

For more descriptions see

Chapter 4, Table 18A
Cole, G. (in Proc. 4th Int. Conf. Mycoses), p. 70
Barron, p. 256
Emmons, 1966
Emmons et al., p. 431 (*Ph. gougerotii*); p. 458 (*Ph. jeanselmei*)
McGinnis, 1977
McGinnis and Padhye, 1977
Nielsen (in Lennette et al.), p. 536 (*Ph. jeanselmei*)
Padhye, A., 1978 (in Proc. 4th Int. Conf. Mycoses), pp. 60–65
Schneidau (in Lennette et al.), p. 525 (*Ph. gougerotii*)
Wang, C.J., 1965

PATHOGENICITY: Mycetoma (*Ph. jeanselmei*), phaeomycotic cyst (*Ph. gougerotii*).

TISSUE FORM: Mycetoma: granules with hyphae and chlamydoconidiumlike cells. Phaeomycotic cyst: hyphae and budding cells in wall of lesion.

Exophiala salmonis (hyphomycete)
This is the first species of the genus *Exophiala* to be described, as established by Carmichael.
For descriptions see

---

*Emmons (1966) describes this as two species of *Phialophora,* separated primarily on clinical differences, but also on the basis of paraffin utilization. *Ph. gougerotii* causes phaeomycotic cysts and utilizes paraffin. *Ph. jeanselmei* causes mycetoma and does not utilize paraffin. McGinnis and Padhye trace the nomenclature and history of both species of *Phialophora* and define them as morphologically identical, placing them in the genus *Exophiala* on the basis of annellide production.

Carmichael, 1966

Cole, G. (in Proc. 4th Int. Conf. Mycoses), p. 73

Ellis, 1971, p. 552

PATHOGENICITY: Not known as a human pathogen but causes disease in trout.

Exophiala spinifera, Phialophora spinifera (hyphomycete)
For descriptions see

Cole, G. (in Proc. 4th Int. Conf. Mycoses), p. 70

Emmons et al., p. 433

McGinnis, 1977

Nielsen (in Lennette et al.), p. 537

PATHOGENICITY: Phaeomycotic cyst (see Ajello, 1978, p. 11).

Exophiala werneckii, Cladosporium werneckii (hyphomycete)

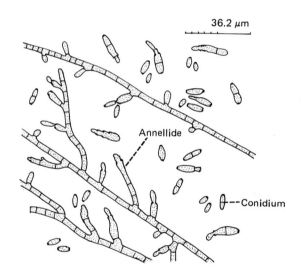

GROSS: Early growth is black, moist, shiny yeastlike. After two weeks, it becomes dark gray-green, with areas of grayish aerial hyphae. Colony may be heaped.

MICRO: Two kinds of conidium production are seen. The first is a simple budding from a single conidium-producing cell. The second is the production of conidia from short (2–3 μm), brown, chunky, scarred conidium-producing cells (annellides). These conidia may occur singly, or as septations (intercalary) within the dark septate hyphae. The conidia may have one to three septations, and they occur singly or in oddly assorted groups. Older hyphae may be large, with thick, pigmented walls.

Annellides: 2 to 3 μm

Conidia: 2.9 × 5 μm

Hyphae: up to 7 μm in diameter.

For more descriptions see

Chapter 4, Table 17

Ajello (in Proc. 4th Int. Conf. Mycoses, 1978), pp. 12–13 and 73

Cole, G. (in Proc. 4th Int. Conf. Mycoses), p. 73

Emmons et al., pp. 172–173

Nielsen, H.S. (in Lennette et al.), pp. 538–539

McGinnis (in Proc. 4th Int. Conf. Mycoses), p. 49

Rippon, p. 90

Wilson and Plunkett, pp. 262 and 378.

PATHOGENICITY: Agent of tinea nigra. Also present as a common mold in organic matter.

TISSUE FORM: Brown septate hyphae and budding cells are easily observed in wet-mount (KOH) preparations.

SERODIAGNOSIS: None are known at present.

Fonsecaea pedrosoi, Phialophora pedrosoi, Hormodendrum pedrosoi
(hyphomycete)

GROSS: Colonies are slow-growing, dark brown, green to black, velvety. This species grows well at 37°C. and it is not inhibited by cycloheximide.

MICRO: Three kinds of conidium production are observed. The first to develop and the most predominant is the *Cladosporium* type, in which conidia are produced in chains with the youngest at the tip (acropetally). When broken apart, attachment points (disjunctors) are observed. Conidia occur in a variety of shapes, including shield cells, which are typical of *Cladosporium* species. The second kind of conidium production is sympodial. Conidia are produced first terminally and then

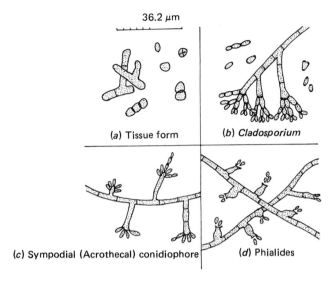

(a) Tissue form

(b) *Cladosporium*

(c) Sympodial (Acrothecal) conidiophore

(d) Phialides

laterally on a conidiophore that enlarges and becomes knobby with the production of each new conidium. The terminal conidium may produce a new conidium. The third kind of conidium production is from phialides and is the last to develop. The conidia are small and usually remain in a loose cluster at the opening of the phialide.

Conidia: 1.5-3 X 3-6 μm.

Phialoconidia: 1.5-3 X 2.5-4 μm.

For more descriptions see

Chapter 4, Tables 16 and 17
Cole, G. (in Proc. 4th Int. Conf. Mycoses), pp. 75-76
Emmons et al., pp. 398-402
Nielsen (in Lennette et al.), pp. 531-533
Rippon, pp. 240-242
Wilson and Plunkett, p. 375

PATHOGENICITY: Agent of chromomycosis.

TISSUE FORM: *Sclerotic* bodies, septate or unicellular, 4-12 μm, and brown septate hyphae may be seen in KOH preparation or with fungal stains.

SERODIAGNOSIS: Complement-fixing antibodies and precipitins have been demonstrated (Buckely and Murray, 1966; Martin et al., 1936).

Fusarium sp. (hyphomycete)

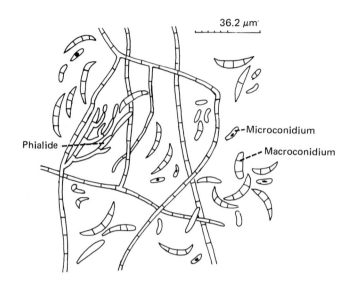

GROSS: Growth is rapid, cottony, white, turning to rose or lavender; may be inhibited by cycloheximide.

MICRO: Two kinds of conidia are observed. Both are produced from phialides. The most characteristic conidia are slender, multicelled, with 2 to 11 septations, and sickle shaped or fusiform, depending on the species. Smaller, one- or two-celled conidia, similar to those of *Acremonium* sp., are also seen.

Macroconidia: 3–8 × 11–100 μm (depending on species).
Microconidia: 2–4 × 4–8 μm.

For more descriptions see

Barnett and Hunter, p. 126
Barron, pp. 164–166
Emmons et al., pp. 520–521
Gillman, pp. 357–372 (species descriptions are given)
Rebell and Forster (in Lennette et al.), pp. 482–490. Some species descriptions are given.
Wilson and Plunkett, p. 384

The *Fusarium* Research Center, Pennsylvania State University, University Park, Pa. 16802, provides an identification service, according to Rebell and Forster.

PATHOGENICITY: Mycotic keratitis (eye invader), onychomycosis, toxin producer.

TISSUE FORM: Septate hyphae are seen in KOH preparation or with fungal stains.

Geotrichum candidum (hyphomycete), *Endomyces geotrichum* (Ascomycotina)

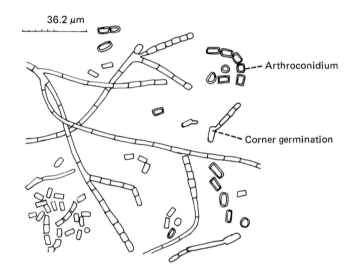

GROSS: Growth is thin, vigorous, waxy or dry with radiating gray-white mycelia, cobwebby. Poor growth or none at 37°C.

MICRO: Hyphae fragment into thin-walled arthroconidia which may be round or square-ended when loose. These are produced in chains with the youngest at the base (basipetally). Some are joined at right angles, producing a bend in a chain of conidia. Loose arthroconidia germinate at the corner of the cell to produce a new hypha. Budding forms are NOT produced.

Arthroconidia: 5-10 X 4 µm.

For more descriptions see

Chapter 4, Table 9
Barnett and Hunter, pp. 62–63
Barron, p. 172
Emmons et al., pp. 204–205
Gillman, p. 206
Rippon, p. 451
Wilson and Plunkett, p. 346

PATHOGENICITY: Agent of geotrichosis; common mold, found in the gastro-intestinal tract of man.

For more information, see

Emmons et al., p. 202
Rippon, pp. 448–451
Bakerspigel, 1978 (in Proc. 4th Int. Conf. Mycoses), p. 144

TISSUE FORM: Arthroconidia 4–8 μm are seen in KOH preparation and with fungal stains.

Gliocladium sp. (hyphomycete)

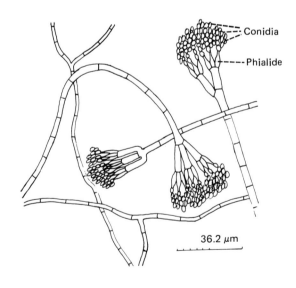

36.2 μm

GROSS: The surface is rough, woolly, or powdery, dark green or, in some species, white to salmon; rapid growth. The reverse is pale to colorless.

MICRO: Simple or branched conidiophores terminating in a whorl of phialides, similar to *Penicillium* sp. Conidia vary in size and color, depending on species, and are produced in chains that are enveloped in a ball of slime.

For more descriptions see

Barnett and Hunter, p. 88
Barron, pp. 177-179
Emmons et al., pp. 522-523
Gillman, pp. 288-291
Wilson and Plunkett, p. 352

PATHOGENICITY: Common mold, not presently known as a pathogenic species.

Helminthosporium sp. (hyphomycete); see also
Drechslera sp.

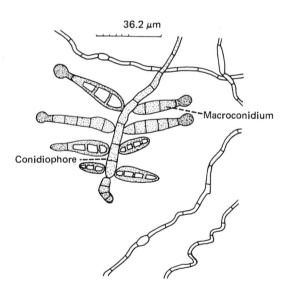

GROSS: Growth is rapid. Surface is gray, sometimes with a slight pink tint in early growth. Surface is woolly with a black reverse.

MICRO: Multiseptate conidia (tretoconidia) are produced through brown smooth-walled conidiophores. (*Drechslera* species are distinguished from *Helminthosporium* species by the knobby conidiophores resulting from the sympodial growth of *Drechslera* species.)

For further descriptions see

Ellis, 1971, pp. 388–393

PATHOGENICITY: See *Drechslera* sp.

Hendersonula toruloidea (coelomycete) (see *Scytalidium*)

Histoplasma capsulatum (hyphomycete), *Ajellomyces capsulata* (Ascomycotina)

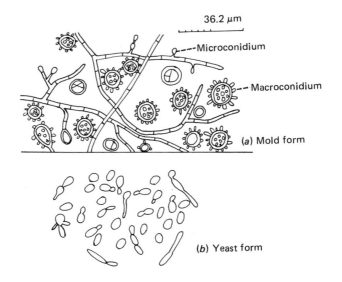

GROSS: Dimorphic fungus.

Mold form: At 22° to 30°C optimal growth is seen on enriched agar, such as brain-heart infusion agar with blood added. Colonies are slow-growing, white to tan, velvety and sometimes cracked at the center. Reverse is tan to brown. Growth occurs on all routine media at 22° to 30°C, including media with cycloheximide added.

Yeast form: At 37°C, yeast form is produced on enriched agar, preferably brain-heart infusion agar with blood and cysteine added. Growth appears as cream to pink pasty, wrinkled colonies. At 37°C growth is inhibited on media with cycloheximide.

MICRO:

Mold form: Characteristic structures are large round or pear-shaped macroconidia that may be smooth or, more characteristically, have fingerlike protuberances. The tuberculate macroconidia are borne on conidiophores at right angles to the hyphae. Oval microconidia are also produced on similar conidiophores.

Tuberculate macroconidia: 8–14 μm

Microconidia: 2–4 μm

Yeast form: Oval budding cells are developed from the hyphae.

Budding cells: 2–3 X 3–4 μm

Special tests: The conversion of the mold form to yeast form and yeast form to mold form is necessary to establish the identification of *H. capsulatum*. The yeast form may be produced most readily by primary inoculation on enriched agar at 37°C.

For more descriptions see

Chapter 4, Table 14

Barnett and Hunter, p. 76

Barron, p. 205

Carmichael, p. 1146

Emmons et al., pp. 328–355

Larsh and Goodman (in Lennette et al.), pp. 514–515

McGinnis and Katz, 1979

Rippon, pp. 340–345

Wilson and Plunkett, p. 359

PATHOGENICITY: Primary systemic pathogen, agent of histoplasmosis.

TISSUE FORM: Small, oval cells, which may or may not bud, are observed loose or intracellularly, within the cytoplasm of macrophages. These cells are seen most easily with the methenamine silver nitrate stain. A Giemsa or Wright stain is often used for observing these cells, particularly in bone marrow smears, but the cells are less easy to see with this method. A KOH wet-mount or a Gram stain is not satisfactory.

Budding cells in tissue: 2–4 μm

SERODIAGNOSIS: Two antigens are used effectively in the serodiagnosis of histoplasmosis. One is merthiolate treated suspension of yeast form cells, and the other, histoplasmin, is a mycelial filtrate produced by cultures of *H. capsulatum* grown on Smith's asparagine medium. Both antigens are used in serologic tests.

Skin tests: A positive skin test indicates past or present exposure to *H. capsulatum* and will be positive for a lifetime. There is some evidence that administration of a histoplasmin skin test causes a rise in antibodies, agglutinins, and precipitins. This factor must be taken into account in interpreting complement fixation and other serological tests.

Complement fixation test: A rising titer indicates progressing disease and a falling titer follows resolution of the disease. Reaction to the yeast-phase antigen is longer than to the mycelial antigen (histoplasmin). Patients with cryptococcosis and blastomycosis also show high titers to histoplasmin.

Immunodiffusion and counterimmunoelectrophoresis: These tests are more useful than the complement fixation test in diagnosing histoplasmosis. Two bands that may be observed are of diagnostic value. The *m* band, which is closest to the antigen well, may occur alone and is present in active or inactive disease or as a result of skin testing. The *h* band usually occurs with the *m* band, is closer to the antibody well, and indicates active infection. A third, *c,* band represents an antigen common to both *H. capsulatum* and *B. dermatitidis.*

Latex agglutination: This test is performed with commercially prepared histoplasmin-sensitized latex particles. A positive latex test indicates acute histoplasmosis. This must be confirmed with a complement fixation test. This test may be negative in cases of chronic histoplasmosis.

Fluorescent antibody: Kaufman (in Lennette et al., p. 564) describes an F.A. technique for recognition of *H. capsulatum* yeast cells, both in culture and in specimens.

Seroidentification of cultures of *H. capsulatum:* An accurate method for the rapid identification of strains of *H. capsulatum* is described by Kaufman and Standard (1978). An immunodiffusion test is performed with antigen prepared from extracts of the culture and antisera of a patient with histoplasmosis. A presumptive identification of *H. capsulatum* can be made two days after growth of the mold is observed. For more information on serodiagnosis see

Emmons et al., pp. 309–310
Kaufman and Standard, 1978
Kaufman (in Lennette et al.), pp. 561–564
Rippon, p. 338 (Preparation of Antigen, p. 554)

Histoplasma capsulatum, var. *duboisii*

GROSS: Mold form and yeast form are similar to *H. capsulatum.*

MICRO: Mold form is like *H. capsulatum.* Yeast form consists of large, round or oval, uninucleate cells with walls 1.5 μm thick. Buds are attached by a narrow neck. Small budding cells are also seen.

Budding cells: 7–15 μm and 2–3 X 3–4 μm

For more descriptions see

Emmons et al., p. 337
Larsh and Goodman (in Lennette et al.), pp. 518–519
Rippon, p. 354

PATHOGENICITY: Agent of African histoplasmosis.

TISSUE FORM: Similar to *B. dermatitidis,* except that bud is narrow-based.

Loboa loboi, Paracoccidioides loboi
Culture form is not known.

PATHOGENICITY: Lobomycosis (keloidal blastomycosis), seen in South America.

TISSUE FORM: Chains of oval budding cells are seen. Some cells may bud at more than one point.

Budding cells: 9 μm in diameter (average)

For more descriptions see

Emmons et al., pp. 384–385
Rippon, p. 283.

Madurella mycetomi (hyphomycete)

GROSS: Growth is slow, leathery to velvety, white to yellow-brown. Grows better at 37°C than at room temperature. Some strains produce a diffusible yellow-brown pigment. Round black bodies (sclerotia) may be seen. Assimilates sucrose but not lactose.

Sclerotia: up to 750 μm.

MICRO: Sclerotia, when present, are made up of polygonal cells, about 10 μm in diameter. On corn meal agar, phialides and phialoconidia may be seen.

For further descriptions see

Chapter 4, Table 18A
Emmons et al., p. 455
Rippon, p. 63
Schneider (in Lennette et al.), pp. 525–526
Wilson and Plunkett, p. 155

PATHOGENICITY: Agent of eumycotic mycetoma.

TISSUE FORM: Firm black grains are composed of brown, pigmented hyphae, with swollen cells and terminal hyphae.

Grains: up to 5 mm
Pigmented hyphae: 1–5 μm in diameter
Swollen cells: up to 30 μm in diameter
Terminal hyphae: 12–15 μm in length

Madurella grisea (hyphomycete)

GROSS: Growth is slow, with raised colonies, 3–5 cm in diameter, velvety, dark gray or gray-green, becoming red-brown with age. It grows better at 30°C than at 37°C. Reverse of colony is black. Red-brown diffusible pigment may be present. This species assimilates lactose but not sucrose.

MICRO: Conidia are not produced. Pycnidia are produced in some strains. Observation of tissue form is needed for identification.

For further descriptions see

Chapter 4, Table 18A
Emmons et al., p. 456
Rippon, p. 64
Schneidau (in Lennette et al.), pp. 525-526
Wilson and Plunkett, pp. 155-156

PATHOGENICITY: Agent of eumycotic mycetoma.

TISSUE FORM: Small, brittle, black grains are observed. Outer edge is brown. Center is clear and composed of hyaline hyphae.

Grains: up to 1 mm.

Microsporum audouini (hyphomycete)

GROSS: Good growth in two weeks. Surface is buff to light reddish brown and very flat. Reverse is reddish brown. On potato dextrose agar a salmon pigment is formed under the thallus. Growth is poor on boiled rice.

MICRO: Terminal chlamydoconidia are typically present. Spindle-shaped, oddly formed macroconidia are seen in rare isolates. Microconidia are not usually seen. "Pectinate" (comblike) hyphae are reported in most isolates.

For further descriptions see

Chapter 4, Table 11
Ajello and Padhye (in Lennette et al.), p. 476
Emmons et al., pp. 143 and 145
Rebell and Taplin, p. 16
Wilson and Plunkett, pp. 369-370

PATHOGENICITY: Anthropophilic agent of tinea capitis and tinea corporis in children. It is rarely seen in adults and rarely invades nails.

TISSUE FORM: Infected hairs fluoresce with a yellow-green color under Wood's light. Ectothrix hair invasion is seen. Segmented hyphae are seen in KOH preparation of skin. See Table 5B.

Microsporum canis (hyphomycete), *Nannizzia*
otae (Ascomycotina)

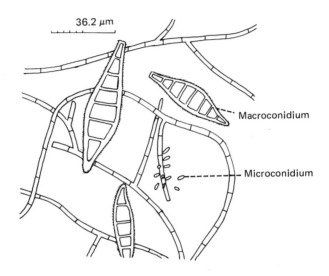

GROSS: Good growth in one week. It has a flat, thin to velvety white surface, radiating border, and pale yellow to deep yellow reverse. It produces good growth on boiled rice.

MICRO: Spindle-shaped macroconidia have thick walls that become roughened, first at the tips and then all over, as culture matures. Microconidia are elongate. Sporulation may be induced by growth on boiled rice.

Macroconidia: 7–15 cells; 15–20 × 60–125 μm; walls up to 4 μm.
Microconidia: 2.5–3.5 × 4–7 μm.

For further descriptions see

Chapter 4, Table 11
Ajello and Padhye (in Lennette et al.), p. 476
Emmons et al., p. 145
Rebell and Taplin, pp. 13–14

Rippon, pp. 152–153
Wilson and Plunkett, p. 370

PATHOGENICITY: Zoophilic, causes tinea capitis and tinea corporis, rarely onychomycosis. Primarily seen in children, but may also be seen in adults. It is associated with infected cats or dogs.

TISSUE FORM: Yellow-green fluorescence of invaded hairs is seen in Wood's light. Ectothrix hair invasion. Segmented hyphae in KOH preparation of skin. See Table 5B.

Microsporum cookei (hyphomycete),
Nannizzia cajetani (Ascomycotina)

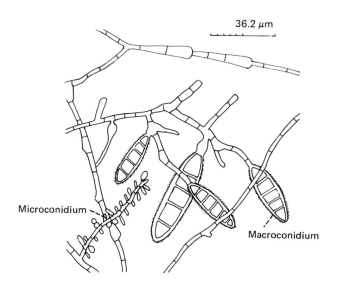

36.2 µm

Microconidium

Macroconidium

GROSS: Surface is coarsely granular tan with deep reddish purple pigment on reverse.

MICRO: Thick, rough-walled macroconidia and microconidia are seen.

Macroconidia: 31–50 × 10–15 µm, walls 5 µm.
Microconidia: 3–8 × 2 µm.

Special tests: Perforates hair in vitro.

For further descriptions see

Emmons et al., p. 153
Rebell and Taplin, p. 29
Rippon, p. 156
Wilson and Plunkett, p. 371

PATHOGENICITY: Geophilic species; not established as a human pathogen.

Microsporum distortum **(hyphomycete)**

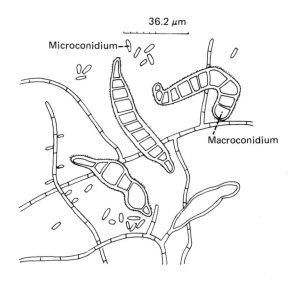

GROSS: Growth is rapid, white, and fluffy. Reverse is bright yellow-orange.

MICRO: Rough-walled macroconidia, similar to those of *M. canis,* are crooked and distorted. Microconidia may be abundant.

For further descriptions see

Emmons et al., p. 153
Rebell and Taplin, p. 15
Rippon, pp. 154–155

PATHOGENICITY: Zoophilic; rare cause of tinea capitis, mainly in New Zealand but also in United States and South America.

TISSUE FORM: Like *M. canis.*

Microsporum ferrugineum, Trichophyton ferrugineum (hyphomycete)

GROSS: Growth is slow (two to three weeks), waxy, compact, furrowed, golden yellow. The edge of the colony is subsurface. White velvety filaments may develop in older colonies.

MICRO: The hyphae are slender and coarse, and occasional chlamydoconidia are seen. Straight hyphae with prominent cross walls (*bamboo* hyphae) are seen. Rough-walled macroconidia have been observed on potato dextrose agar with charcoal.

For further descriptions see

Emmons et al., p. 151
Rebell and Taplin, p. 19
Rippon, p. 153
Wilson and Plunkett, pp. 367–368

PATHOGENICITY: Anthropophilic, causes tinea capitis in the Orient.

TISSUE FORM: Ectothrix, Wood's light positive.

Microsporum fulvum (hyphomycete), *Nannizzia fulva* (Ascomycotina)

GROSS: Growth is similar to *M. gypseum.*

MICRO: Macroconidia, with up to five septations, are similar to those of *M. gypseum.* Spirals may be seen. Microconidia, also similar to *M. gypseum,* are seen.

Macroconidia: 25-60 × 8.5-15 μm, up to five septations.
Microconidia: 2-3.5 × 3-8 μm.

For further descriptions see

Ajello and Padhye (in Lennette et al.), p. 477
Emmons et al., p. 148
Rebell and Taplin, p. 25
Rippon, p. 154

PATHOGENICITY: Similar to *M. gypseum,* but possibly less virulent.

TISSUE FORM: See *M. gypseum.*

Microsporum gallinae, Trichophyton gallinae (hyphomycete)

GROSS: This species produces moderate white, velvety, folded growth in two weeks. Diffusible, pale red pigment is produced.

MICRO: On routine media short, branched hyphae and a few slender micro-conidia are seen. Sporulation increases on media with thiamine or yeast extract added, and macroconidia with smooth or roughened walls are seen. This species is differentiated from *T. megnini* by its ability to grow without histidine, by the production of rough-walled macroconidia, and by the production of diffusible pigment in the medium.

Rare macroconidia: $15-150 \times 6-8$ μm, 2–10 septations.

For further descriptions see

Emmons et al., p. 151
Rebell and Taplin, p. 21
Rippon, p. 155
Wilson and Plunkett, p. 368

PATHOGENICITY: Zoophilic, causes chicken favus. Rare agent of tinea capitis and tinea corporis.

Microsporum gypseum (Hyphomycete); *Nannizzia gypsea, Nannizzia incurvata* (Ascomycotina)

GROSS: Colony is buff to cinnamon-brown, powdery to velvety with good growth in two weeks. Reverse may produce thin veins of deep red-brown color.

36.2 μm

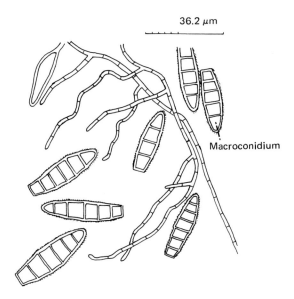

Macroconidium

MICRO: Abundant, thin-walled macroconidia with rounded ends are observed. Microconidia are also seen.

Macroconidia: 25–60 X 7.5–16 μm, walls, 1–3 μm, cells, 4–6 septations
Microconidia: 2.5–3 X 4–6 μm.

Special test: Perforates hair in vitro.
For further descriptions see

Ajello and Padhye (in Lennette et al.), p. 476
Emmons et al., p. 146
Rebell and Taplin, pp. 23–24
Rippon, p. 153
Wilson and Plunkett, pp. 333 and 370

PATHOGENICITY: Geophilic and zoophilic, causes tinea capitis, tinea corporis, and tinea favosa.

TISSUE FORM: Ectothrix hair invasion, may produce favuslike crusts (scutula). Segmented hyphae seen in KOH preparation of skin scales. Greenish yellow fluorescence of invaded hair is seen under Wood's light.

Microsporum nanum (hyphomycete),
Nannizzia obtusa (Ascomycotina)

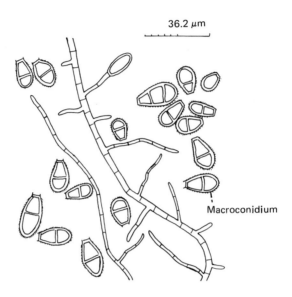

Macroconidium

GROSS: Growth is white, velvety, becoming buff and finely granular at two weeks. Reverse is pale yellow to red-brown.

MICRO: Pear-shaped macroconidia, rough walled with one to three septations, rarely four, and most commonly two. Thin microconidia are also seen.

Macroconidia: 12–18 X 5–7 μm, 1–3 septae.
Microconidia: 2 X 5 μm.

Special tests: Perforates hair in vitro.
For further descriptions see

Ajello and Padhye (in Lennette et al.), p. 477
Emmons et al., p. 148
Rebell and Taplin, p. 26
Rippon, p. 154
Wilson and Plunkett, pp. 332 and 370

PATHOGENICITY: Zoophilic, causes ringworm in pigs. Rare cases of tinea corporis and tinea capitis.

TISSUE FORM: Nonfluorescent, ectothrix, thin hyphal threads.

Microsporum persicolor (hyphomycete),
Nannizzia persicolor (Ascomycotina)

GROSS: This species is similar to *T. mentagrophytes;* flat, velvety to finely powdered, white to peach to light buff. On defined cereal, Ajello and Padhye report most isolates turn peach to rose or even deep red.

MICRO: Microconidia, slender or round, are abundant and resemble those of *T. mentagrophytes.* Spiral hyphae are common. Macroconidia are scarce, usually six celled, with some roughness at the tip.

Special test: Perforates hair in vitro.
For further descriptions see

Ajello and Padhye (in Lennette et al.), p. 477
Emmons et al., p. 151
Rebell and Taplin, p. 27
Rippon, p. 155

PATHOGENICITY: Zoophilic, associated with small rodents; rare pathogen.

Microsporum vanbreuseghemii (Hyphomycete),
Nannizzia grubyea (Ascomycotina)

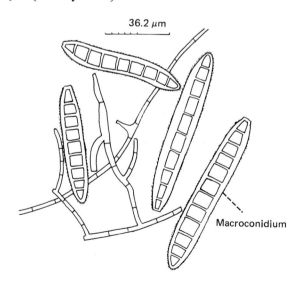

36.2 μm

Macroconidium

GROSS: Growth is rapid, granular, pink to deep rose, with yellow reverse.

MICRO: Multiseptate, thick, rough-walled macroconidia are slender with rounded ends. Microconidia are oval.

Macroconidia: 58–61 X 0.4–10.6 μm.
Microconidia: 9.2 X 4.4 μm.

Special tests: Perforates hair in vitro.
For further descriptions see

Emmons et al., p. 148
Rebell and Taplin, p. 30
Rippon, p. 156
Wilson and Plunkett, pp. 333 and 370

PATHOGENICITY: Rare cause of ringworm.

Monilia **sp. (hyphomycete): See** *Neurospora* **sp. (Ascomycotina)**
In medical literature, the genus name *Monilia* has long been used incorrectly for the group of yeasts that belong to the genus *Candida*. The term *Monilia* is correctly descriptive of the imperfect genus of *Neurospora* species.

Monosporium apiospermum **(hyphomycete):**
See *Petriellidium boydii* **(Ascomycotina)**

Mortierella **sp. (Class, Zygomycete; Order, Mucorales)**

GROSS: Colony is gray or yellowish, dense, velvety, flat.

MICRO: Sporangiophores are thin, simple or branched, becoming threadlike at the tip. Sporangia are round, terminal, and with a thin membrane. Columellae are lacking. Conidia (called stylospores) are round, one celled and borne on short branches.

For further descriptions see

Emmons et al., p. 277
Greer (in Lennette et al.), p. 544
Gillman, pp. 49 and 63
Rippon, p. 445

PATHOGENICITY: Subcutaneous mucormycosis. Isolated from cases of abortion and fatal pneumonia in cattle.

TISSUE FORM: Marked eosinophilia. Scarce, wide, aseptate hyphae.

Mucor sp. (Class, Zygomycete; Order, Mucorales)

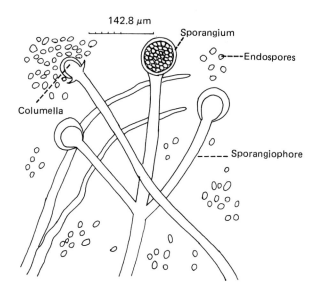

GROSS: Growth is rapid, dense, cottony, tan to gray. Fills tube or plate. Mature sporangia may be seen with the naked eye.

MICRO: Sporangiophores are branched. Sporangia containing endospores are round. A collarette may be seen at the base of a columella. Rhizoids are lacking. Chlamydospores are often present.

For further descriptions see

Emmons et al., p. 275

Greer (in Lennette et al.), p. 544

Gillman, pp. 26–45

Rippon, p. 443

Wilson and Plunkett, p. 326

PATHOGENICITY: Mucormycosis, (zygomycosis, phycomycosis).

TISSUE FORM: Wide aseptate hyphae.

Neurospora sitophila (**Ascomycotina**),
Monilia sitophila (**hyphomycete**)

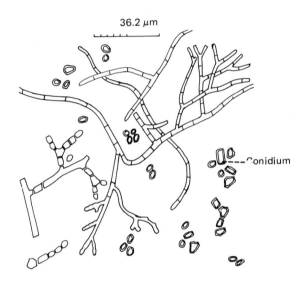

GROSS: Rapid growing, cobweb like colony (gray, white or orange) fills tube or plate with an "ungroomed" appearance. Clumps of orange or pink tufts are seen.

MICRO: Oval conidia are produced in chains that may branch, with the youngest at the tip (acropetal). In the perfect stage, perithecia are observed.

For further descriptions see

Barnett and Hunter, p. 66
Barron, p. 227
Emmons et al., p. 521
Gillman, pp. 207–209
Rippon, pp. 480 and 514
Wilson and Plunkett, pp. 345–346

PATHOGENICITY: Rare pathogen, reported in keratitis.

Nigrospora sp. (hyphomycete)

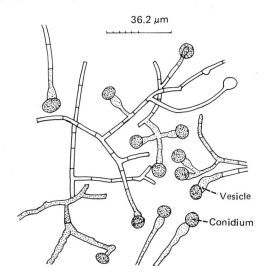

36.2 μm

Vesicle

Conidium

GROSS: Colony is woolly, dirty gray and rapid growing. Reverse is black.

MICRO: Hyphae are hyaline. Conidiophores are dark with end cell inflated to form a round or flattened vesicle. Conidia are terminal, black, and round.

For further descriptions see

Barnett and Hunter, p. 78
Barron, pp. 235-237
Ellis, 1971, pp. 319-320
Gillman, p. 324
Wilson and Plunkett, p. 374

PATHOGENICITY: Soil isolate, not known to be a pathogen.

Nocardia asteroides **(Actinomycetales)**

GROSS: Orange colonies have a chalky white surface, dry, pasty, and wrinkled. Growth is inhibited by antibacterial antibiotics. This species does not hydrolize casein, xanthine, or tyrosine.

MICRO: Freely branching filaments, 1 μm in diameter, may be partially acid-fast.

For further descriptions see

Chapter 4, Table 18B
Emmons et al., pp. 112–114, 455, and 554
Gordon (in Lennette et al.), pp. 175–183
Rippon, pp. 37–38
Wilson and Plunkett, pp. 147 and 154

PATHOGENICITY: Nocardiosis, actinomycotic mycetoma.

TISSUE FORM: Gram-positive, irregularly stained, thin (1 μm or less in diameter), broken bacillary forms are seen. These are partially acid-fast and may appear to branch.

Nocardia brasiliensis (Actinomycetales)

GROSS: Colonies are white, dull yellow, or orange-brown with a chalky white surface and crumbly or mealy in consistency. Growth is inhibited by antibacterial antibiotics. This species hydrolizes casein and tyrosine but not xanthine.

MICRO: Identical to *N. asteroides.*

For further descriptions see

Chapter 4, Table 18B
Emmons et al., p. 454
Gordon (in Lennette et al.), pp. 175–183
Rippon, p. 60
Wilson and Plunkett, p. 154

PATHOGENICITY: Agent of actinomycotic mycetoma.

TISSUE FORM: White to yellowish granules, less than 1 mm, are made up of Gram-positive, irregularly stained, thin (1 μm), branching filaments. Club-shaped radiating filaments may be present. These may be partially acid-fast.

Nocardia caviae (Actinomycetales)

GROSS: Similar to *N. asteroides.*

MICRO: Similar to *N. asteroides.* Hydrolizes xanthine but not casein and tyrosine.

For further descriptions see references given for *N. brasiliensis.*

PATHOGENICITY: See *N. brasiliensis.*

TISSUE FORM: See *N. brasiliensis.*

Paecilomyces sp., Acremonium sp., Spicaria sp. (hyphomycete)

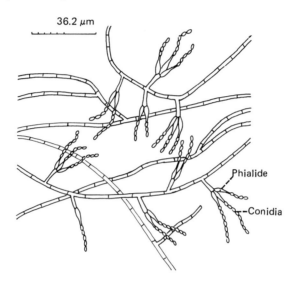

GROSS: Colonies are greenish brown to grayish brown to pink, powdery to velvety or woolly, rapid, irregular growth. Isolates are rarely green, a characteristic that helps to distinguish these from *Penicillium* species, which are more generally green.

MICRO: Graceful phialides with bent axis develop in whorls or singly on hyphae. Lemon-shaped phialoconidia are produced basipetally in chains. The looseness of the phialides and the chains of lemon-shaped conidia help to distinguish the species of this genus from those of *Penicillium.* This genus is similar to *Verticillium* and *Acremonium.*

For more descriptions see

Barnett and Hunter, p. 90

Barron, p. 245

Emmons et al., pp. 521-522

Gillman, pp. 308-309

Kendrick and Carmichael (in Ainsworth, Vol. IVA), pp. 438 and 442

Wilson and Plunkett, pp. 352-353

PATHOGENICITY: Rare cause of endocarditis, keratomycosis, and pulmonary disease. Also isolated from pulmonary disease of tortoises. (See Rippon, pp. 471 and 487, and Wilson and Plunkett, p. 352.) Isolated as a laboratory contaminant.

TISSUE FORM: Fungal elements, 1.5 to 3 μm, and rounded bodies have been reported in autopsy section following the death of a patient who had had valve replacements (Rippon, p. 471).

Paracoccidioides brasiliensis, Blastomyces brasiliensis (hyphomycete)

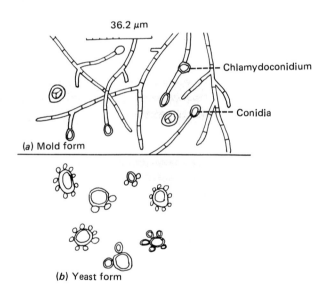

GROSS: Dimorphic fungus.

Mold form: At room temperature this form is slow growing, with primary growth seen in two or three weeks, membranous or velvety, white to cream, becoming brown with age.

Yeast form: On enriched agar at 37°C the yeast form is pasty and wrinkled. Growth is inhibited by cycloheximide.

MICRO:

Mold form: Hyphae and chlamydoconidia are seen. Sporulation is usually lacking on isolates received by our laboratory and others. Thick-walled arthroconidia and pear-shaped conidia, 3 to 4 μm, may be produced on yeast extract agar as described by Emmons et al. and by Rippon.

Yeast form: Round to almost round cells, 1 to 25 μm in diameter, with multiple buds, 1 to 10 μm in diameter distinguish this from *B. dermatitidis,* which has single buds only in the yeast phase.

For more descriptions see

Chapter 4, Table 14

Carmichael, p. 1148

Emmons et al., pp. 376–377

Rippon, pp. 402–403

Wilson and Plunkett, p. 385

PATHOGENICITY: Paracoccidioidomycosis (see Chapter 3). The disease occurs in South America.

TISSUE FORM: Multiple budding yeast cells of various sizes, as described in yeast form above, are seen.

SERODIAGNOSIS: Tests have been fairly well developed by South American workers. Both yeast-phase and mold-form antigens are used.

Skin tests: These tests are useful in epidemiological surveys.

Complement fixation tests: These tests are positive in 84% to 95% of patients, with the yeast-phase antigen giving better results than the mycelial-phase antigen.

Immunodiffusion tests: These tests are comparable to complement fixation tests.

Fluorescent antibody tests for in vivo and in vitro diagnosis have also been developed. A common antigen with *B. dermatitidis* and *H. capsulatum* has been demonstrated.

For more information on serodiagnosis see

Kaufmann (in Lennette et al.), pp. 563 and 565

Rippon, p. 400

Penicillium sp. (hyphomycete), *Talaromyces*
vermiculatus, Biverticullata symmetrica
(Subdivision, Ascomycotina; Class,
Plectomycetes)

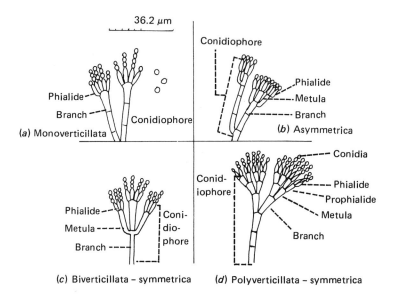

(a) Monoverticillata
(b) Asymmetrica
(c) Biverticillata – symmetrica
(d) Polyverticillata – symmetrica

GROSS: Colony is rapid-growing, powdery, flat. Most isolates are bluish green, becoming grayish brown with age. Colors may vary from white to pink to brown. Reverse may be colorless to deep red or brown.

MICRO: Conidiophores (penicillus) are stiff and may be branched or unbranched. The conidiogenous (conidium-bearing) cells are groups of flask-shaped phialides, produced directly on a single conidiophore or on a central branch of a conidiophore called a metula. Phialoconidia are usually round and may be rough; they are produced in basipetal chains.

The *Penicillium* species are separated by Gillman, after the method of Thom, by the kinds of branching of the conidiophore.

Monoverticillata: Whorls of phialides are borne on a single branch. See Figure 86(*a*).
Asymmetrica: Branches and metulae may occur in one or more series, branching
          asymmetrically. See Figure 86(*b*).
Biverticillata-symmetrica: A symmetrical whorl of metulae produce symmetrical
          whorls or phialides. See Figure 86(*c*).

Polyverticillata-symmetrica: Conidiophore (penicillus) consists of three or more
                        symmetrical series of branches. See Figure 86(*d*).

For more descriptions see

Barnett and Hunter, p. 90

Barron, p. 247

Emmons et al., pp. 491, 519–520

Gillman, pp. 235–284

Raper, Thom, and Fennell, 1949

Wilson and Plunkett, pp. 351–352

PATHOGENICITY: Primarily isolated as a laboratory contaminant. Certain
species are known to cause farmer's lung (Rippon, p. 503) and some cause peni-
cillosis (Emmons et al., p. 491; Rippon, p. 456). Some are recognized as toxin
producers (Emmons et al., pp. 52–53; Rippon, p. 500).

TISSUE FORM: Intracellular forms, markedly like the tissue-form cells of *H.
capsulatum*, are described and illustrated in tissues invaded by *P. marneffei* (Emmons et al., pp. 491–492).

INHIBITORY QUALITIES: *Penicillium* species are well known as inhibitors of
other microorganisms. The antibiotic, penicillin, and the antifungal, griseofulvin,
are produced by *Penicillium* species (Rippon, p. 538; Wilson and Plunkett, p. 239).
A species of *Penicillium* has been reported to inhibit *C. immitis* (Rippon, p. 359).

Petriellidium (Allescheria) boydii
(Ascomycotina, pyrenomycete);
Monosporium apiospermum
(hyphomycete)

GROSS: Culture grows rapidly, producing gray, cottony aerial mycelia, with
gray-green reverse. It is inhibited by cycloheximide and grows well at 37°C.

MICRO: Oval pale brown conidia are borne on long or short, thin conidiophores.
Tufts of conidiophores (coremia), each bearing a conidium, may occur. On potato
dextrose agar or on corn meal agar, thin-walled perithecia containing asci and
ascospores with pointed ends are developed.

Conidia: 8–10 $\times$ 5–7 μm

Perithecia: 100–200 μm

Ascospores: 4–5 $\times$ 7–8 μm

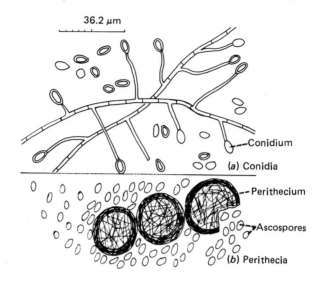

36.2 μm

—Conidium

(a) Conidia

--Perithecium

--Ascospores

(b) Perithecia

For more descriptions see

Chapter 4, Table 18A

Emmons et al., pp. 457–458

Gillman, p. 296

Müller and von Arx (in Ainsworth et al., IVA), p. 100

Rippon, p. 62

Schneidau (in Lennette et al.), pp. 523–524

Wilson and Plunkett, p. 335

PATHOGENICITY: Most common agent of eumycotic mycetoma in the United States. Isolated from mycotic keratitis (Rippon, p. 476). Systemic infections are reported by Lutwick et al. (1976).

TISSUE FORM: Dark brown, branching, segmented hyphae and round budding cells are seen. In chromomycosis, single or septate sclerotic bodies are also seen.

Phialophora sp. (hyphomycete); see also *Exophiala, Fonsecaea* and *Wangiella* sp.

GROSS: Colonies are dark gray to dark brown or brownish green, waxy to velvety. Reverse is black to dark brown.

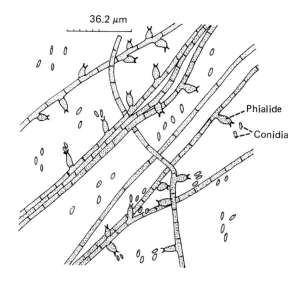

36.2 µm

Phialide

Conidia

MICRO: Short or somewhat elongate flask-shaped pigmented phialides, usually with a distinct collarette, producing conidia that may be light or pigmented and resemble a vase of small flowers.

For more descriptions see

Barnett and Hunter, p. 82
Barron, p. 256
Ellis, 1976, p. 524

For species differentiation see

Emmons et al., pp. 433–436
McGinnis, 1977 (in Proc. 4th Int. Conf. Mycoses), pp. 49–54
Rippon, pp. 244–245, p. 473

PATHOGENICITY: *Ph. verrucosa* is an agent of chromomycosis. Phaeomycotic cyst may be caused by *Ph. parasitica, Ph. repens,* or *Ph. richardsiae.* Keratomycosis may be caused by *Ph. verrucosa.*

TISSUE FORM: Dark brown, branching, segmented hyphae and round budding cells are seen. In chromomycosis, single or septate sclerotic bodies are also seen.

Phoma sp. (coelomycete)

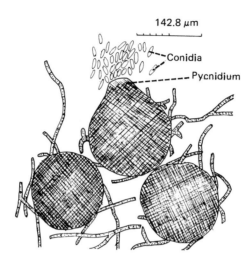

GROSS: Colony is gray to tan, or pink, red or yellow, velvety to woolly. Reverse is black.

MICRO: Dark-colored, flask-shaped pycnidia (characteristic of Coelomycetes) are filled with one-celled hyaline conidia. It is not always easy to distinguish the pycnidia of the Coelomycetes from the perithecia and cleistothecia of the Ascomycotina.*

Pycnidia: 60-150 $\times$ 500-600 μm

Conidia: 3-4 $\times$ 5-12 μm

For more descriptions see

Barnett and Hunter, p. 166

Emmons et al., p. 534

Gillman, p. 198

Wilson and Plunkett, p. 338

---

*It is common practice in a medical laboratory to identify any mold that produces saclike structures as *Phoma* sp. Such an isolate may, in fact, be any one of a number of plant pathogens in the coelomycete class, or in the Ascomycotina. Significant isolates are referred to an agricultural research center for a definitive identification.

PATHOGENICITY: Plant parasite, rare cause of phaeomycotic cyst (Emmons et al., pp. 425 and 433) and of phomamycosis (Rippon, p. 470).

Piedraia hortai (Ascomycotina)

36.2 μm

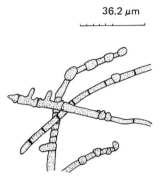

GROSS: Colonies are greenish black to black with the appearance of soot. Some strains are white to cream colored. Growth is extremely slow, raised or flat, velvety or waxy. Growth is aided by addition of thiamine and is inhibited by cycloheximide.

MICRO: Dark, thick-walled, closely septate hyphae with numerous swollen and irregularly shaped cells. Asci and ascospores are rarely seen in culture. Identification depends on demonstration of tissue form.

For more descriptions see

Ajello and Padhye (in Lennette et al.), p. 469
Beneke and Rogers, p. 54
Conant et al., p. 635
Emmons et al., p. 182
Rippon, p. 93
Wilson and Plunkett, p. 338

PATHOGENICITY: Black piedra of scalp or beard, seen in Africa and South America.

TISSUE FORM: Hard, gritty nodules, composed of cemented mycelium, containing asci and from two to eight ascospores, average 25 to 55 μm, surrounding a hair shaft. These nodules must be differentiated from nits.

Pityrosporum furfur, Pityrosporum orbiculare,
Malasezzia furfur (blastomycete)

36.2 µm

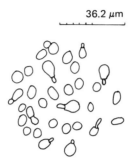

GROSS: Pasty white colonies that grow well at 37°C on cycloheximide media or Sabouraud agar with olive oil added as an oleic acid source. These colonies do not grow on routine media. Identification is made from microscopic preparations of tissue form and from clinical appearance.

MICRO: Budding cells are seen, which have been variously described as appearing like a bowling pin, a jumping bean, or a medicine capsule. The cells are one-celled phialides that produce a single phialoconidium.

For more descriptions see

Ajello and Padhye (in Lennette et al.), pp. 470–471
Emmons et al., pp. 176–180
Rippon, p. 87
Wilson and Plunkett, pp. 341–342

PATHOGENICITY: Agent of tinea versicolor. *Pityrosporum* species are isolated as normal skin inhabitants. Eye-lid infection may occur (Rippon, p. 487).

TISSUE FORM: Clusters of round cells, up to 8 µm, which occasionally can be seen to bud, and short, crescent-shaped or long and thin hyphae are easily seen on KOH preparations. These hyphae and clusters of cells are stained dramatically with the methenamine silver nitrate or periodic acid-Schiff stains (Chap. 4, Plate 2).

Prototheca sp. (green alga)

GROSS: Pasty white, yeastlike colony grows on routine media.

For descriptions see

Emmons et al., pp. 515–516
Kaplan, W. (in Proc. 4th Int. Conf. Mycoses, 1978), pp. 218–232
Rippon, p. 461

PATHOGENICITY: Agent of protothecosis.

TISSUE: Round to oval endosporulating cells, 1.3 to 25.0 μm, which are produced by cleavage.

Rhinosporidium seeberi **(Subdivision, Mastigomycotina;**
Class, Chytridomycete)
Culture form is not known.

PATHOGENICITY: Agent of rhinosporidiosis.

TISSUE FORM: "Sporangia," 100 to 350 μm, may discharge up to 2,000 endospores. These range from minute to 6 or 7 μm at point of discharge.

For more descriptions see

Emmons et al., pp. 256, 464, and 470
Rippon, pp. 292–293
Wilson and Plunkett, pp. 208 and 322

Rhizopus **sp. (Class, Zygomycete;**
Order, Mucorales)

GROSS: Growth is rapid, dense, cottony, gray, fills tube. Reverse is colorless or pale.

MICRO: Round, black sporangia are filled with endospores. The sporangia are usually unbranched, rising from a runner called a stolon. Rhizoids develop from the stolon at a point opposite the sporangiophore.

For more descriptions see

Emmons et al., pp. 273–275
Gillman, p. 20
Green (in Lennette et al.), pp. 543–544

Rippon, pp. 443-444
Wilson and Plunkett, p. 324

PATHOGENICITY: Mucormycosis (zygomycosis), most frequently caused by *R. arrhizus*. *R. rhizopodiformis* has recently been implicated (Bottone et al.).

TISSUE FORM: Wide, 10 to 20 μm, aseptate hyphae, stain well with H & E stain.

SERODIAGNOSIS: Immunodiffusion tests have given promising preliminary results (Jones and Kaufman, 1978).

Rhizopus arrhizus (Class, Zygomycete;
Order, Mucorales)

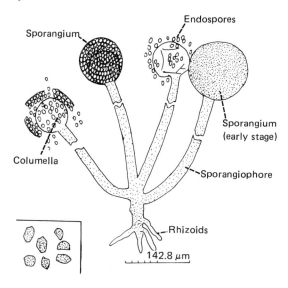

GROSS: Growth is more dense and velvety than *R. nigricans.*

MICRO: Sporangiophores are brown, rarely single and may be branched. Sporangia are round. Columellae are round and flattened at the termination of the sporangiophore, with a smooth brown membrane. Spores are grayish brown with longitudinal striations, varied in shape. Rhizoids are pale.

Sporangiophore: 0.5-2.0 mm in length
Sporangia: 120-150 μm

Columellae: 40-75 × 60-100 μm

Endospores: 4.8-7.0 × 4.8-5.6 μm

Special tests: Grows well at 37°C and will grow at temperatures up to 42°C. Will not grow at 52°C.

PATHOGENICITY: This species may cause mucormycosis.

Rhizopus nigricans (Class, zygomycete; Order, Mucorales)

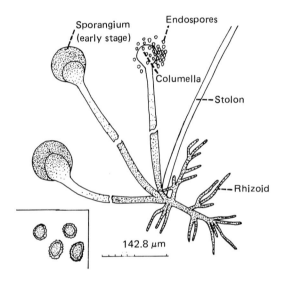

GROSS: See *Rhizopus* sp.

MICRO: Sporangiophores are usually in groups of two, three, or more. Columellae are hemispheric. Sporangia are hemispheric. Gray-blue endospores are unequal in size and shape. Rhizoids are well developed and deep yellow or brown.

Sporangiophores: 0.5-2 mm in length

Sporangia: 100-350 μm

Columellae: 70-90 μm

Endospores: 9-12 × 7-8 μm

Special test: No growth at 37°C.

PATHOGENICITY: Common mold, not pathogenic.

Rhizopus rhizopodiformis (Class, Zygomycete; Order, Mucorales)

GROSS: Rapid, dense, cottony, gray growth, fills the tube within three days. Reverse is colorless or pale yellow. Grows well from 22° to 52°C.

MICRO: Short sporangiophores may occur singly or in groups on an arched stolon above the rhizoids and may be branched. These are hyaline (clear) or brown.

Sporangiophore: 120-125 μm

Sporangia: 66.6-140 μm (average 92 μm)

Endospores: 4.5-6.7 μm (average 5-6 μm)

Special tests: Grows well at 37°C and will grow at temperatures up to 52°C, helping to distinguish this from *R. arrhizus,* which will not grow at temperatures over 44°C.

For further descriptions see

Bottone et al., pp. 531-533

Emmons et al., p. 275

PATHOGENICITY: Subcutaneous and systemic infections were reported in a hospital unit where *R. rhizopodiformis* was also isolated from adhesive bandages (Bottone et al.). Skin infections have been reported in postoperative wound infections (Sheldon and Johnson).

Rhodotorula sp. (blastomycete, Cryptococcacaea)

GROSS: Colony is pink or orange, creamy (Plate 3).

MICRO: Single budding cells and occasional pseudohyphae are seen.

Special test: Urease produced, as in the *Cryptococcus* species; inositol-negative, which separates *Rhodotorula* species from *Cryptococcus* species, which are inositol-positive.

   For differentiation of *R. rubra* and *R. glutinis,* see Table 9.

For more descriptions see

Chapter 4, Table 9

Barron, p. 271

Emmons et al., p. 527

Rippon, p. 227

Silva-Hutner and Cooper (in Lennette et al.), pp. 497 and 504

Wilson and Plunkett, p. 342

PATHOGENICITY: May be isolated from severely traumatized tissue, probably as a colonizer or as transient in the blood stream (fungemia). Frequently cultured from sinks and shower curtains in bathrooms.

Saccharomyces **sp. (Ascomycotina)**

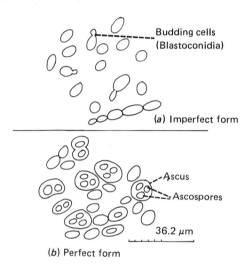

(a) Imperfect form

(b) Perfect form

GROSS: Colonies are white to cream colored, buttery. On bromcresol green agar, colonies are glistening and bluish green. (See Plate 3.)

MICRO: Unicellular, budding conidia, oval or round, which may form short chains and may elongate into pseudohyphae. Free asci, containing one to four ascospores, are produced on special media such as ascospore agar.

Conidia: $3 \times 5\ \mu$m

Special tests: Strong fermenters; see Table 9. Production of ascospores on special media (see Chap. 4).

For further descriptions see

Chapter 4, Table 9

Silva-Hutner and Cooper (in Lennette et al.), p. 497 and pp. 504-505

Rippon, p. 515, diagram of life cycle

Wilson and Plunkett, p. 329

PATHOGENICITY: Rarely a pathogen. It has been isolated from paronychia (Wilson and Plunkett, p. 270), rare cause of oral thrush (Emmons et al., p. 24), pulmonary disease in brewers (Rippon, p. 228).

Industrial use: These are the yeasts that are used in making bread, wine, and beer.

Scopulariopsis sp. (hyphomycete)

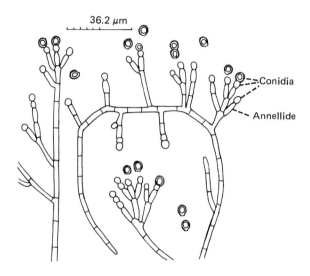

GROSS: Growth may start as a white, waxy, wrinkled, and spaghettilike colony, becoming velvety and then powdery, light tan, or brown. White tufts appear after two weeks. Colonies are never green.

MICRO: Conidiophores may branch in a manner similar to *Penicillium* sp. The conidium-producing (conidiogenous) cells are annellides, elongating slightly before the production of each new conidium. A scarred tip, which is not always easy to see, remains after the release of each conidium. The conidia are blown out basipetally into chains that break apart easily. The conidia are lemon-shaped to round, become rough-walled and are flattened at the basal edge where they are released from the annellide.

Conidia: 4-2 × 3.5-7 μm

For more descriptions see

Barnett and Hunter, p. 94
Barron, p. 275
Ellis, pp. 326-327
Emmons et al., pp. 491, 493, 521-522
Gillman, pp. 286-288
Wilson and Plunkett, p. 353

PATHOGENICITY: Established as a primary agent in onychomycosis and as an opportunist in keratitis and in otitis (Rippon, pp. 130 and 488-489). Common soil mold.

TISSUE FORM: Hyphae, 2 to 10 μm in diameter, and occasionally conidia are seen. (See Plate 1.)

Scytalidium sp. (hyphomycete); *Scytalidium*
state of *Hendersonula toruloidea* (coelomycete)

GROSS: Colonies appear in four to six days. These are white at first, becoming dark green to black in 10 to 15 days. They are inhibited by cycloheximide. The surface growth is woolly, with scattered tufts and filaments. The reverse is dark brown to black. No diffusion occurs. Grows well from 20° to 37°C.

MICRO: Short hyaline hyphae with aseptate terminal extensions. Pigmented hyphae are septate and break up into long chains of arthroconidia. In addition, some hyphal septations are round or oval, or swollen. These filaments take a curled form, sometimes in two or three concentric rings. Some of the swollen septations are divided longitudinally and transversely.

Septate hyphae: 5-10 X 5-25 μm
Aseptate terminal extensions: 30-40 μm
Arthroconidia: 2-5 X 7 μm
Hyphal septations: 6-7 to 20 μm in diameter

For further descriptions see

Ellis, 1971, p. 28
Ellis, 1976, p. 16
Mariat et al., 1978
Sutton, B.C. (in Ainsworth, IVA), pp. 524 and 567

PATHOGENICITY: Opportunistic agent of onychomycosis and verrucous dermatitis.

TISSUE FORM: Single cells with occasional septations, false buds, or hyphal extensions are seen.

Sepedonium sp. (hyphomycete)

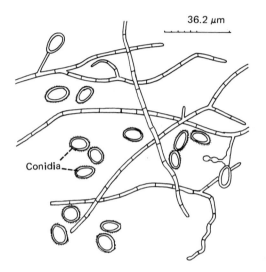

GROSS: Colonies are white or buff or tan, powdery. These may become fluffy after tufts develop. Moderate rate of growth.

MICRO: Large hyaline or yellow, round conidia are rough walled, single, borne on slender conidiophores. These conidia must be distinguished from those of *H. capsulatum* by demonstrating no growth at 37°C, no growth on cycloheximide media at room temperature, and no microconidia. Phialides, similar to those of *Verticillium* sp., are also reported.

Conidia: average 15 μm

For more descriptions see

Barnett and Hunter, p. 76
Barron, pp. 278-279

Carmichael, p. 1149
Gillman, p. 301
Wilson and Plunkett, p. 359

PATHOGENICITY: Not reported as a pathogen.

Sporothrix schenckii, Sporotrichum
schenckii (hyphomycete)

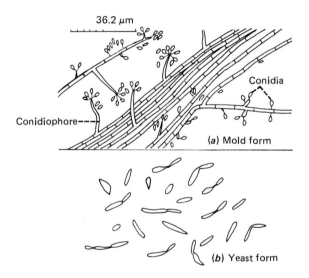

36.2 μm

Conidia

Conidiophore

(a) Mold form

(b) Yeast form

GROSS: Dimorphic fungus.

Mold form: At room temperature initial growth appears in three to seven days and is waxy, white to cream colored, becoming brown or black. Older cultures become leathery, flat, or wrinkled, with elevated center. They resemble dirty candle wax. Reverse is light-colored. Growth is not inhibited by cycloheximide.

Yeast form: At 35°C growth is moist, white to cream colored. At 37°C, some isolates fail to grow. These isolates which fail to grow at 37°C have been shown by Kwon-Chung (1979) to be isolated from fixed cutaneous lesions. Those that do grow at 37°C were isolated from deeper infections.

MICRO:

Mold form: Conidia may be hyaline or dark walled. The conidia are borne sympodially on thin short branches called denticles, at the terminal end of a conidiophore, or they may form a "sleeve" of conidia along the sides of the hyphae. Hyphae are delicate.

Conidia: 2-3 X 3-6 μm

Hyphae: 1-2 μm in diameter

Yeast form: Conidia convert to elongated budding cells.

Budding cells: 1-3 X 3-10 μm

Special test: Growth is not inhibited by cycloheximide.
For more descriptions see

Chapter 4, Table 14
Barnett and Hunter, p. 94
Barron, p. 284
Carmichael, pp. 1149-1150
Emmons et al., pp. 416-423
Neilsen (in Lennette et al.), pp. 528-530
Rippon, pp. 262-263
Wilson and Plunkett, pp. 354-355

PATHOGENICITY: Subcutaneous or systemic sporotrichosis. Strains that fail to grow at 37°C are isolated from fixed cutaneous lesions. Strains that are able to grow at 37°C are isolated from lymphangitic, subcutaneous, and deep body areas (Kwon-Chung, 1979).

TISSUE FORM: Elongated budding yeast cells are seen in periodic acid-Schiff stain when tissues are first treated with malt diastase or with the methenamine silver nitrate stain.

SERODIAGNOSIS:

Skin test: Delayed hypersensitivity reaction to killed conidial or yeast cells indicates exposure to *S. schenckii* or present or past infection.
Tube and latex agglutination tests: These use whole yeast antigen, demonstrate present infection, and are helpful in diagnosing systemic sporotrichosis.

Precipitins can be demonstrated by immunodiffusion in 75% of culturally confirmed cases.

Complement fixation is less satisfactory.

Immunofluorescent tests can be useful.

For more information about serodiagnosis see

Kaufman (in Lennette et al.), pp. 563 and 565

Nielson (in Lennette et al.), pp. 529-530

Rippon, pp. 261-262; preparation of antigen, p 554

Roberts and Larsh, 1971

Streptomyces **sp. (Actinomycetales);**
see also *Actinomadura* **sp.**

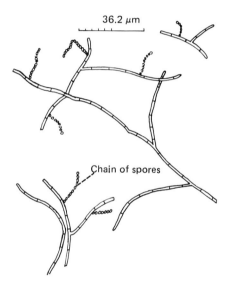

GROSS: Characteristic earthy odor is produced. Growth is slow, heaped, dry, chalky or waxy, usually white or gray, but may be other colors.

MICRO: Finely branched filaments are 1 µm in diameter or less. Tiny spores are borne in chains. These spores may be enhanced by growth on Czapek-Dox agar. Tight, spiraling filaments may also be present.

Spores: Less than 1 µm

For more descriptions see

Chapter 4, Table 18B
Emmons et al., pp. 15, 29, and 454
Gordon (in Lennette et al.), pp. 175–178, 180–184
Rippon, pp. 13–15
Wilson and Plunkett, pp. 154, 361–362

PATHOGENICITY: Agent of actinomycotic mycetoma; also a common soil isolate.

TISSUE FORM: Granules 5 to 7 mm; colors representative of the color of filaments may be in exudate of sinus. Filaments stain well with Gram's stain or methenamine silver nitrate stain.

Syncephalastrum sp. (Class, Zygomycete, Order, Mucorales)

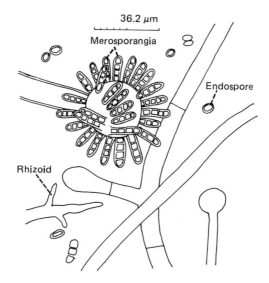

GROSS: Growth is rapid, dense, cottony, or woolly, gray, fills tube.

MICRO: Tubular *merosporangia* containing a row of any number from three or five to 10 or 18 round endospores borne in petal fashion on the swollen vesicle at the tip of a sporangiophore. Hyphae are aseptate, developing simple septations with age. Rudimentary rhizoids are formed.

Merosporangia: 4–6 × 9–60 μm

Endospores: 3–5 μm

Vesicle: 10–40 μm

Hyphae: 4–8 μm

For more descriptions see

Barnett and Hunter, p. 60

Emmons et al., pp. 525–526

Gillman, p. 67

Wilson and Plunkett, pp. 315, 327–328

PATHOGENICITY: Common soil isolate, recently reported in nail invasion (see chapter 3).

Torula sp. (hyphomycete)

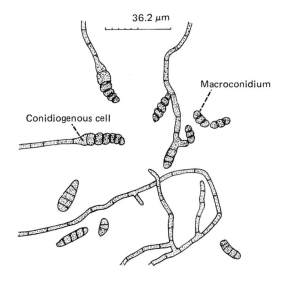

GROSS: Black, slow growth builds up into a wrinkled mound at maturity.

MICRO: Sporulation is enhanced on corn meal agar. Brown hyphae are wide (up to 5 μm). Long chains of dark conidia have the appearance of heavily segmented hyphae. Conidiogenous cell is usually polyblastic and round. Fertile end is thin walled and clear. Sterile (basal end) is thick walled and dark colored.

For more descriptions see

Barron, pp. 301–302
Ellis, 1971, p. 336
Gillman, p. 318

PATHOGENICITY: Not known as a pathogen.

Torulopsis glabrata (blastomycete)

GROSS: Colonies are moist white to gray or pale cream, glistening. On bromcresol green agar, colonies are intense green to deep yellow-green and are usually 1 to 2 mm in diameter (see Plate 3). Growth is inhibited by cycloheximide.

MICRO: Small budding cells are produced on all media. No hyphae are produced on corn meal agar.

Budding cells: 1.5–4.5 μm

For more descriptions see

Plates 3 and 4
Chapter 4, Table 9
Emmons et al., pp. 488–489
Rippon, p. 226
Silva-Hutner (in Lennette et al.), pp. 497 and 505
Wilson and Plunkett, pp. 339–340

PATHOGENICITY: Opportunistic pathogen; may cause urinary tract infection. See Sekhon, A.S., 1978 (in Proc. 4th Int. Conf. Mycoses), pp. 167–175; Rippon, pp. 224-226. Isolated as normal flora from sputum and genital specimens.

TISSUE FORM: Budding yeast, 2.5-4 $\times$ 6 μm.

SERODIAGNOSIS: Immunodiffusion and latex agglutination tests are positive using *C. albicans* antigen (Sekhon, p. 170).

Trichoderma sp. (hyphomycete)

GROSS: Fast, thin, white hyphal growth, develops into compact woolly tufts, turning green at maturity. Production of green tufts is enhanced by growth on Czapek-Dox or potato dextrose agar.

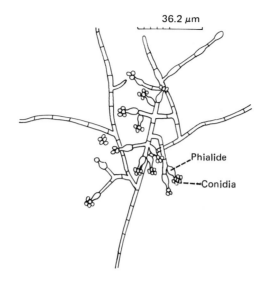

MICRO: Branched conidiophores bear short phialides singly or in groups. Hyaline or green phialoconidia remain in terminal clusters at the tip of the phialide.

Phialoconidia: 2.5-3.2 × 1.5-2 μm

For more descriptions see

Barnett and Hunter, p. 88
Emmons et al., pp. 522-523
Gillman, pp. 212-215
Wilson and Plunkett, pp. 348-349

Trichophyton ajelloi, Keratinomyces ajelloi
(hyphomycete); *Arthroderma uncinatum*
(Ascomycotina)

GROSS: Good growth occurs in one week. The surface is flat, heaped, or folded, granular to powdery or downy, cream colored or light tan with a slight orange tint. The reverse may be colorless in early growth, turning deep purple or bluish red. Pigment diffuses into the medium.

MICRO: Multicelled, smooth-walled macroconidia are abundant. Microconidia are pear shaped to slender.

Macroconidia: 5 to 12 cells; 20-65 × 5-10 μm

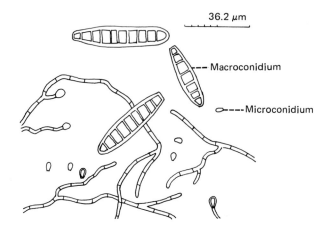

Special tests: Penetrates hair in vitro.
For more descriptions see

Ajello, 1968, pp. 147-159
Rebell and Taplin, p. 31
Rippon, p. 168
Wilson and Plunkett, pp. 331 and 372

PATHOGENICITY: Isolated from soil and from small animals. Rarely reported as a pathogenic species.

Trichophyton concentricum (hyphomycete)

GROSS: This species is similar to *T. schoenleinii*. The surface is white to honey colored, glabrous to fine velvety, heaped and folded. The reverse is very light yellowish brown.

MICRO: Short branched hyphae, abnormal swellings, and chlamydoconidia are produced. Macroconidia and microconidia are lacking on routine media but have been reported on bean pod media (Rippon, p. 164).

Special tests: Some strains are stimulated by addition of thiamine.
For more descriptions see

Emmons et al., p. 159
Rebell and Taplin, p. 61

Rippon, p. 164
Wilson and Plunkett, p. 366

PATHOGENICITY: Tinea imbricata, which occurs in the South Pacific.

TISSUE FORM: A pattern of circinate skin lesions composed of concentric rings is unique to this disease.

Trichophyton equinum (hyphomycete)

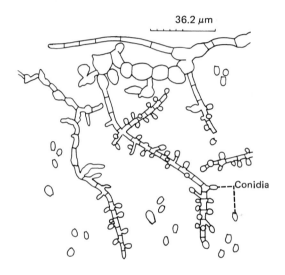

GROSS: Growth is moderate to fast. The surface is white at first, becoming yellow to yellowish brown, velvety, and folded. The reverse is yellow to reddish brown, with a diffusible pigment.

MICRO: Many microconidia are borne laterally on hyphae, rarely clustered. These are thin, elongate or round. Macroconidia are rare.

Special tests: Most isolates require nicotinic acid, but strains isolated in Australia and in New Zealand do not require nicotinic acid (see Table 12).
For more descriptions see

Ajello and Padhye (in Lennette et al.), p. 478
Emmons et al., p. 161

Rebell and Taplin, p. 45
Wilson and Plunkett, p. 369

PATHOGENICITY: Agent of horse ringworm, occasionally pathogenic to humans.

TISSUE FORM: Large ectothrix spores, 3 to 7 μm, are seen on horse hair.

Trichophyton fischeri (hyphomycete)

GROSS: This species is similar to *T. rubrum*. The surface exhibits a moderate rate of growth, velvety or cottony, white. The reverse, on Sabouraud agar, is colorless to deep red. No color is produced on corn meal agar with 0.2% dextrose and Tween-80 or on erythritol albumen agar.

MICRO: Structures are similar to *T. rubrum* but the macroconidia may be longer.

Microconidia: 2×5 μm or 2–3×3–4 μm
Macroconidia: 3×50 μm

Special tests: No red reverse color is produced on corn meal agar with 0.2% dex-trose and Tween-80 or on erythritol albumen agar. There is no hair penetration. Urease production is slow or negative.
For more descriptions see

Kane pp. 231–241

PATHOGENICITY: Not a pathogenic species.

NOTE: This species may easily be misidentified as the common pathogenic derma-tophyte *T. rubrum*. The two species may be differentiated by the longer macroconidia of *T. fischeri* and by the lack of color production by *T. fischeri* on either corn meal agar with 0.2% dextrose or on erythritol albumen agar.

Trichophyton megninii, Trichophyton roseum (hyphomycete)

GROSS: Good growth occurs in two weeks. The surface of the colony is white at first, becoming pale rose to violet, velvety, and folded. The reverse is deep rose.

MICRO: Microconidia are small, pear shaped, or elongate and borne on the sides of hyphae or in chains or clusters. Sporulation is enhanced by addition of histidine.

Macroconidia are rarely seen. These may be produced on trypticase soy agar (Emmons, p. 161).

Macroconidia: 3-6 × 10-35 μm; 2- to 8-celled
Special tests: Requires histidine (Trichophyton agar #7) for growth (see Chap. 4, Table 12).
For more descriptions see

Emmons et al., p. 161
Rebell and Taplin, p. 49
Rippon, p. 165
Wilson and Plunkett, p. 368

PATHOGENICITY: Rare species, found in Europe and Africa. Agent of tinea barbae, occasionally tinea corporis and tinea capitis.

TISSUE FORM: Ectothrix.

Trichophyton mentagrophytes (hyphomycete), *Arthroderma*
benhamiae (Ascomycotina); *T. mentagrophytes* var.
mentagrophytes (zoophilic), *T. mentagrophytes* var.
interdigitale (anthropophilic)

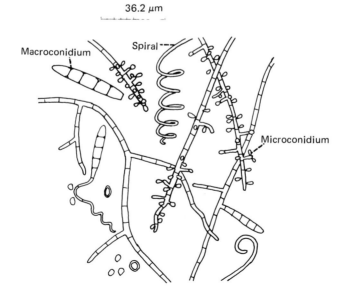

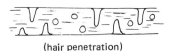
(hair penetration)

GROSS: The surface is flat or furrowed, velvety or finely powdery or granular, white to cream or tan. White cottony growth typically has a central velvety or powdery cream-color depression. The reverse varies from colorless to dark reddish brown.

MICRO: Microconidia are abundant and usually round but may be elongate, particularly in anthropophilic strains. The microconidia are borne on the sides of hyphae, singly or in clusters. Spiral hyphae, when present, are an identifying characteristic of this species. Macroconidia are not present in the anthropophilic variety but are usually abundant in zoophilic strains. These may have a taillike appendage, in contrast to *T. rubrum* macroconidia which do not. *Nodular* organs (knotted hyphae) may be seen in some species.

Macroconidia: Single-celled, 4–8 μm; 2- to 5-celled 6–8 $\times$ 20–50 μm.

Special tests: Penetrates hair in vitro; usually urease-positive within four days. No red-color pigmentation is produced on corn meal agar; no vitamin requirements; stellate colonies on potato dextrose agar.

For more descriptions see

Chapter 4, Table 11
Ajello and Padhye (in Lennette et al.), p. 478
Emmons et al., p. 154
Rebell and Taplin, pp. 40–43
Rippon, pp. 157–158
Wilson and Plunkett, pp. 363–365

PATHOGENICITY: Invades skin and nails. Zoophilic variety may invade the scalp hairs. *T. mentagrophytes* var. *mentagrophytes,* the zoophilic strain, is granular in culture, and causes an extremely inflammatory infection. *T. mentagrophytes* var. *interdigitale,* the anthropophilic strain, is more downy in culture and produces less conidia. It causes a more benign and chronic infection.

TISSUE FORM: Segmented hyphae are seen in KOH preparations. Invasion of hair shaft is ectothrix, with small spores surrounding the hair shaft. *T. mentagrophytes* var. *quinckeanum,* which is the agent of mouse favus, may produce an endothrix infection.

Trichophyton rubrum (hyphomycete); no perfect stage known.

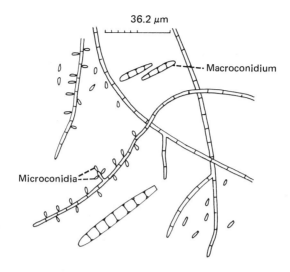

36.2 µm

Macroconidium

Microconidia

GROSS: The surface growth at one week is small, white, usually fluffy with a waxy edge. At two weeks, colonies are white, fluffy, sometimes with thin waxy areas. Granular species may be powdery and tan. The reverse is often colorless, becoming yellow or light brown on routine media. It may develop rings of deep purplish red-brown or deep ruby red. This pigment does not diffuse. The ruby-red color is characteristic of this species and gives it the name *rubrum.*

MICRO: Slender microconidia are borne laterally at various angles on the hyphae. The microconidia may be scarce on routine media but usually will develop in abundance on potato dextrose agar. In granular strains the microconidia are numerous, and may be oval and bulging. Macroconidia are also produced in granular strains. These macroconidia may produce microconidia and also may break up into arthroconidia.

Microconidia: 2–3 X 3–5 µm

Macroconidia: 2- to 8-celled, 4–6 X 15–30 µm

Special tests: No hair penetration. Urease production is slow or negative, except in granular strains. Red color produced on corn meal agar with 0.2% dextrose and on erythritol albumen agar within one month. No vitamin requirements.

For more descriptions see

Chapter 4, Table 11
Ajello and Padhye (in Lennette et al.), pp. 478–479
Emmons et al., p. 156
Rebell and Taplin, pp. 50–51
Rippon, pp. 158–160
Wilson and Plunkett, p. 365

PATHOGENICITY: Anthropophilic, most common agent of tinea corporis, tinea pedis, and onychomycosis. Rare cause of tinea capitis. A rare subcutaneous disease, Majocchi's granuloma, is caused by *T. rubrum*. Also, rare systemic invasion may occur (see Chap. 3).

TISSUE FORM: Septate hyphae and arthroconidia are seen in KOH preparations and with special fungal stains.

Trichophyton schoenleinii (hyphomycete)

36.2 μm

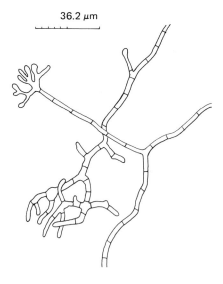

GROSS: Growth is moderately slow; at one week small and compact, developing into a 2-cm colony at two to three weeks. The surface is white at first, becoming brown-white, thin and velvety, heaped and wrinkled with age. The reverse is colorless to light brown. A cracking of the agar may be observed.

MICRO: Branched hyphae with terminal *nail head* swollen tip is characteristic of this species. Branching, which is likened to chandeliers or to deer antlers, is also described. Microconidia, which are rarely seen, are varied in size and shape. Macroconidia are not produced.

Special tests: Microconidia may be developed on boiled rice. Grows well at 37°C.
               No vitamin requirements.
For more descriptions see

Ajello and Padhye (in Lennette et al.), p. 479
Emmons et al., p. 159
Rebell and Taplin, pp. 59-60
Rippon, pp. 163-164
Wilson and Plunkett, p. 367

PATHOGENICITY: Agent of favus of the scalp. Also may infect skin and nails (see Chap. 3).

TISSUE FORM: Long, segmented hyphae are seen within hair shaft on KOH. Air bubbles are commonly seen.

Trichophyton soudanense (hyphomycete)

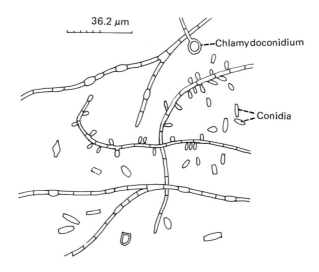

GROSS: Growth is slow. The surface is yellow to light orange, velvety, flat or folded, with a fringed or radiating border. The reverse is deep yellow. A violet variant is reported (Rippon, p. 166).

MICRO: Abundant arthroconidia and chlamydoconidia are seen. Microconidia, similar to those of *T. tonsurans*, are produced only on potato dextrose agar. Characteristic reflexive and right-angled branching is described.

Special tests: Trichophyton agars #6 and #7, no growth. These media are ammonium nitrate and ammonium nitrate with histidine agars (Chap. 4, Table 12). Löwenstein-Jensen medium, dark colony.
For more descriptions see

Rebell and Taplin, p. 56
Rippon, p. 166

PATHOGENICITY: Common cause of ringworm in Africa, and may now be spreading to other countries.

TISSUE FORM: Endothrix, similar to *T. tonsurans.*

***Trichophyton terrestre* (hyphomycete), *Arthroderma quadrifidum, Arthroderma lenticularum* (Ascomycotina)**

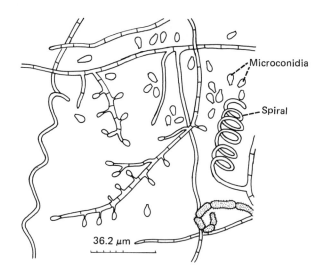

GROSS: The soil isolate exhibits rapid growth, is downy and creamy to white. The reverse is yellow to salmon-color. The animal isolate shows slow growth, flat to furrowed, white to tan. The surface is granular. The reverse is deep red, diffusing into the medium.

MICRO: Microconidia, larger than those of *T. mentagrophytes* and *T. rubrum*, are square based and have a prominant attachment scar when released. Macroconidia vary from one or two to nine cells. Spirals may be present.

Microconidia: 4-6 X 3-4 μm

Special tests: Penetrates hair in vitro (aiding in distinguishing this from *T. rubrum*). May produce deep red color on corn meal and potato dextrose agar which aids in distinguishing it from *T. mentagrophytes*.
For more descriptions see

Emmons et al., p. 163
Rebell and Taplin, pp. 33-34
Wilson and Plunkett, p. 369

PATHOGENICITY: Soil isolates and animal (hedgehogs) isolates are reported. Not known as a human pathogen.

Trichophyton tonsurans (hyphomycete)

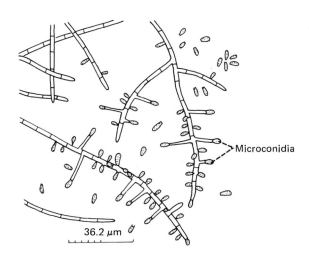

GROSS: Surface growth at one week is compact, granular or powdery, yellow to buff or red-brown, often with a radiating border. At three weeks the colony may be flat, with a central folded depression, or heaped and irregular. The reverse is yellow to dark brown, or reddish brown.

MICRO: Bulging microconidia are varied in size and shape and are borne at right angles, either directly on the side of the hyphae or on short pedicels which may branch at right angles. Macroconidia may be present. Spirals are occasionally seen. Intercalary and terminal chlamydoconidia are often seen.

Microconidia: 2-5 X 3-7 μm

Special tests: Growth is enhanced by addition of thiamine (see Chap. 4, Table 12). For more descriptions see

Chapter 4, Table 11
Ajello and Padhye (in Lennette et al.), pp. 479–480
Emmons et al., pp. 156 and 159
Rebell and Taplin, p. 52
Rippon, p. 162
Wilson and Plunkett, p. 365

PATHOGENICITY: Anthropophilic; black dot ringworm, tinea corporis, rare onychomycosis.

TISSUE FORM: Endothrix hair invasion.

Trichophyton verrucosum (hyphomycete)

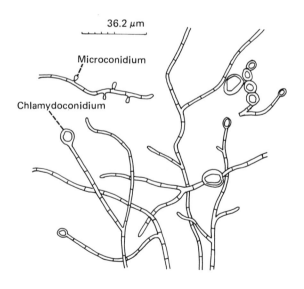

36.2 μm

Microconidium

Chlamydoconidium

GROSS: Growth is extremely slow, usually not appearing for three to four weeks on primary isolation. Colonies remain small, usually not becoming more than 1 to 3 cm in diameter after several months. The surface is dull white or gray. Occasional strains are yellow, velvety or waxy, heaped. The reverse is colorless and penetrates deeply into the agar.

MICRO: Chains of chlamydoconidia and occasionally small microconidia are produced. Macroconidia are rarely seen.

Special tests: All strains require thiamine for growth and in addition many require inositol. Growth is better at 37°C than at 22° to 30°C. Chlamydoconidium production is enhanced at 37°C.

For more descriptions see

Chapter 4, Table 11

Ajello and Padhye (in Lennette et al.), p. 480

Emmons et al., p. 161

Rebell and Taplin, pp. 47–48

Rippon, pp. 162-163

Wilson and Plunkett, p. 368

PATHOGENICITY: Zoophilic, highly inflammatory scalp and skin infection, may cause scarring. Causes ringworm in cattle.

TISSUE FORM: Large ectothrix (5-10 μm) spores.

Trichophyton violaceum (hyphomycete)

GROSS: The surface is slow growing, velvety or waxy, buff to lavender to deep violet. The reverse is colorless to deep purple.

MICRO: Chlamydoconidia and, rarely, microconidia and macroconidia (2- to 5-celled) are seen.

Special tests: Partially thiamine dependent (see Chap. 4, Table 12).

For more descriptions see

Ajello and Padhye (in Lennette et al.), p. 480

Emmons et al., p. 159

Rebell and Taplin, p. 54

Rippon, pp. 161–162
Wilson and Plunkett, p. 366

PATHOGENICITY: Anthropophilic; tinea capitis, similar to *T. tonsurans* infections. Seen most often in Europe, Africa, and Asia.

TISSUE FORM: Endothrix hair invasion.

Trichophyton yaoundei (hyphomycete)

GROSS: Growth is very slow. In primary culture colony is small, yellow, waxy, buttonlike and may become brown. Medium turns dark brown. Subcultures are waxy, dull white, heaped at the center, and slow growing.

MICRO: Slender microconidia are rarely seen. Macroconidia are not formed.

Special tests: *T. yaoundei* grows well on all vitamin media, with and without vitamins (Trichophyton agars #1 through #7). This helps to distinguish *T. yaoundei* from *T. verrucosum, T. violaceum,* and *T. tonsurans,* all of which have a vitamin requirement (see Chap. 4, Table 12).

For more descriptions see

Rebell and Taplin, p. 58
Rippon, p. 167

PATHOGENICITY: Anthropophilic, major cause of tinea capitis in equatorial Africa.

TISSUE FORM: Endothrix hair invasion.

Trichosporon cutaneum, Trichospron beigelii (blastomycete)

GROSS: Colonies are dull white or cream, heaped, wrinkled, waxy, translucent.

MICRO: True hyphae break up into arthroconidia, which may produce budding cells.

Arthroconidia: 2–4 X 3.5–9 μm

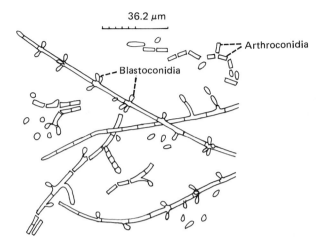

Special tests: Growth is inhibited by cycloheximide. Carbohydrate assimilations
are described in Chap. 4, Table 9. On bromcresol green agar, colonies
are gray-green, heaped and wrinkled (see Plate 3).

For more descriptions see

Plates 3, 4, and 5

Chapter 4, Table 9

Barron, p. 308

Emmons et al., p. 183

Rippon, pp. 93-94

Silva-Hutner and Cooper (in Lennette et al.), pp. 497, 505-506

Wilson and Plunkett, p. 345

PATHOGENICITY: *T. beigelii* is described by Emmons (p. 183) as the agent of
white piedra. *T. cutaneum* (which is culturally identical to *T. beigelii*) is referred
to by Emmons (p. 183) as the agent of subcutaneous and systemic fungal infection.

TISSUE FORM: In white piedra, white nodules composed of tangled hyphae and
spores are attached to the hairs of the scalp or beard or in genital areas. In KOH
preparation it is seen that these groups of spores are surrounded by a thick capsule,
which may make the etiologic agent difficult to isolate.

Trichothecium sp. (hyphomycete)

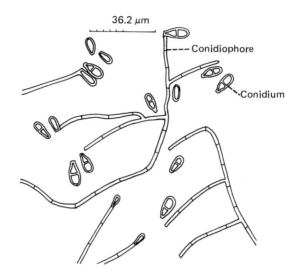

36.2 μm

---- Conidiophore

·Conidium

GROSS: The surface of *T. roseum* grows rapidly and is woolly and salmon-pink. The reverse is pale to tan.

MICRO: Slender conidiophores produce large two-celled, smooth-walled, pear-shaped conidia at the terminal end, one below the next (acrogenously). In routine microscopic mounts, a single conidium is usually observed on the tip of a conidiophore giving the structure a golf-club appearance. These conidia may be distinguished from those of *M. nanum* by the presence of attachment points, which can be seen on both the conidium and the conidiophore. Also, the conidia of *M. nanum* are rough walled. An interesting discussion on the development of these conidia is found in Kendrick's *Taxonomy of the Fungi Imperfecti*, p. 170.

Conidia: 12–18 × 8–10 μm

For more descriptions see

Chapter 2, Figure 28
Barnett and Hunter, p. 104
Barron, pp. 309–310
Emmons, pp. 526–527

Gillman, p. 310
Wilson and Plunkett, pp. 362–363

PATHOGENICITY: Soil isolate, not known as a pathogenic fungus.

Ustilago sp. (Basidiomycotina)

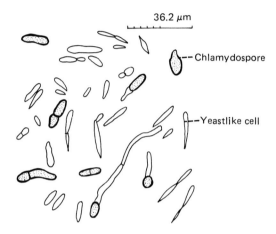

GROSS: Pasty white to cream to tan colony may become covered with large, black, waxy clumps, due to chlamydospore production.

MICRO: Irregular yeastlike cells are seen. Black chlamydospores may develop.

For more descriptions see

Conant et al., pp. 688–689
Wilson and Plunkett, p. 385

PATHOGENICITY: Plant pathogen (corn smut fungus), usually occurs as a contaminant in a medical laboratory. This fungus has been reported in brain lesions but has not been confirmed culturally (Emmons et al., p. 506; and Rippon, p. 459).

Verticillium sp. (hyphomycete)

GROSS: The surface shows rapid growth and is white, velvety to cottony, and flat. The reverse is colorless to pale yellow.

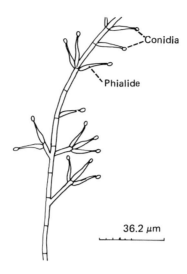

MICRO: Slender phialides are borne singly or in whorls on simple or branched hyaline or pigmented conidiophores. Phialoconidia are held in slime in a cluster at the tip of the phialide.

For more descriptions see

Barnett and Hunter, p. 88
Barron, pp. 321–322
Gillman, pp. 302–304
Wilson and Plunkett, pp. 353–354

PATHOGENICITY: Plant parasite, destructive to peppermint fields. Rare pathogen, mentioned by Rippon, p. 480, as agent of keratitis.

Wangiella (*Phialophora*) *dermatitidis*,
Fonsecaea dermatitidis (hyphomycete)

GROSS: Early growth is black, glistening, and moist. Colonies at three weeks are leathery, velvety, and black. The reverse is black.

MICRO: Early growth consists almost entirely of budding cells. As culture matures, hyphal growth develops with pale brown conidiophores which may be simple or branched. The conidium-bearing (conidiogenous) cell is terminal or intercalary

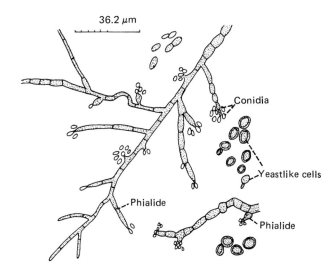

36.2 μm

Conidia

Yeastlike cells

Phialide

Phialide

and is a phialide without a collarette. Round or oval conidia are hyaline and remain in a mass at the point of extrusion from the phialide. Pale brown or clear-colored yeastlike cells are also present.

Conidia: 2.0-3.8 × 2.5-6.1 μm.

Special tests: Grows well at 25° to 40°C, with best growth at 37° to 40°C. For more descriptions see

Chapter 4, Table 17

In Proceedings of the Fourth International Conference on Mycoses, 1978:

Ajello, pp. 13-14

Cole, pp. 67-68

McGinnis, pp. 55-57

Emmons et al., pp. 402-403

Neilson (in Lennette et al.), pp. 532-535

Padhye, McGinnis, and Ajello, 1978

Rippon, p. 242

Wilson and Plunkett, p. 184

PATHOGENICITY: Chromomycosis; phaeomycotic cyst; systemic opportunistic mycosis, with dissemination to the brain (Emmons, p. 480). Occasionally isolated as a laboratory contaminant.

TISSUE FORM: In chromomycosis sclerotic bodies: unicellular or septate cells (Emmons et al., p. 391), and brown, branched, segmented hyphae. In phaeomycosis, brown, branched segmented hyphae are seen.

BIBLIOGRAPHY

Ajello L: The black yeasts as disease agents: Historical perspective, in Proceedings of the Fourth International Conference on the Mycoses. Scientific Publication No. 356. Washington DC: Pan American Health Organization, 1978, p 9.

Ajello L: Taxonomic review of dermatophytes. *Sabouraudia* 6:147, 1968.

Ajello L, Padhye AA: Dermatophytes and the agents of superficial mycoses, in Lennette EH, Spaulding EH, Truant JP (eds): *Manual of Clinical Microbiology,* ed 2. Washington DC: American Society for Microbiology, 1974, p 469.

Al-Doory Y, Gordon MA: Application of fluorescent antibody procedures to the study of pathogenic dematiaceous fungi. I. Differentiation of *Cl. carrionii* and *Cl. bantianum. J Bacteriol* 86:332, 1963.

Bakerspigel A: Medically important species of yeasts isolated in Ontario Canada, in Proceedings of the Fourth International Conference on the Mycoses. Scientific Publication No. 356. Washington DC: Pan American Health Organization, 1978, p 141.

Bardana EJ Jr, McClatchy JK, Farr RS, et al: The primary interaction of antibody to components of Aspergilli. I. Immunologic and chemical characteristics of a nonprecipitating antigen. *J Allergy and Clin Immunol* 50:222, 1972.

Bardana EJ Jr: Measurement of humoral antibodies to Aspergilli. *Ann NY Acad Sci* 221:64, 1974.

*Barnett HL, Hunter BB: *Illustrated Genera of Imperfect Fungi.* Minneapolis: Burgess Publishing Co, 1972.

*Barron GL: *The Genera of Hyphomycetes from the Soil.* Huntington NY: Robert E Krieger Publishing Co, 1968 (reprint 1971).

Beneke ES, Rogers AL: *Medical Mycology Manual,* ed 3. Minneapolis: Burgess Publishing Co, 1970.

Bottone EJ, Weitzman I, Hanna BA: *Rhizopus rhizopodiformis:* Emerging etiological agent of mucormycosis. *J Clin Microbiol* 9:530, 1979.

Buckley HR, Murray IG: Precipitating antibodies in chromomycosis. *Sabouraudia* 5:78, 1966.

*Useful in the identification of odd fungal isolates (see Chap. 5).

*Carmichael JW: Chrysosporium and some other aleuriosporic Hyphomycetes. *Can J Bot* 40:1137, 1962.

Carmichael JW: Cerebral mycetoma of trout due to Phialophora-like fungus. *Sabouraudia* 5:120, 1966.

Cole GT: Conidiogenesis in the black yeasts, in Proceedings of the Fourth International Conference on the Mycoses. Scientific Publication No. 356. Washington DC: Pan American Health Organization, 1978, p 66.

Conant NF, Smith DT, Baker RD, et al; *Manual of Clinical Mycology,* ed 3. Philadelphia: WB Saunders Co, 1971.

Dolan CT, Roberts GD: Mycology, Section III in Washington JA (ed): *Laboratory Procedures in Clinical Microbiology.* Boston, Little, Brown & Co, 1974.

Dowell VR, Sonnenwirth AC: Gram-positive, nonsporeforming anaerobic bacilli, in Lennette EH, Spaulding EH, Truant JP (eds): *Manual of Clinical Microbiology,* ed 2. Washington DC: American Society for Microbiology, 1974, p 396.

*Ellis MB: *Dematiaceous Hyphomycetes.* Kew, Surrey, Commonwealth Mycological Institute, 1971.

*Ellis MB: *More Dematiaceous Hyphomycetes.* Kew, Surrey, Commonwealth Mycological Institute, 1976.

*Emmons CW, Binford CH, Utz JP, et al: *Medical Mycology,* ed 3. Philadelphia: Lea and Febiger, 1977.

Emmons CW: Pathogenic dematiaceous fungi. *Japanese J Med Mycol* 7:233, 1966.

Estes SA, Merz WG, Maxwell LG: Primary cutaneous phaeohyphomycosis caused by *Drechslera spicifera. Arch Dermatol* 113:813, 1977.

Fiese MJ: *Coccidioidomycosis.* Springfield IL: Charles C Thomas, 1958.

Gerber J, Chomicki J, Brandsberg JW, et al: Pulmonary aspergillosis caused by *Aspergillus fischeri* var. *spinosus.* Report of a case and value of serological studies. *Am J Clin Pathol* 60:861, 1973.

*Gillman JC: *A Manual of Soil Fungi,* ed 2. Ames, IA: The Iowa State University Press, 1957 (fourth printing, 1971).

Greer DL: Fungi of phycomycosis, in Lennette EH, Spaulding EH, Truant JP (eds): *Manual of Clinical Microbiology,* ed 2. Washington DC: American Society for Microbiology, 1974, p 541.

Gordon MA: Aerobic pathogenic actinomycetaceae, in Lennette EH, Spaulding EH, Truant JP (eds): *Manual of Clinical Microbiology,* ed 2. Washington DC: American Society for Microbiology, 1974, p 175.

Halde C, Padhye AA, Haley LD, et al: *Acremonium falciforme* as a cause of mycetoma in California. *Sabouraudia* 14:319, 1976.

Haley LD, Callaway CS: *Laboratory Methods in Medical Mycology,* ed 4. US Department of Health Education and Welfare. HEW Publication No. (CDC) 78–8361, 1978.

Harold W, Snyder M: Scheme for cultural identification of *Candida* species of medical importance. Difco Technical Information Bulletin No. 0615, 1969.

Huppert M, Sun SH, Bailey JW: Natural Variability in *Coccidioides immitis,* in Ajello L (ed): *Coccidioidomycosis.* Tucson: The University of Arizona Press, 1967, p. 323.

Huppert M, Sun SH, Rice E: Specificity of exoantigen for identifying cultures of *Coccidioides immitis. J Clin Microbiol* 8:346, 1978.

Jones KW, Kaufman L: Development and evaluation of an immunodiffusion test for diagnosis of systemic zygomycosis (mucormycosis): Preliminary report. *J Clin Microbiol* 7:97, 1978.

Kane J: *Trichophyton fischeri* sp. Nov: A saprophyte resembling *Trichophyton rubrum, Sabouraudia* 15:231, 1977.

Kaplan W: Prototheosis and infection caused by morphologically similar green algae, in Proceedings of the Fourth International Conference on the Mycoses. Scientific Publication No. 356. Washington DC: Pan American Health Organization, 1978, p 218.

Kaplan W, Kaufman L: Specific fluorescent antiglobulins for the detection and identification of *Blastomyces dermatitidis* yeast phase cells. *Mycopathologia* 19:173, 1963.

Kaufman L: Serodiagnosis of fungal diseases, in Lennette EH, Spaulding EH, Truant JP (eds): *Manual of Clinical Microbiology,* ed 2. Washington DC: American Society for Microbiology, 1974, p 557.

Kaufman L, McLaughlin DW, Clark MJ, et al: Specific immunodiffusion test for blastomycosis. *Appl Microbiol* 26:244, 1973.

Kaufman L, Standard P: Improved version of exoantigen test for identification of *Coccidioides immitis* and *Histoplasma capsulatum* cultures. *J Clin Microbiol* 8:42, 1978.

Kendrick B (ed): *Taxonomy of Fungi Imperfecti.* Proceedings of the First International Specialists Workshop-Conference on Criteria and Terminology in the Classification of Fungi Imperfecti Held at the Environmental Sciences Center of the University of Calgary, Kananskis, Alberta, Canada. Toronto: University of Toronto Press, 1971.

*Kendrick WB, Carmichael JW: Hyphomycetes, in Ainsworth GC, Sparrow FK, Sussman AS (eds): *The Fungi IVA.* New York: Academic Press, 1973, p 323.

Kwon-Chung KJ: Description of a new genus, *Filobasidiella,* the perfect state of *Cryptococcus neoformans. Mycologia* 67:1197, 1975.

Kwon-Chung KJ: Morphogenesis of *Filobasidiella neoformans,* the sexual state of *Cryptococcus neoformans. Mycologia* 68:821, 1976.

Kwon-Chung KJ: A new species of *Filobasidiella,* the sexual state of *Cryptococcus neoformans* B and C serotypes. *Mycologia* 68:942, 1976.

Kwon-Chung KJ: Comparison of isolates of *Sporothrix schenckii* from fixed cutaneous lesions with isolates from other types of lesions. *J Infect Dis* 1393:424, 1979.

Larsh HW, Goodman NL: Fungi of systemic mycoses, in Lennette EH, Spaulding EH, Truant JP (eds): *Manual of Clinical Microbiology,* ed 2. Washington DC: American Society for Microbiology, 1974, p 508.

Lodder J, Kreger-Van Rij NJW: *Yeasts, A Taxonomic Study,* ed 2. Amsterdam, North Holland Publishing Co, 1970.

Lutwick LI, Galgiani JN, Johnson RH, et al: Visceral fungal infections due to *Petriellidium boydii. Am J Med* 61:37, 1976.

Mariat F, Liautaud B, Liautaud M, et al: *Hendersonula toruloidea,* agent d'une dermatite verruqueuse mycosique observee en Algerie. *Sabouraudia* 16:133, 1978.

Martin DS, Baker RD, Conant NF: A case of verrucous dermatitis caused by *Hormodendrum pedrosoi* (chromomblastomycosis) in North Carolina. *Amer J Trop Med* 16:593, 1936.

*McGinnis MR: *A Laboratory Handbook of Medical Mycology.* NY Academic Press, in press.

McGinnis MR: Human pathogenic species of *Exophiala, Phialophora* and *Wangiella,* in Proceedings of the Fourth International Conference on the Mycoses. Scientific Publication No. 356. Washington DC: Pan American Health Organization, 1978, p 37.

McGinnis MR, Katz B: *Ajellomyces* and its synonym *Emmonsiella. Mycotaxon* 8:157, 1979.

McGinnis MR, Padhye AA, *Exophiala jeanselmei*, a new combination for *Phialophora jeanselmei. Mycotaxon* 5:341, 1977.

McGinnis MR: *Exophiala spinifera*, a new combination for *Phialophora spinifera. Mycotaxon* 5:337, 1977.

McGinnis MR: *Wangiella*, a new genus to accommodate *Hormiscum dermatitidis. Mycotaxon* 5:353, 1977.

Muchmore HG, Felton FG, Scott EN: Rapid presumptive identification of *Cryptococcus neoformans. J Clin Microbiol* 8:166, 1978.

Müller E, von Arx JA: Pyrenomycetes: Melioles, Coronphorales, Sphaeriales, in Ainsworth GC, Sparrow FK, Sussman AS (eds): *The Fungi* IVA. New York: Academic Press, 1973, p 87.

Nielsen HS Jr: Dematiaceous fungi, in Lennette EH, Spaulding EH and Truant JP (eds): *Manual of Clinical Microbiology*, ed 2. Washington DC: American Society for Microbiology, 1974, p 528.

Nielsen HS, Conant NF: Practical evaluation of antigenic relationships of yeast-like dematiaceous fungi. *Sabouraudia* 5:283, 1968.

Padhye A: Comparative study of *Phialophora jeanselmei* and *P. gougerotii* by morphological, biochemical and immunological methods, in Proceedings of the Fourth International Conference on the Mycoses. Scientific Publication No. 356. Washington DC: Pan American Health Organization, 1978, p 60.

Padhye AA, McGinnis MR, Ajello L: Thermotolerance of *Wangiella dermatitidis. J Clin Microbiol* 8:424, 1978.

Proceedings of the Fourth International Conference on Mycoses. Scientific Publication No. 356. Washington DC: Pan American Health Organization, 1978.

*Raper KB, Fennell DI: *The Genus Aspergillus.* Huntington NY: Robert E Krieger Publishing Co, 1973.

Raper KB, Thom C, Fennell DI: *A Manual of Penicillia.* Baltimore, The Williams and Wilkins Co, 1949.

Ray LF, Campbell MC: *A Syllabus on Fungi for Dermatologists.* Portland: University of Oregon Medical School, 1973.

Rebell GC, Forster RK: Fungi of keratomycosis, in Lennette EH, Spaulding EH, Truant JP (eds): *Manual of Clinical Microbiology,* ed 2. Washington DC: American Society for Microbiology, 1974, p 482.

*Rebell G, Taplin D: *Dermatophytes, Their Recognition and Identification.* Coral Gables, FL: University of Miami Press, 1974.

Rippon JW: *Medical Mycology.* Philadelphia, WB Saunders Co, 1974.

Rippon JW, Anderson DN, et al.: Blastomycoses: Specificity of antigens reflecting the mating types of *Ajellomyces dermatitidis.* Abstracts of the Annual Meeting of the American Society for Microbiology, 1972, p 131.

Roberts GD, Larsh HW: The serologic diagnosis of extracutaneous sporotrichosis. *Amer J Clin Pathol* 56:597, 1971.

Schneidau JD: Fungi of maduromycosis, in Lennette EH, Spaulding EH, Truant JP (eds): *Manual of Clinical Microbiology,* ed 2. Washington DC: American Society for Microbiology, 1974, p 522.

Sekhon AS: *Bacterioides fragilis* and *Torulopsis glabrata* in a patient with gastrointestinal ulcers and chronic renal failure, with review of literature on torulopsis, in Proceedings of the Fourth International Conference on the Mycoses. Scientific Publication No. 356. Washington DC: Pan American Health Organization, 1978, p 167.

Silva-Hutner M, Cooper BH: Medically important yeasts, in Lennette EH, Spaulding EH, Truant JP (eds): *Manual of Clinical Microbiology,* ed 2. Washington DC: American Society for Microbiology, 1974, p 491.

Smith CD, Goodman NL: Improved culture methods for the isolation of *Histoplasma capsulatum* and *Blastomyces dermatitidis* from contaminated specimens. *Am J Clin Pathol* 63:276, 1974.

Sutton BC: Coelomycetes, in Ainsworth GC, Sparrow FK, Sussman AS (eds): *The Fungi IVA.* New York: Academic Press, 1973, p 513.

Wang CJK: Annellophores in *Torula jeanselmei. Mycologia* 58:614, 1966.

*Wilson JW, Plunkett OA: *The Fungous Diseases of Man.* Berkeley, University of California Press, 1974.

Glossary

Acervulus: Saucer-shaped mass of hyphae on which conidia are borne.

Acroauxic: Growth in length of conidiophores is restricted to apical branches (Ellis, p. 10).

Acrogenous: Contents pass through conidiogenous cell and conidium takes form immediately outside, as in *Epicoccum* sp. (Ellis, p. 12).

Acropetal: A chain of conidia with the youngest at the tip.

Acropleurogenous: Produced apically and on the sides.

Acrothecal: See **Sympodial.**

Adiaspore: "A fungus spore which, when introduced into an animal or incubated *in vitro* at elevated temperature, increases greatly in size without eventual reproduction or replication" (Emmons, p. 571).

Aleurioconidia: Conidia that are borne directly on a hypha, on short pedicels, or on undifferentiated conidiophores.

Aleuriophore: Conidiophore bearing an aleurioconidium.

Aleuriospores: See **aleurioconidia.**

Amerospores: Nonseptate conidia.

Ampulla: Swollen apex of a sporogenous cell.

Annellation: Vegetative remnant forming a scar as a result of conidium production from an annellidic conidiogenous cell.

Annellide: Conidiogenous cell that produces conidia in a basipetal fashion. A scarred tip remains after the production of each conidium.

Annellidic: Descriptive of a conidiogenous cell that elongates at the tip as each new blastic conidium is produced from within the cell.

349

Annelloconidia: Conidia produced from an annellide.

Annellospores: See **annelloconidia**.

Apophysis: A swelling, often just below the sporangium, as in the Mucorales.

Arthric: A form of thallic conidium production characterized by conversion and disarticulation of a preexisting determinate hyphal element.

Arthroconidia: Conidia that are produced in a chain by septation and breaking up, in a basipetal fashion from a conidiogenous hypha.

Arthrospores: See **Arthroconidia**.

Ascocarp: Fungal structure containing asci and ascospores.

Ascospore: An endogenous spore produced within an ascus as a result of sexual union of two fungal elements.

Ascus (plural: asci): Fungal structure containing one or more ascospores.

Asexual reproduction: The production of conidia by vegetative growth.

Asperate: Rough.

Basauxic: "Conidiophores each consist of a mother cell and an extensible filament arising from within it which may be conidiogenous" (Ellis, p. 11).

Basidiocarp: Structure containing basidiospores.

Basidiospores: Spores produced in the basidiomycotina as a result of sexual union of two to four fungal elements.

Basipetal: Conidia produced in a chain with the youngest at the base.

Biseriate: Phialide is borne on a prophialide. This term is used in describing some *Aspergillus* species.

Blastic: Method of conidium production in which conidium is formed before septating wall is formed.

Blastoconidia: Conidia that are blown out from a mother cell, are capable of budding, produce new blastoconidia or pseudohyphae, and are capable of producing germ tubes that develop into hyphae.

Blastospores: See **Blastoconidia**.

Botryoblastoconidia: Conidia that are produced simultaneously from an ampulla of a conidiogenous cell, on short denticles, singly, or in acropetal chains.

Botryoblastospores: See **Botryoblastoconidia**.

Bulbils: Irregular groups of cells that form a reproductive unit in the mycelia sterila.

Bulla: Clinical description of a large blister.

Catenulate: In a chain.

Chlamydoconidium: Descriptive of chlamydospores in Fungi Imperfecti.

Chlamydospore: Large, double-walled resting spore.

Clavate: Club shaped.

Cleavage: Development of spores by cleavage planes progressing inwardly from the periphery of a sporangium (e.g., *Mucor* or *Rhizopus* species); also in tissue phase (spherule or sporangium) of *Coccidioides immitis* (Wilson and Plunkett, p. 285).

Cleistothecium: A closed ascocarp.

Coenocytic: Having many nuclei and few or no septa, as in the hyphae of the Zygomycetes.

Collarette: Cup-shaped structure at the opening of a conidiogenous or sporogenous cell.

Columella (plural: columellae): Sterile inflated end of a sporangophore extending into the sporangium (Gillman, p. 436).

Conidiogenous cell: Cell that produces conidia.

Conidiophore: Conidiogenous cell and branches of specialized hyphae on which conidiogenous cells are borne.

Conidium (plural: conidia): Asexual fruiting body of a fungus, not formed by cleavage (Kendrick, p. 47).

Dematiaceous: Descriptive of fungi with dark-colored conidia and conidiophores.

Denticle: Short, thin projection bearing a spore.

Determinate: Adjective applied to conidiophore or conidiogenous cell that ceases extension growth at or before onset of conidium production (Kendrick, p. 255).

Deuteromycotina: See **Fungi Imperfecti**.

Dichotomous: Branching in two equal parts.

Didymospores: One-septate conidia.

Dictyospores: Longitudinally and transversely septate conidia.

Dimorphic: Two forms, as *yeast form* and *mold form,* or *spherule form* and *arthroconidium form.*

Disjunctor: Attachment point on a conidium or conidiophore that remains as a dark scar after the conidium is released.

Ectothrix invasion: Spores surround the hair shaft.

Endospore: Spore produced within a membrane called a spherule or a sporangium.

Endothrix invasion: Spores are contained within the hair shaft.

Eukaryotic cells: Cells distinguished from prokaryotic cells by presence of a nuclear membrane and other more complex cellular organizations.

Exogenous: Conidium borne free on a conidiogenous cell, not enclosed in a sporangium.

Fission: Method of conidium separation from a parent cell in which a natural break occurs at a double septum between the walls of the conidium and the conidiogenous cell.

Fracture: Method of conidium separation in which the walls of the cell adjacent to the conidium are ruptured by mechanical stress to release the conidium.

Fungi Imperfecti: Taxonomic form subdivision of fungi established to accommodate species in which a sexual (perfect) form is not present; also called *Deuteromycotina.*

Fusiform: Spindle shaped.

Gametangium: Sexual hypha.

Geniculate: Bent-kneelike, as in *Curvularia.*

Germ tubes: Tubules produced from a spore or conidium without constriction at the production point.

Glabrous: Waxy, smooth.

Globose: Round.

Gymnocarp: An ascocarp that is a loose mesh of hyphae containing asci and ascopores.

Helicospores: Spiral-formed conidia.

Hyaline: Light-colored.

Hyalo-: Prefix denoting *light-colored.*

Hypha (plural: hyphae): Tubular cells, which grow by elongation or branching; corresponding to the stems of plants.

Imperfect form: Asexual form of fungal growth. See also **Fungi Imperfecti.**

Indeterminate: Descriptive of conidiogenous cell that continues extension growth during or between formation of successive conidia, as an annellide.

Intercalary: Between two undifferentiated cells.

Keratitis: Inflammation of the cornea.

Keratomycosis: Fungal disease of the cornea.

Macronematous: Conidiophores that are morphologically different from vegetative hyphae. These are usually erect. Compare with **Micronematous.**

Meristem: Any place on a hypha, conidiogenous cell, or conidium where growth occurs that results in an increase in volume.

Meristem arthroconidia: Conidia produced basipetally in chains from the base of a conidiophore that increases in length as conidia are produced.

Meristem arthrospores: See **Meristem arthroconidia.**

Meristem blastoconidia: "Conidia borne singly at the apex, or singly at the apex and laterally, and often in regular whorls on conidiophores which elongate from the base" (Barron p. 35).

Meristem blastospores: See **Meristem blastoconidia.**

Merosporangium: Tubular cell growing from swollen vesicle, containing endospores; seen in *Syncephalastrum* sp.

Metula (plural: metulae): In *Penicillium* sp. the branches of a conidiophore on which the phialides are borne.

Micronematous: Conidiophores that are morphologically similar to hyphae.

Mold: A general term used to describe a fungus characterized by a tangled mass of mycelium resulting in a leathery to granular to cottony colony. Also spelled *mould.*

Monoblastic: Conidiogenous cell that blows out at one point.

Mononematous: Conidiophore solitary.

Mutation: A yeast or mold that has undergone a change of characteristic structures. A sterile mutant is a mold that no longer produces characteristic spores.

Mycelium: A mass of hyphae.

Onychomycosis: Fungal disease of nails.

Penicillus: Branched conidiophore forming a brush, seen in *Penicillium* species.

Percurrent: Descriptive of conidiogenous cell that continues growth through opening from which a conidium has been released.

Perfect form: Sexual form of fungal growth.

Perithecium: An ascocarp with an opening at one end.

Phaeo-: Prefix denoting *dark colored.*

Phialide (n.), phialidic (adj.): Conidiogenous cell from which blastic conidia are produced in basipetal succession, each with newly laid walls that are not derived from the wall of the conidiogenous cell. Collarette may be observed at point of opening.

Phialoconidia: Conidia that are produced from a phialide.

Phialospores: See **Phialoconidia**.

Phragmospores: Multiseptate conidia.

Pleomorphism: See **Mutation** (sterile).

Polyblastic: Conidiogenous cell that blows out at more than one point (as in *Cladosporium* sp.).

Polytretic: Conidiogenous cell with several channels through which conidia are produced.

Poroconidia: Conidia that are produced through minute pores in the wall of a conidiophore or a previously formed conidium. Term has been replaced by word *tretoconidium.*

Porospores: See **Poroconidia**.

Probasidium: Hyphal structure that bears basidiospores.

Prokaryotic cells: Cells distinguished from eukaryotic cells by a lack of a nuclear membrane and a more simple cellular organization.

Prophialide: Structure that bears a phialide (in *Aspergillus* species).

Pseudohyphae: Elongated blastoconidia.

Pycnidium: Saclike structures containing conidia (asexual).

Pyriform: Pear shaped.

Retrogressive: Defines a conidiogenous cell or hypha that may be converted into a conidium.

Sclerotic body: Round, deeply pigmented bodies seen in tissue form of chromomycosis.

Sclerotium: A hard mass of hyphae or pseudoparenchyma that forms a reproductive unit.

Scoleoscoporae: Threadlike conidia.

Scutulum: Cuplike structure formed by masses of hyphae and epithelial debris.

Semiendogenous: Conidia that form partly inside the tip of a phialide.

Sessile: Borne directly on the side of a hypha, or undifferentiated conidiophore.

Shield cell: Shield-shaped cells seen in *Cladosporium* species, with one growth point (disjunctor) at one end and two disjunctors at the other end.

Spherule: Sporangiumlike structure containing endospores that are produced by cleavage; seen in tissue phase of *Coccidioides immitis.*

Sporangiophore: Specialized hypha that bears a sporangium.

Sporangium (plural: sporangia): Membrane containing endospores produced by cleavage.

Spore: Fruiting body of a fungus, generally used to describe a body produced as a result of a sexual union, or asexual cells produced by cleavage.

Sporodochium: Cushion-shaped mass of hyphae bearing conidiophores and conidia.

Sporogenous: Spore bearing.

Stable: Determinate conidiogenous cell that is not retrogressively converted into a conidium.

Staurospores: Star shaped conidia.

Sterigma (plural: sterigmata): Commonly applied to the phialides and prophialides of *Aspergillus* and the phialides and metullae of *Penicillium.* Properly applied to the denticle on which a basidiospore is produced in the Basidiomycotina.

Stolon: Hypha from which sporangiophores and rhizoids are produced.

Subglobose: Almost round.

Sympodial: Growth of a conidiogenous cell beneath or beside a previous conidium that pushes the conidium to one side (synonym: **Acrothecal**).

Sympodioconidia: Conidia that are blown out successively from a conidiophore that enlarges as each new conidium is produced (see **Sympodial**).

Sympodulospores: See **Sympodioconidia**.

Thallic: Method of conidium production in which the septating wall of the conidium is developed before the swelling of the conidium occurs (if it occurs at all).

Thallospore: An asexual spore produced from a hypha, e.g., arthroconidium or chlamydoconidium.

Thallus: Vegetative body of a fungus.

Tinea: Superficial or cutaneous fungal infection. (See Chap. 3 for different forms of tinea.)

Tretic: Cells produced from inner wall of conidiogenous cell.

Uniseriate: Phialide attached directly on vesicle (in *Aspergillus* species); see also **Biseriate**).

Vesicle: (1) Clinical: A small blister formed in a cutaneous fungal infection; (2) Culture: A swollen conidiophore tip on which conidiophores and conidia are borne.

Yeast: A fungus characterized by budding cells and producing a moist to pasty colony.

Zygospore: Sexual spore produced from the union of two gametangia.

BIBLIOGRAPHY

Barron GL: *The Genera of Hyphomycetes from the Soil.* Huntington NY: Robert E Krieger Publishing Co, 1968 (reprint, 1971).

Ellis MB: *Dematiaceous Hyphomycetes.* Kew, Surrey, Commonwealth Mycological Institute, 1971.

Emmons CW, Binford CH, Utz JP, et al: *Medical Mycology,* ed 3. Philadelphia: Lea and Febiger, 1977.

Gillman JC: *A Manual of Soil Fungi,* ed 2. Ames IA: The Iowa State University Press, 1957 (fourth printing, 1971).

Kendrick B (ed): *Taxonomy of Fungi Imperfecti.* Toronto: University of Toronto Press, 1971.

Appendix

Instruments and Applicances

Laminar flow safety hood with electric burner for sterilizing inoculating blades
Microscope
Incubators
  35° to 37°C with 5–10% CO_2
  30°C (optional, room temperature 22° to 25° is satisfactory)
  40°C for some temperature requirements
  42°C with 20% CO_2 for *Coccidioides immitis* identification
  45°C for nitrate-Zephiran swab test
Oven or water bath
  50°C for API suspension media
  95°C for methenamine silver nitrate test
Refrigerator
Scales for preparing reagents
Bunsen burner
Hot plate or tripod with asbestos mat
Autoclave

Tools

Stiff sharp blade or needle on handle (Bard-Parker #7 handle with a good supply of #11 blades is recommended)

Dissecting needles

Inoculating loops

Firm forceps, 4 to 5 inches

Hemostat

Scissors

Glassware or Clear Plastic

Flasks, beakers, and funnels for media preparation

Graduated cylinders — 10 ml, 25 ml, 100 ml, and 500 ml

Graduated pipettes, 5 ml and 10 ml

Sterile capillary pipettes

Thermometers for daily recording of temperatures

Homogenizers for grinding of specimens

Dropper bottle for staining reagents

Coplin jars for staining procedures

Screw-capped bottles for stock reagents

Screw-capped tubes for media

Screw-capped bottles for media (optional, see discussion to follow)

Sterile Petri dishes

Glass microscope slides

Glass cover slips, 22 $\times$ 22 mm and 22 $\times$ 30 mm

Miscellaneous

Wooden sticks, with and without cotton swabs

Rubber bulbs for pipettes

Flow pen with waterproof ink

Wax marking crayon
Tape for labels and for sealing plates
Clear nail polish for sealing microscopic mounts
Discard containers
Disinfectant solution
Record books and file boxes and file cards
Distilled water

Reagents for Microscopic Preparations (see Chap. 4)

REAGENTS USED ONLY IN A MYCOLOGY LABORATORY

10% KOH
KOH-DMSO (optional)
India ink or nigrosin
Lactophenol cotton blue
Glycerine

REAGENTS AVAILABLE IN OTHER LABORATORIES

Gram's stain (Bacteriology)
Modified acid-fast stain (Bacteriology)
Giemsa stain (Hematology)
Methenamine silver nitrate stain (Pathology)
Periodic acid-Schiff stain (Pathology)
Mayer's mucicarmine stain (Pathology)
Hematoxylin and eosin stain (Pathology)
Papanicolaou's stain (Cytology)

Media

Media for primary isolation (see Chap. 4, Table 4)
Media for differential tests (see Chap. 4, Table 6)

REAGENTS, STAINS, AND MICROSCOPIC MOUNTS

All reagents are stored at room temperatures in screw-capped glass bottles, unless other directions are given. Bottles are labeled with the formula, date of preparation, expiration date, and initials of the person preparing the formula. For most reagents an expiration date of one year is given. In general usage it may be determined that a longer or even an indefinite time is satisfactory.

10% KOH (Potassium Hydroxide)

Potassium hydroxide	10 g
Distilled water	100 ml

1. Add potassium hydroxide crystals to distilled water slowly and with stirring.
2. Mix by stirring until crystals are completely dissolved.

KOH (Potassium Hydroxide)-DMSO

Potassium hydroxide	20 g
Distilled water	60 ml
Dimethyl sulfoxide (DMSO)	40 ml

1. Add potassium hydroxide crystals to distilled water slowly, with stirring.
2. Mix, by stirring, until crystals are completely dissolved.
3. Add DMSO and stir thoroughly.

See Zaias and Taplin, p. 608.

India Ink

India ink is purchased in art supply stores. Pelican Drawing Ink, 17 Black, Gunther Wagner, Germany, is recommended by Paik and Suggs, p. 945.

Giemsa Stain

Giemsa stain, powdered (certified)	0.75 g
Methyl alcohol, pure	65.0 ml
Glycerol, pure	35.0 ml

Shake well in bottle with glass beads. Keep tightly closed and stoppered at all times. Filter if necessary.

Lactophenol Cotton Blue

Phenol crystals	20 g
Lactic acid	20 ml
Glycerine	40 ml
Distilled water	20 ml
Cotton blue, 1% aqueous (Poirrier's blue)	2 ml

1. Add lactic acid and glycerine to the distilled water and mix thoroughly.
2. Add phenol crystals and mix. Heat gently in hot water with frequent agitation until crystals are completely dissolved.
3. Add 2 ml of 1% cotton blue solution and mix thoroughly.

Reagents for Mayer's Mucicarmine Stain

WEIGERT'S IRON HEMATOXYLIN

1. Solution A
Hematoxylin	1.0 g
Alcohol 95%	100.0 ml
2. Solution B
Ferric chloride, 29% aqueous solution	4.0 ml
Distilled water	95.0 ml
Hydrochloric acid, concentrated	1.0 ml
3. Working solution
   Equal parts A and B prepared fresh.

METANIL YELLOW SOLUTION

1. Metanil yellow	0.25 g
2. Distilled water	100.0 ml
3. Glacial acetic acid	0.25 ml

MUCICARMINE STAIN

1. Carmine	1.0 g
2. Aluminum chloride, anhydrous	0.5 g
3. Distilled water	2.0 ml

Mix stain in test tube. Heat in water bath for 2 minutes. Liquid becomes almost black and syrupy. Dilute with 100 ml of 50% alcohol and let stand for 24 hours. Filter. Dilute 1 to 4 with tap water for use. Expiration: 1 month.
See Emmons et al. p. 481.

Methenamine Silver Nitrate Staining Reagents (Rapid Method)

1. 10% chromic acid (chromium trioxide)

Chromic acid	10.0 g
Distilled water	100 ml

2. 1% sodium metabisulfite

Sodium bisulfite	1.0 g
Distilled water	100 ml

3. 5% silver nitrate

Silver nitrate	5.0 g
Distilled water	100 ml

Store in dark colored bottle in 4°C refrigerator; use as needed.

4. 3% aqueous methenamine (hexamethylenetetramine)

Methenamine	3.0 g
Distilled water	100 ml

5. 5% aqueous borax

Borax (sodium borate)	5.0 g
Distilled water	100 ml

6. 1% aqueous gold chloride

    Gold chloride   15 grain vial

    Distilled water   100 ml

7. 5% sodium thiosulfate (hypo) solution

    Sodium thiosulfate   5.0 g

    Distilled water   100 ml

8. Light green working solution

    a. 0.2% light green (stock solution)

        Light green, SF yellowish   0.2 g

        Distilled water   100 ml

        Glacial acetic acid   0.2 ml

    b. 10 ml of (a) is added to 50 ml distilled water

9. 70% alcohol

10. 95% alcohol   } used in plastic squirt bottles as needed

11. Absolute alcohol

12. Xylol, used from dropper bottle

13. Histoclad, Permount, or other mounting medium

See Mahan and Sale, p. 102.

Reagents for Modified Acid-Fast Stain (Hank's Method)

CARBOLFUCHSIN REAGENT

1. Solution 1

    Basic fuchsin   3 gm

    95% ethyl alcohol   100 ml

2. Solution 2

    Phenol (concentrated)   5 ml

    Distilled water   95 ml

Add 90 ml of solution 2 (phenol solution) to 10 ml of solution 1 (carbolfuchsin solution). Store at 37°C in a tightly sealed bottle.

SULFURIC ACID–METHYLENE BLUE REAGENT

1. Solution 3

Methylene blue	1 gm
Distilled water	100 ml

2. Solution 4

Sulfuric acid (concentrated)	5 ml
Distilled water	95 ml

Add 20 ml of solution 3 (methylene blue) to 80 ml of solution 4 (sulfuric acid). Store at room temperature in a tightly sealed bottle.
See Haley and Callaway, p. 48.

Nitrate-Zephiran Treated Swabs

NITRATE-ZEPHIRAN BUFFERED REAGENT

KNO_3	2.0 g
$Na_2H_2PO_4 \cdot H_2O$	11.7 g
Na_2HPO_4	1.14 g
Zephiran chloride (17% solution)	1.2 ml
Distilled water	200 ml

1. Weigh and measure all ingredients carefully.
2. Add 1.2 ml Zephiran chloride to 200 ml distilled water.
3. Add dry chemicals and mix to dissolve completely.

PREPARATION OF SWABS

1. Place 0.1 ml of reagent in each of desired number of straight-sided, clean test tubes (13 cm $\times$ 150 cm).
2. Place a standard cotton swab (Johnson and Johnson, 6-inch, 15 cm) in each tube so that fluid will be absorbed.
3. Allow swabs to dry in tubes overnight at room temperature.
4. Remove swabs from tubes. Place in a large screw-top test tube (25 $\times$ 200 mm).
5. Sterilize by autoclaving at 15 pounds pressure for 15 minutes.

Swabs are stored in refrigerator at 4°C. Warm to room temperature before using.
See Hopkins and Land, p. 497.

Reagents for Periodic Acid-Schiff Stain

1. Formal-ethanol mixture

   40% formaldehyde   10 ml

   Absolute alcohol   90 ml

2. Periodic acid, 1%

   Periodic acid   1 g

   Distilled water   100 ml

3. Schiff's reagent (commercially available*)

   Boiling distilled water   200 ml

   Basic fuchsin   1 g

   a. Cool to 50°C and filter.

   b. Add 20 ml 1N HCl (83 ml concentrated HCl/1,000 ml distilled water). Cool to 25°C.

   c. Add sodium bisulfite, 1 g; store in screw-top bottle in dark for two days.

   d. Add activated charcoal, 0.5 g; shake intermittently for one hour.

   e. Filter.

   f. Store in dark-colored, tightly closed bottle, in refrigerator (5 years); pour into a Coplin jar for use. Solution may be reused until it turns pink, at which time it must be discarded.

4. Light green working solution (see reagents for methenamine silver nitrate stain)

5. 70% alcohol

6. 95% alcohol   } use in plastic squirt bottles

7. Absolute alcohol

8. Xylol — use from dropper bottle.

9. Mounting medium (Histoclad, Permount, or other mounting medium).

See Emmons et al., p. 566.

*Harelco #2818, 480 Democrat Rd., Gibbstown, NJ 08027

Swartz-Medrek Contrast Stain for Fungi*

Swartz-Lamkins stain   0.2 ml
0.5% rose bengal in buffered Shear's mounting fluid   0.1 ml
Watch glass

1. Just before staining, solutions are mixed in a watch glass.
2. Material is examined as in procedure for KOH preparation.
3. Fungal elements appear blue against a pink background.

See Swartz and Medrek, p. 494.

Vaspar

1:1 wt/wt: petrolatum jelly and paraffin (melting point, 48° to 56°C)
See Huppert, Harper, Sun, et al. p. 21.

FORMULAE FOR MEDIA

Media described in the following pages are those in use in our laboratories. Formulae are given for those that are prepared from raw materials. Complete formulae for commercial mixtures will be found in the references given.

Plate media may generally be kept in sealed containers for three weeks in the refrigerator. Tube media in slants may be kept, tightly sealed, for six months. Tube media in deeps may be kept, tightly sealed, for one year.

---

*Ingredients are commercially available from Muro Pharmacal Laboratories Inc., 890 East Street, Tewksbury, MA 01876.

Ascospore Agar

Potassium acetate	10.0 g
Yeast extract	2.5 g
Dextrose	1.0 g
Agar	30.0 g
Distilled water	1000 ml

1. Mix thoroughly to give a uniform suspension.
2. Heat to boiling and boil for one minute, with agitation.
3. Dispense 8 ml in screw-top tubes.
4. Autoclave at 121°C, 15 lbs pressure for 15 minutes.
5. Cool in slanted position.
6. Final pH: 6.5.

See Vera and Dumoff, p. 925.

Biphasic Medium for Blood Culture

1. Agar

   Brain-heart infusion agar (commercially available)   52 g

   Distilled water   1000 ml

   a. Suspend 52 g in 1 liter of distilled water; heat to boiling to dissolve.
   b. Distribute 25 ml into 3-ounce bottles with screw-top caps fitted with rubber diaphragms.
   c. Autoclave at 15 lb pressure (121°C) for 15 minutes.
   d. Cool to room temperature, allowing agar to harden on side of bottle.

2. Broth (on the day after the agar is hardened)

   Brain-heart infusion (commercially available)   37 g

   Distilled water   1 liter

   a. Suspend and dissolve 37 g of brain-heart infusion in 1 liter of water.
   b. Autoclave at 15 lb pressure (121°C) for 15 minutes.
   c. Add 30 ml to each bottle, aseptically.
   d. Final pH: 7.4.

See *BBL Manual of Products and Laboratory Procedures,* p. 95; *Difco Manual,* pp. 77–79, 90–91; Roberts and Washington, pp. 309–310.

Brain-Heart Infusion Agar

Brain-heart infusion agar	52 g
Distilled water	1000 ml

1. Suspend 52 g of dehydrated medium in a liter of distilled water; mix thoroughly.
2. Heat with frequent agitation and boil for one minute.
3. Slants:*
   a. Dispense 8 ml in screw-capped tubes.
   b. Sterilize by autoclaving at 121°C (15 lbs pressure) for 15 minutes.
   c. Cool to room temperature in a slanted position (deep slants).
4. Petri dishes:
   a. Sterilize by autoclaving at 121°C (15 lbs pressure) for 15 minutes.
   b. Dispense 36 ml into sterile Petri dishes.
5. Final pH: 7.4.

See *BBL Manual of Products and Laboratory Procedures,* p. 95; *Difco Manual,* p. 90.

Brain-Heart Infusion Agar with 5% Sheep Blood

Brain-heart infusion agar (BBL)	26 g
Distilled water	500 ml
Sheep blood	25 ml

1. Suspend 26 g of dehydrated medium in 500 ml of distilled water; mix thoroughly.
2. Heat with frequent agitation and boil for one minute.
3. Sterilize by autoclaving at 121°C (15 lbs pressure) for 15 minutes.

---

*Moisture is necessary at base of slant. If agar is dry, medium is not effective.

4. Cool to 48°C.
5. Add 25 ml sheep blood.
6. Dispense 8 ml aseptically into sterile screw-capped tubes.
7. Cool in slanted position.
8. Final pH: 7.4.

See *BBL Manual of Products and Laboratory Procedures*, p. 95; *Difco Manual*, p. 91.

Bromcresol Green-Agar Medium

Candida BCG agar base (Difco)	66 g
Distilled water	1000 ml
Neomycin (sterile)	500 μg/ml medium

1. Add 66 g of BCG agar base to 1,000 ml of distilled water and mix.
2. Heat to boiling with frequent agitation at 121°C (15 lb pressure) for 15 minutes.
3. Cool to 50°C in a water bath.
4. When medium has cooled to 50°C, aseptically add neomycin to give 500 μg per ml of medium.
5. Mix thoroughly by swirling.
6. Pour into sterile Petri dishes and allow to solidify at room temperature.
7. Final pH is 6.1 at 25°C (room temperature).

See Harold and Snyder, p. 7.

Caffeic Acid Agar Medium

Agar	15 g
Inositol	10 g
Urea	5 g
Yeast nitrogen base without amino acids and ammonium sulfate (Difco)	1.45 g
Caffeic (3,4 dihydroxycinnamic) acid	0.2 g

Ferric citrate	0.01 g
Gentamicin	40 mg
Distilled water	1,000 ml

1. Fifteen grams agar (Difco), autoclaved with 900 ml distilled water at 15 lb for 15 minutes; cool to 80° to 90°C.
2. Stock solution of ferric citrate is prepared by dissolving one gram of ferric citrate in 100 ml distilled water.
3. One ml of stock ferric citrate is added to 100 ml distilled water, to which the inositol, yeast nitrogen base without amino acids and ammonium sulfate (Difco), caffeic acid and gentamicin have been added; heat to dissolve, then cool to 80° to 90°C.
4. Add urea. DO NOT HEAT FURTHER.
5. Filter sterilize with a 0.45 μm membrane filter.
6. Combine cooled autoclaved agar with filtered, sterilized ingredients.
7. Dispense into sterile tubes for pouring later or into Petri dishes.
8. Final pH: 6.2 ± 0.3.

See Healey, Dillavou, and Taylor, p. 387.

Carbohydrate Assimilation Media for Yeasts (Wickerham Tubes)

Yeast nitrogen base (Difco or BBL)	3.35 g
Distilled water (deionized)	500.0 ml
Carbohydrate desired	2.5 g

YEAST NITROGEN BASE

1. Suspend 3.35 g yeast nitrogen base in 400 ml of distilled water. Mix thoroughly until medium is completely dissolved.
2. Sterilize by autoclaving at 121°C (15 lb pressure) for 15 minutes.
3. Cool to room temperature.

CARBOHYDRATE SOLUTION

1. Suspend 2.5 g of desired carbohydrate in 100 ml distilled water.
2. Sterilize by filtration (Seitz or Millipore).

**COMBINED CARBOHYDRATE SOLUTION
AND YEAST NITROGEN BASE**

1. Add 100 ml sterilized carbohydrate solution to 400 ml autoclaved, cooled yeast nitrogen base. Final carbohydrate concentration is 0.5%.
2. Aseptically, dispense 2 ml aliquots in sterile screw-capped tubes.
3. Final pH is 5.6 at room temperature.

See *BBL Manual of Products and Laboratory Procedures,* p. 158; *Difco Manual,* p. 252.

Carbohydrate Assimilation Media for Yeasts
(Agar for Auxanographic Plates)

Yeast nitrogen base (BBL or Difco)	0.67 g
Noble's or washed agar	20.0 g
Distilled water	1,000 ml

1. Suspend ingredients in water and mix thoroughly to give a uniform suspension.
2. Heat to boiling and boil gently for one minute with agitation.
3. Tube in 20 ml aliquots in screw-capped tubes.
4. Autoclave at 121°C, 15 lb pressure for 15 minutes.
5. Allow to solidify as deeps. Melt in boiling water bath and pour plates as needed.

See *BBL Manual of Products and Laboratory Procedures,* p. 158; *Difco Manual,* p. 252; Haley and Callaway, p. 196.

Carbohydrate Fermentation Broth

Heart infusion broth base (BBL)	25 g
Bromthymol blue (1% aqueous solution)	3 ml
Distilled water	1,000 ml

Sugar solution (5–10% aqueous solution) filter-sterilized (the sugars used include dextrose, maltose, sucrose, lactose)

PREPARATION OF BASIC MEDIUM

1. Dissolve 25 g of infusion broth base in 1000 ml distilled water.
2. Add 3 ml of 1% solution of Bromthymol blue (final concentration of indicator in medium is 0.003%).
    a. Dissolve 1 g of bromthymol blue in 20 ml of 0.1 N sodium hydroxide (Na OH). Be sure that all except a slight residue is dissolved before proceeding to the next step.
    b. Add 80 ml of distilled water and mix thoroughly.
    c. This is the stock 1% solution. Store in the dark at room temperature.
3. Check pH; adjust the pH to 7.2 to 7.3 at room temperature.
4. Dispense in 9-ml amounts in tubes into which inverted Durham tubes have been placed.
5. Sterilize by autoclaving at 121°C (15 lb pressure) for 15 minutes.

ADDITION OF SUGAR

Aseptically, add the filter-sterilized sugar stock solution to each tube of the base medium. Glucose, lactose, and sucrose are added to give a final concentration of 1%. Maltose is added in a final concentration of 0.5%.

See *BBL Manual of Products and Laboratory Procedures,* p. 114; *UOHSC Microbiology Division Procedure* No. 330 a-46.

Casein Agar

SKIMMED MILK SUSPENSION

Skimmed milk powder (BBL or Difco)	75 g
Distilled water	500 ml

1. Add powdered milk to the distilled water, a little at a time, with constant stirring. Do not leave lumps.
2. Stir until completely dissolved.
3. Sterilize by autoclaving at 115°C (10 lb pressure) for 20 minutes.
4. Cool to 50° to 55°C in a water bath.

AGAR SOLUTION

Agar   2.0 g
Distilled water   500 ml

1. Suspend agar in distilled water.
2. Heat to boiling with frequent agitation until agar is completely dissolved.
3. Sterilize by autoclaving at 121°C (15 lb pressure) for 15 minutes.
4. Cool to 50° to 55°C in a water bath.

COMPLETE MEDIUM

1. When both parts are at 50° to 55°C, aseptically pour the agar solution into the skimmed milk suspension.
2. Swirl to mix thoroughly.
3. Pour 20 ml into sterile screw-capped tubes.
4. Final pH: 7.0 ± 0.1.

See Vera and Dumoff, p. 897.

Christensen's Urea Agar

UREA AGAR BASE

Urea agar base (BBL)   29 g
Distilled water   100 ml

1. Dissolve 29 g of urea agar base in 100 ml distilled water.
2. Sterilize by filtration.

MELTED AGAR

Agar   15 g
Distilled water   900 ml

1. Suspend agar in water, heat with gentle mixing to boiling.
2. Autoclave at 121°C at 15 lb pressure for 15 minutes.
3. Cool to 50°C.

COMBINED INGREDIENTS

1. Add sterile urea agar base to melted cooled agar.
2. Mix thoroughly.
3. Dispense in sterile screw-capped tubes and cool as slants.
4. Final pH is 6.9 ± 0.1.

See *BBL Manual of Products and Laboratory Procedures*, p. 154.

Converse Liquid Medium (Modified by Levine)

1	M Glucose (MW 180.16)	22.0 ml
1	M Ammonium acetate (MW 77.08)	16.0 ml
1	M Monopotassium phosphate (MW 137.99)	3.75 ml
1	M Dipotassium phosphate (MW 141.96)	3.0 ml
1	M Magnesium sulfate (MW 246.48)	1.6 ml
0.01 M Zinc sulfate (MW 287.54)		1.24 ml
0.01 M Sodium chloride (MW 58.45)		24.0 ml
0.01 M Sodium bicarbonate (MW 84.01)		14.0 ml
0.01 M Calcium chloride (MW 147.03)		2.0 ml
Distilled water, bring to volume		1000 ml

1. Combine ingredients and bring to 1,000-ml volume with distilled water.
2. Dispense 10 ml per screw-capped tube.
3. Autoclave at 120°C at 15 lb pressure for 15 minutes.
4. Final pH is 6.6 at room temperature.

See Converse, pp. 784–792; Levine, Cobb, and Smith, pp. 436–449.

Corn Meal Agar with Tween-80

Powdered corn meal agar (commercially available)	17 g
Distilled water	1,000 ml
Tween-80 (polysorbate 80)	10 ml

1. Add powdered corn meal agar to the distilled water and mix.
2. Heat to boiling with frequent agitation until the medium is completely dissolved.
3. Remove from heat and add 10 ml of Tween-80; mix thoroughly.
4. Deeps: Dispense 15-ml amounts in screw-top tubes.
5. Slants: Dispense 18-ml amounts in screw-top tubes.
6. Sterilize by autoclaving at 121°C (15 lb pressure) for 15 minutes.
7. Allow to solidify at room temperature as deeps. Plates are poured as needed.
8. Final pH is 5.6–6.2 at 25°C (room temperature).

See *Difco Manual,* p. 246; Vera and Dumoff, p. 899.

Corn Meal Agar with Tween-80 and 0.2% Dextrose

Powdered corn meal agar with 0.2% dextrose (Difco)*	17 g
Distilled water	1,000 ml
Tween-80	10 ml

1. Add powdered corn meal agar with 0.2% dextrose to the distilled water and mix.
2. Heat to boiling with frequent agitation until the medium is completely dissolved.
3. Remove from heat and add 10 ml Tween-80; mix thoroughly.
4. Dispense 8-ml amounts in screw-top tubes.
5. Sterilize by autoclaving at 121°C (15 lb pressure) for 15 minutes.
6. Allow to solidify at room temperature as slants.
7. Final pH is 6.2 at 25°C (room temperature).

See *Difco Manual,* p. 246; Vera and Dumoff, p. 899.

Czapek-Dox Agar

Czapek-Dox agar (commercially available)	50 g
Distilled water	1000 ml

*Bacto Corn meal agar with dextrose (Difco) is specified for this formula.

1. Suspend 50 g of dehydrated material in 1000 ml of distilled water and mix thoroughly.
2. Heat with frequent agitation and boil for one minute.
3. Dispense 18 ml into screw-top tubes.
4. Autoclave at 121°C (15 lb pressure) for 15 minutes.
5. Final pH is 7.5.

See *BBL Manual of Products and Laboratory Procedures,* p. 102; *Difco Manual,* p. 245; Vera and Dumoff, p. 899.

Dermatophyte Test Medium (DTM)

Phytone peptone (BBL)	10 g
Dextrose	10 g
Agar	20 g
Distilled water	1,000 ml
Phenol red (0.5% aqueous solution)	40 ml
Cycloheximide	0.5 g
Gentamicin sulfate	100,000 units
Sterile chlortetracycline HCl	100,000 units
0.8M HCl	6 ml

1. Suspend phytone, dextrose, and agar in 100 ml of distilled water and mix thoroughly.
2. Heat to boiling with frequent agitation until all ingredients are completely dissolved; remove from heat.
3. While medium is still hot and with stirring:
   a. Add 40 ml of phenol red (0.5% aqueous solution).
   b. Add 6 ml of 0.8M HCl.
   c. Add cycloheximide (dissolve 0.5 g cycloheximide in 2 ml of acetone before addition).
   d. Add gentamycin sulfate (dissolve gentamycin in a 2 ml aliquot of distilled water prior to addition).
4. Sterilize by autoclaving at 118°C (12 lb pressure) for 10 minutes.
5. Cool media to 47° to 50°C in a water bath.
6. Aseptically, dissolve chlortetracycline in 25 ml of sterile distilled water and add to melted medium with stirring.

7. Aseptically, dispense medium in 8 ml aliquots to sterile screw-capped tubes.

8. Allow to solidify in a slant position (deep slants) at room temperature. The medium should be yellow in color.

9. Final pH is 5.5 at room temperature.

See Taplin, Zaias, Rebell et al., pp. 203–214.

Eosin–Methylene Blue Agar with Tetracycline

Eosin-methylene blue (BBL)	37.4 g
Distilled water	1000 ml
Tetracycline	100.0 mgm

1. Suspend 37.4 g of BBL powder in 1 liter of distilled water. Mix until a uniform suspension is made.

2. Heat with frequent agitation and boil for one minute.

3. Autoclave at 121°C (15 lbs pressure) for 15 minutes.

4. Cool to about 45°C, add tetracycline, and agitate gently.

5. Pour plates.

See *BBL Manual of Products and Laboratory Procedures,* p. 117; Walker and Huppert, pp. 551–558.

Erythritol Albumin Agar

Bactocasamino acid	3.0 g
$KgSO_4$	0.1 g
KH_2PO_4	1.8 g
Erythritol	10.0 g
Fresh albumin (egg white)	10.0 ml
Bactoagar	20.0 g
Distilled water	950.0 ml

1. All ingredients, except erythritol and fresh albumin, are mixed and heated until dissolved, autoclaved at 15 lb pressure for 15 minutes, and cooled to 50°C.

2. Preparation of albumin

   Soak eggs in 95% ethyl alcohol for 15 minutes

   Clean hands with alcohol

   Crack eggs with a sterile knife and drain egg white into a sterile blender

   Switch the blender on and then off immediately to make an even consistency of the egg white. (Do not leave blender on any longer or too much froth will be formed)

   Pour egg white into a sterile flask and store at 4°C.
3. Erythritol is dissolved in 50 ml of distilled water.
4. Albumin and erythritol are sterilized by Seitz filtration, added to cooled agar, and carefully mixed.
5. Medium is dispensed into sterile screw-capped tubes and cooled in slanted position.
6. Final pH is 5.4 ± 0.1

See Fischer and Kane, pp. 167-182.

0.4% Gelatin for Differentiation of *Nocardia* and *Streptomyces* Species

Gelatin   4.0 g

Distilled water   1,000 ml
1. Suspend gelatin in water and heat to boiling.
2. Dispense into screw-capped tubes.
3. Autoclave 121°C at 15 lb pressure for 10 minutes.
4. Final pH is 7.0.

See Wolf, Russell, and Shimoda, p. 358.

12% Gelatin for Demonstration of Proteolytic Activity

Heart infusion broth (Difco)   25 g

Gelatin   120 g

Distilled water   1,000 ml

1. Suspend powdered broth and gelatin in distilled water and heat to boiling.
2. Dispense into screw-capped tubes.
3. Autoclave for 10 minutes at 15 lb pressure.
4. Final pH is 7.2-7.4.

See *Difco Manual* pp. 80, 154; Wolf, Russell, and Shimoda, p. 358.

Glucose Yeast Extract Agar

Glucose	10 g
Yeast extract	5 g
Agar	15 g
Distilled water	1,000 ml

1. Suspend ingredients in 1,000 ml distilled water and mix thoroughly.
2. Heat to boiling with frequent agitation until medium is completely dissolved.
3. Dispense in 8-ml amounts into screw-capped tubes.
4. Sterilize by autoclaving at 121°C at 15 lb pressure for 15 minutes.
5. Cool to room temperature in slanted position.
6. Final pH is 6.6 ± 0.2 at room temperature.

See Sun, Huppert, and Vukovich, pp. 186-190.

Hair Penetration Medium

1. Sterilized human hair that has had no chemical treatment (hair from a child less than 5 years of age is recommended).
2. Ten milliliters sterile distilled water in screw-top tube.
3. One drop of sterile 10% yeast extract.

Ingredients are combined in screw-top tube or in sterile Petri dish at time of use.
See Ajello and Georg, pp. 3-17.

380   Doing It

5% Hog Gastric Mucin

1. Put 5 g of gastric mucin in 95 ml distilled water; emulsify with a Waring blender for 5 minutes.
2. Autoclave for 15 minutes at 120°C; cool.
3. Adjust pH to 7.3 with NaOH (sterile).
4. Check for sterility and store in refrigerator.
5. Use equal parts of the gastric mucin and the fungus suspension and inject the mixture (1 ml) intraperitoneally into the laboratory animal.

See Beneke and Rogers, p. 49.

Inhibitory Mold Agar
(Enriched Fungus Isolation Medium with Chloramphenicol)

Inhibitory mold agar (BBL)   36 g
Distilled water   1,000 ml

1. Suspend 36 g of powdered inhibitory mold agar in 1,000 ml of distilled water. Mix and let stand at room temperature for five minutes.
2. Heat to boiling with frequent agitation until the medium is completely dissolved.
3. Slants.
    a. Dispense, while hot, 8 ml in screw-top tubes.
    b. Sterilize by autoclaving at 121°C (15 lb pressure) for 15 minutes.
    c. Cool to room temperature in a slanted position (deep slants).
4. Final pH is 6.7 at room temperature.

See *BBL Manual of Products and Laboratory Procedures*, p. 114.

Ionagar #2

Ionagar #2*   10 g
Distilled water 1,000 ml

*Ionagar is obtained from the Oxoid Company, 145 Bentley Avenue, Ottawa, Ontario X2E 677, Canada; telephone number: (613) 226–1318. Substitutions are not recommended.

1. 10 g of Ionagar* is added to 1,000 ml distilled water.
2. Soak for 15 minutes.
3. Dissolve agar by placing in boiling water bath or by flowing steam.
4. Dispense 10 ml per screw-capped tube.
5. Sterilize by autoclaving for 15 minutes at 15 lb pressure, 121°C.
6. Cool as slants.

See *Oxoid Manual,* p. 55.

Löeffler's Serum

Löeffler medium powder (BBL or Difco)	80 g
Distilled water 45°C	1,000 ml

1. Powder is added gradually with mixing to flask of warmed distilled water.
2. Uniform suspension is added to screw-capped tubes.
3. Medium is coagulated and sterilized by inspissation (see references below).
4. Final pH 7.2 ± 0.1.

See *BBL Manual of Products and Laboratory Procedures,* p. 118, *Difco Manual,* pp. 128, 339.

Middlebrook and Cohn 7 H 10 Agar (Oleic Acid Albumin Agar)

Middlebrook and Cohn 7 H 10 agar (BBL)	18 g
Distilled water	900 ml
Glycerol	5 ml
BBL 11886 Middlebrook O A D C enrichment	100 ml

1. Five milliliters of glycerol is added to 900 ml of distilled water.
2. Powdered Middlebrook and Cohn 7 H 10 agar base is added to water and glycerol.
3. Mixture is gently swirled to make a uniform suspension. Do not boil.
4. Suspension is divided into five 180-ml amounts and autoclaved at 121°C, 15 lb pressure for 15 minutes.
5. Cool to 50°C.

6. 20 ml of BBL 11886 Middlebrook O A D C enrichment is added to each 180 ml of cooled agar and swirled gently to mix.

7. Agar is dispensed into sterile tubes for slants or into sterile Petri dishes.

8. Final pH is 6.6 ± 0.1.

See *BBL Manual of Preducts and Laboratory Procedures,* p. 124.

Mycosel Agar or Mycobiotic Agar
(Fungus Selection Agar With Cycloheximide And Chloramphenicol)

Mycosel agar (BBL), or Mycobiotic agar (Difco)   36 g

Distilled water   1,000 ml

1. Suspend 36 g of powdered mycosel or mycobiotic agar in 1,000 ml of distilled water and mix thoroughly. Let stand at room temperature for five minutes.

2. When suspension is uniform, heat to boiling with frequent agitation until medium is completely dissolved. Do not overheat.

3. Slants
   a. Dispense 8 ml in screw-capped tubes
   b. Sterilize by autoclaving at 118°C (12 lb pressure) for 15 minutes
   c. Cool to room temperature in a slanted position.

4. Petri dishes
   a. Sterilize by autoclaving at 118°C (12 lb pressure) for 15 minutes
   b. Dispense 36 ml in sterile Petri dishes.

5. Final pH is 6.9 at room temperature.

See *BBL Manual of Products and Laboratory Proecedures,* p. 128, *Difco Supplementary Literature,* p. 263.

Pharmamedia

Pharmamedia*   2 g

Dextrose   2 g

*Available from Trader's Protein Division, P.O. Box 1837, Fort Worth, Texas.

Agar   2 g
Distilled water   100 ml

1. Mix thoroughly.
2. Heat to boiling.
3. Dispense into screw-top tubes.
4. Autoclave at 120°C at 15 lb pressure for 15 minutes.
5. Cool in slanted position.
6. pH 6.5-7.0.

See Dolan and Roberts, p. 144; Weeks, p. 153-156.

Potato Dextrose Agar (PML)

Diced potatoes (avoid new potatoes)   333 g
Deionized H_2O 1,000 ml
Dextrose   25 g
Agar   20 g

1. Wash potato with the peel; dice finely.
2. Boil potatoes gently for 30 minutes.
3. Strain through cheese cloth, squeezing out all liquid.
4. Bring volume up to 1,000 ml.
5. Add dextrose and agar; heat to dissolve.
6. Slants
   a. Dispense 8 ml in screw-capped tubes
   b. Autoclave at 121°C, 15 lb pressure, for 15 minutes
   c. Cool in slanted position.
7. Pour tubes
   a. Dispense 18 ml in screw-capped tubes
   b. Autoclave at 121°C, 15 lb pressure, for 15 minutes.
8. Final pH is 5.6 ± 0.1.

See *American Type Culture Collection Catalogue*, p. 180.

Rice (Boiled) for Identification of *Microsporum Audouini*

Rice grains, white, unenriched, uncooked   about 20 grains
Tap water   5 ml

1. To 5 ml of tap water in a screw-capped tube, add about 20 grains of white rice (uncooked). Make as many tubes as desired.
2. Sterilize by autoclaving at 121°C, 15 lb pressure, for 15 minutes.
3. Cool to room temperature.

See Conant et al., p. 416.

Sabouraud Agar (Emmons Modification, pH 6.9)

Sabouraud dextrose agar Emmons (BBL)   47 g
Distilled water   1,000 ml

1. Suspend 47 g of powdered medium in 1,000 ml of distilled water and mix thoroughly to give a uniform suspension.
2. Heat to boiling with frequent agitation until medium is completely dissolved.
3. Slants
   a. Dispense 8 ml in screw-capped tubes
   b. Sterilize by autoclaving at 121°C, 15 lb pressure, for 15 minutes
   c. Cool to room temperature in a slanted position.
4. Petri dishes
   a. Sterilize by autoclaving at 121°C, 15 lb pressure, for 15 minutes
   b. Dispense 36 ml in sterile Petri dishes.
5. Final pH is 6.5-7.0 at room temperature.

See *BBL Manual of Products and Laboratory Procedures,* p. 135; Emmons et al., p. 535.

Sabouraud Broth

Sabouraud liquid broth powder (BBL)   30 g
Distilled water   1,000 ml

1. Suspend the powdered Sabouraud broth in distilled water.
2. Mix thoroughly until medium is completely dissolved.
3. Adjust pH to 5.7 at room temperature if necessary.
4. Dispense 7.5 ml aliquots in screw-capped tubes.
5. Sterilize by autoclaving at 121°C, 15 lb pressure, for 15 minutes. Do not overheat.
6. Final pH is 5.7 at room temperature.

See *BBL Manual of Products and Laboratory Procedures,* p. 135.

Sabouraud Dextrose Agar (pH 5.6)

Sabouraud dextrose agar (BBL or Difco)   65 g
Distilled water   1,000 ml

1. Suspend 65 g of powdered medium in 1,000 ml of distilled water and mix thoroughly to give a uniform suspension.
2. Heat to boiling with frequent agitation until medium is completely dissolved.
3. Slants
   a. Dispense 8 ml in screw-capped tubes
   b. Sterilize by autoclaving at 121°C, 15 lb pressure, for 15 minutes
   c. Cool to room temperature in slanted position.
4. Petri dishes
   a. Sterilize by autoclaving at 121°C, 15 lb pressure, for 15 minutes
   b. Dispense 36 to 40 ml in sterile Petri dishes.
5. Final pH 5.6 at room temperature.

See *BBL Manual of Products and Laboratory Procedures,* p. 135; *Difco Manual,* p. 238.

Seed Agar (Staib's Medium, Niger Seed Agar)

Pulverized *Guizotia abyssinica* seed*	50 g
Dextrose	1 g
KH_2PO_4	1 g
Creatinine	1 g
Agar	15 g
Chloramphenicol	1 g
Distilled water	1000 ml

1. Add the seed to about 100 ml of distilled water and pulverize in a blender.
2. Add this to approximately 1,000 ml of distilled water and boil for one hour.
3. Strain through cheese cloth and add enough distilled water to the extract to make 1,000 ml.
4. Add the remaining ingredients and boil until dissolved.
5. Dispense 18 ml into screw-top tubes.
6. Autoclave at 121°C, 15 lb pressure, for 15 minutes.
7. pH is 6.5.

See Dolan and Roberts, p. 469.

Simplified Seed Agar Medium†

Guizotia abysinica seed	50 g
Agar	15 g
Distilled water	1000 ml
Chloramphenicol	50 mg

1. Pulverize *G. abysinica* seed in electric mixer. Boil for 25 to 30 minutes in 1,000 ml of water. Filter through gauze and filter paper.
2. Add 15 g of agar. Make up volume to one liter with distilled water.

*The seed is available from The Philadelphia Seed Company, P.O. Box 230, Plymouth Meeting, PA 19462 in 1-lb, 2-lb, 5-lb, and 10-lb lots.
†Preliminary tests using this simplified formula have been satisfactory in our Laboratory.

3. Autoclave 110°C for 25 minutes.
4. Cool to 50°C. Add chloramphenicol that has been dissolved in 10 ml of absolute alcohol.

See Paliwal and Randhawa, p. 346.

Sterile Distilled Water for Preservation of Stock Cultures

Distilled water

1. Dispense distilled water (10 ml) into screw-top tubes.
2. Autoclave at 15 lb pressure, 121°C for 15 minutes.

See Castellani, pp. 147–206.

Trichophyton Agar (Numbers 1–7)

Trichophyton agar (desired number − Difco)   59 g
Distilled water   1,000 ml

1. Suspend desired Trichophyton agar medium in 1,000 ml distilled water and mix thoroughly.
2. Heat to boiling with frequent agitation until medium is completely dissolved.
3. Dispense in 8 ml amounts in *chemically clean* screw-capped tubes.
4. Sterilize by autoclaving at 121°C, 15 lbs pressure, for 12 minutes.
5. Cool to room temperature in a slanted position (deep slants).

Difco Trichophyton agar 1 (no vitamins):

Casamino acids, vitamin free	2.5 g
Dextrose	40.0 g
Monopotassium phosphate	1.8 g
Magnesium sulfate	0.1 g
Agar	15.0 g

Difco Trichophyton agar 2: Trichophyton agar 1 with 50 mg inositol.

Difco Trichophyton agar 3: Trichophyton agar 1 with 50 mg inositol and 200 μg thiamine.

Difco Trichophyton agar 4: Trichophyton agar 1 with 200 μg thiamine.

Difco Trichophyton agar 5: Trichophyton agar 1 with 2 mg nicotinic acid.

Difco Trichophyton agar 6: (no vitamins)

Ammonium nitrate	1.5 g
Dextrose	40.0 g
Magnesium sulfate	0.1 g
Monopotassium phosphate	1.8 g
Agar	15.0 g

Difco Trichophyton agar 7: Trichophyton agar 6 with 30 mg histidine HCl.

See *Difco Supplemental Literature,* pp. 76–77; Georg and Camp, p. 113.

Tyrosine Agar

Nutrient agar	23 g
Tyrosine	5 g
Distilled water	1,000 ml

1. Nutrient agar:
   a. Add 900 ml distilled water to the nutrient agar and mix
   b. Apply heat and swirl frequently until the agar is completely dissolved
   c. Cool to 55°C.
2. Tyrosine:
   a. Add the tyrosine to 100 ml distilled water and mix
   b. Be sure water is at room temperature or hotter.
3. Complete medium:
   a. To the nutrient agar at 55°C, add the tyrosine suspension and mix
   b. Be sure the tyrosine crystals are evenly distributed
   c. Dispense 18 ml per screw-capped tube
   d. Sterilize by autoclaving at 121°C, 15 lb pressure, for 15 minutes
   e. Cool to room temperature in a butt.
4. Final pH 7.0 ± 0.1.

See *Vera and Dumoff,* p. 923.

Urea Dextrose Agar

AGAR

Agar   15 g
Distilled water   900 ml

1. Suspend 15 g of agar in 900 ml of distilled water.
2. Heat to boiling with frequent agitation until agar is completely dissolved.
3. Sterilize by autoclaving at 121°C, 15 lb pressure, for 15 minutes.
4. Cool to 50° to 55°C in a water bath.

BASAL MEDIUM

Urea agar base (Difco)   29 g
Dextrose   4 g
Distilled water   100 ml

1. Suspend 29 g of urea agar base in 100 ml of distilled water.
2. Mix thoroughly until medium is completely dissolved.
3. Add 4 g of dextrose and mix thoroughly until dissolved.
4. Sterilize by filtration (Millipore).

COMPLETE MEDIUM

1. To 900 ml of sterile melted agar at 50° to 55°C, aseptically add 100 ml of the filter sterilized basal medium.
2. Mix thoroughly.
3. Aseptically, dispense 8 ml per sterile screw-capped tube.
4. Cool to room temperature, in a slanted position.
5. Final pH is 6.5-6.8.

See *Difco Supplemental Literature,* p. 428; Philpot, p. 189.

Xanthine Agar

Nutrient agar   23 g
Xanthine   4 g
Distilled water   1,000 ml

NUTRIENT AGAR

a. Add 900 ml distilled water to the nutrient agar and mix.
b. Apply heat and swirl frequently until the agar is completely dissolved.
c. Cool to 55°C.

XANTHINE

a. Add the xanthine to 100 ml distilled water.
b. Mix to distribute the crystals evenly.
c. Be sure the water is at room temperature or hotter.

COMPLETE MEDIUM

a. To the nutrient agar at 55°C, add the xanthine suspension.
b. Mix until the crystals are evenly distributed.
c. Dispense 18 ml per screw-capped tube.
d. Sterilize by autoclaving at 121°C, 15 lb pressure, for 15 minutes.
e. Cool to room temperature in a butt.
f. pH 7.0 ± 0.1.

See Vera and Dumoff, p. 923.

Yeast Extract Phosphate Medium with Ammonia
for *Histoplasma capsulatum* and *Blastomyces dermatitidis* Isolation from Contaminated Specimens

Yeast extract (Difco)	1.0 g
Phosphate buffer	2.0 ml
Bactoagar	20.0 g
Chloramphenicol	0.5 g
Distilled water	1,000.0 ml

1. Suspend ingredients in distilled water and mix thoroughly.
2. Heat to boiling with frequent agitation.
3. Dispense 18 ml in screw-top tubes.
4. Sterilize by autoclaving at 121°C, 15 lb pressure, for 15 minutes.
5. Final pH 6.0 at room temperature.

PHOSPHATE BUFFER PREPARATION

1. Dissolve 40 g Na_2HPO_4 in 300 ml distilled water.
2. Add 60 g KH_2PO_4.
3. Adjust pH to 6.0 with HCl or NaOH if necessary.
4. Adjust volume to 400 ml.

USE WITH AMMONIA

1. Two tubes (36 ml) are poured in sterile Petri dishes at time of use.
2. Specimens are inoculated onto medium by spreading 0.5 to 1.0 ml on surface of medium.
3. Immediately after inoculation, one drop (approximately 0.5 ml) of concentrated NH_4OH (ammonia) is dropped (off center) onto agar surface, and allowed to diffuse, without being spread. (Higher concentrations of ammonia will inhibit pathogenic fungi.)

See Smith and Goodman, p. 63; UOHSC Microbiology Division Procedure No. 330d-30.

QUALITY CONTROL

A good quality control program is essential in a well run clinical laboratory. The following suggested tests are based on those in use at the University of Oregon Health Sciences Center.

Instrument and Appliance Quality Control

Laminar safety hoods are regularly inspected and regulated by the company that produces the hood.

Microscopes are kept covered when not in use and are regularly cleaned and centered.

Daily temperature records are kept for all refrigerators, water baths, ovens, and incubators (including room temperature).

Scales are calibrated for correct weights.

Reagent Quality Control Tests

10% KOH (Potassium hydroxide): Fungal elements in sputum are observed for clarity.

KOH-DMSO: Fungal elements in skin scales are observed for clarity.

India ink: A wet mount of culture or specimen demonstrating capsules of *Cr. neoformans* is observed.

Methenamine silver nitrate, periodic acid-Schiff, and Giemsa stains: A slide demonstrating fungal elements in sputum, biopsy tissue, or other clinical specimen is included each time stain is performed.

Lactophenol cotton blue: Fungal structures from a mold culture are observed for clarity.

Modified acid-fast stain: A slide demonstrating a positive reaction (*N. asteroides*) and a negative reaction (*Streptomyces* sp.) is included each time test is performed.

Nitrate-Zephiran, treated swabs: A positive control (*Cr. albidus*) and a negative control (*Cr. neoformans*) is included each time the test is performed. For testing red yeasts, the positive control is *Rhodotorula glutinis* and the negative control is *R. rubra*.

Mayer's mucicarmine stain: A slide demonstrating capsules of *Cr. neoformans* is included each time stain is performed.

Swartz-Medrek stain: Fungal elements in thin skin scales are observed.

SUGGESTIONS FOR MAINTAINING POSITIVE
CONTROL MATERIAL FOR QUALITY
CONTROL OF REAGENTS.

Sputum with fungal elements: Formalin may be added to a sputum specimen containing fungal elements. This may be stored indefinitely at $4°C$ in a tightly closed screw-capped container.

Skin scales with fungal elements: Scrapings of skin scales with fungal hyphae are stored in a dry clean container at room temperature.

Slides demonstrating fungal elements in clinical specimens. A collection of extra heat-fixed slides or slides with sections of paraffin-embedded tissue containing fungal elements is kept in good supply.

Modified acid-fast stain: Heat-fixed smears are made from fresh (3 to 7-day cultures) of *N. asteroides* and *Streptomyces* sp.

Cr. neoformans capsules: Capsules are enhanced in culture by successive subcultures on enriched agar at 37°C. These may be maintained indefinitely in suspension in sterile distilled water, to which formalin has been added, in a tightly capped container.

Media Quality Control Tests

Media are inoculated and incubated in the manner given in procedures in Chapter 4. A sterility test is included for each medium. The pH is checked, as given in formulae for each medium.

Ascospore agar: Ascospores are produced by *S. cerevisiae.*

Biphasic medium for blood cultures: *C. albicans,* suspended in 4 ml of blood, grows within two days.

Brain-heart infusion agar: *H. capsulatum* or *B. dermatitidis* grow within one week at 35° to 37°C.

Brain-heart infusion agar with sheep blood: The yeast phase of *H. capsulatum* grows within four weeks.

Bromcresol green agar: *C. albicans* colonies are pale. *Staphylococcus* (coagulase positive) is inhibited.

Caffeic acid agar medium: *Cr. neoformans* colonies are brown.

Staphylococcus (coagulase positive) is inhibited.

Carbohydrate assimilation media for yeasts (Wickerham tubes and auxanographic plates):

Dextrose:	*Tr. cutaneum* grows in three days
Galactose:	*Tr. cutaneum* grows in three days
	T. glabrata does not grow in three days
Inositol:	*Cr. neoformans* grows in seven days
	Rhodotorula species do not grow in seven days
Lactose	
Maltose	*Tr. cutaneum* grows in three days
Raffinose	*T. glabrata* does not grow in three days
Sucrose	
Trehalose:	*T. glabrata* grows in three days
	C. krusei does not grow in three days

Xylose: *Tr. cutaneum* grows in three days

                T. glabrata does not grow in three days

YNB control: *Tr. cutaneum* does not grow in three days.

Carbohydrate fermentation broth:

Dextrose: *C. tropicalis* produces acid and gas within one week

Lactose: *C. pseudotropicalis* produces acid and gas within three weeks

               T. glabrata does not produce acid and gas within three weeks

Maltose ⎫ *C. tropicalis* produces acid and gas within three weeks

Sucrose ⎭ *T. glabrata* does not produce acid or gas within three weeks

Casein agar: *N. brasiliensis* hydrolyzes casein.

Christensen's urea agar: *Cr. neoformans* produces a deep magenta color in medium within three days.

Converse liquid medium, modified: *C. immitis* spherules are produced.

Corn meal agar with Tween-80: *C. albicans* produces hyphae and blastoconidia within three days.

Corn meal agar with Tween-80 and 0.2% dextrose: *T. rubrum* colony develops a deep red color within one month. *T. mentagrophytes* colony does not develop red color.

Czapek-Dox agar. *A. fumigatus* colony is blue-green within one week.

                N. asteroides colony is orange with chalky surface within one week.

                Streptomyces species produce chains of tiny spores within three weeks.

Dermatophyte Test Medium (DTM):

T. rubrum (or other dermatophyte) produces red color change in medium in one week.

C. albicans grows but does not produce a color change in medium.

T. glabrata does not grow in one week (inhibition by cycloheximide).

Staphylococcus (coagulase positive) does not grow within one week (inhibition by tetracycline).

Escherichia coli, or *Pseudomonas* sp. does not grow in one week (inhibition by gentamicin).

Eosin–methylene blue agar with tetracycline:

Fresh *C. albicans* isolate produces hyphae and blastoconidia within 24 hours.

Staphylococcus (coagulase positive) is inhibited.

Erythritol albumen agar:

T. rubrum colony develops a deep red reverse color within one month.

T. mentagrophytes colony does not develop a deep red color.

12% gelatin: *Cladosporium* (common species) liquefies gelatin within three weeks.

0.4% gelatin: *N. brasiliensis* grows at 35° to 37°C in 10 days.

Glucose yeast extract agar: *C. immitis* arthroconidia are produced within two weeks.

Hair penetration medium:

  T. mentagrophytes produces wedge-shaped penetrating holes within four weeks.

  T. rubrum does not penetrate hair.

5% hog gastric mucin: See procedure for animal inoculation.

Inhibitory mold agar:

  H. capsulatum grows within one week.

  Staphylococcus (coagulase positive) is inhibited at one week.

Ionagar #2: See procedure for conversion of Arthroconidium form to spherule form of *C. immitis.*

Löeffler's serum: *Cladosporium* (common species) liquefies slant within three weeks.

Middlebrook and Cohn 7 H 10 agar: *N. asteroides* grows well.

Mycobiotic agar (Difco), Mycosel agar (BBL):

  C. albicans grows well in three days.

  T. glabrata is inhibited in three days by cycloheximide.

  Staphylococcus (coagulase positive) is inhibited in three days by chloramphenicol.

Pharmamedia: *B. dermatitidis* is produced in yeast form within three weeks at 35° to 37°C.

Potato dextrose agar: *T. rubrum* microconidia are produced within one week.

Rice (boiled) for identification of *M. audouini:*

  M. audouini grows poorly or not at all in two weeks.

  M. canis grows well in two weeks.

Sabouraud agar (Emmons modification): *M. audouini* grows well.

Sabouraud broth:

  C. tropicalis produces a narrow film and gas in three days.

  C. krusei produces a wide surface film and gas in three days.

  C. albicans produces no surface growth.

Sabouraud dextrose agar:

  C. albicans grows well in three days.

  Staphylococcus (coagulase positive) growth is retarded in three days compared with growth on Sabouraud agar (Emmons modification).

Seed agar (Staib's medium, Nigerseed agar):

   Cr. neoformans colonies are brown in three days.

   Staphylococcus (coagulase positive) is inhibited in three days.

Trichophyton agar #1 (casein agar):

   T. mentagrophytes grows within two weeks

   T. equinum does not grow within two weeks

Trichophyton agar #2 (casein agar with inositol):

   T. mentagrophytes grows within two weeks

   T. equinum does not grow within two weeks

Trichophyton agar #3 (casein agar with inositol and thiamine):

   T. verrucosum grows within four weeks

   T. equinum does not grow within four weeks

Trichophyton agar #4 (casein agar with thiamine):

   T. tonsurans grows in two weeks

   T. equinum will not grow in two weeks

Trichophyton agar #5 (casein agar with nicotinic acid):

   T. equinum will grow within four weeks.

   T. verrucosum will not grow within four weeks.

Trichophyton agar #6 (ammonium nitrate agar):

   M. gallinae grows within two weeks

   T. megnini will not grow within two weeks

Trichophyton agar #7 (ammonium nitrate agar with histidine):

   T. megnini grows within two weeks

   T. soudanense will not grow within two weeks

Tyrosine agar: *N. brasiliensis* hydrolyzes tyrosine.

Urea dextrose agar:

   T. mentagrophytes produces a deep magenta color in medium within four days

   T. rubrum does not produce a color change in medium within four days (granular strains of *T. rubrum* may produce a pink color in four days)

Xanthine agar: *N. caviae* hydrolyzes casein.

Yeast extract phosphate agar with ammonia added (see directions for formula preparation):

   H. capsulatum grows in two weeks

   C. albicans is inhibited

Internal Quality Control

Laboratory procedures and the proficiency of laboratory workers are tested regularly, usually once a month, with an "unknown" fungal isolate. These isolates may be chosen from the cultures maintained for quality control, from clinical isolates, or from a teaching culture collection.

Self-evaluation and review questions are helpful, particularly for a technologist newly assigned to work in a mycology unit. Suggested review questions will be found at the end of this section.

MAINTENANCE OF STOCK CULTURE COLLECTION

A minimal stock culture collection for quality control of media will be maintained. In addition, it is usually wise to maintain interesting isolates that may be needed for further studies. Teaching laboratories will make a particular effort to collect several strains of each of the primary pathogens as well as those that are isolated as opportunists.

Quality Control Cultures

Fresh isolates of proven identity are preferable to old stock strains of yeasts or molds for quality control tests. These are labeled with the name of the isolate and the identifying laboratory number. They may be maintained in the following manner.

YEASTS

A barely turbid suspension is made in sterile distilled water from a three-day colony (on noncycloheximide medium) of the yeasts listed below. These suspensions are stored in sterile screw-capped containers for no longer than one year and may be used directly for quality control tests.

C. albicans	*Cr. neoformans*
C. krusei	*Rh. glutinis*
C. pseudotropicalis	*Rh. rubra*
C. tropicalis	*Sa. cerevisiae*
Cr. albidus, var.	*T. glabrata*
albidus	*T. cutaneum*

MOLDS

Storage Cultures on Distilled Water

The easiest, most effective and efficient way to maintain mold isolates indefinitely is on sterile distilled water. A pure culture is grown, usually on potato dextrose agar slant subcultured from original isolate. (Successive subcultures tend to produce sterile mutant strains.) When the culture is producing good colony growth with typical spore production, several milliliters of sterile distilled water are pipetted from a sterile screw-capped tube over the surface of the slant. The surface is gently scraped with the pipette or a sharp sterile blade to make a suspension of broken mycelium and spores in the water. This suspension is transferred back to the original tube of distilled water. The screw cap is tightly closed, sealed, and labeled with the name of the isolate and identifying laboratory number and date. Cultures are revived by pipetting one or two milliliters of suspension onto an agar slant. Distilled water cultures will usually remain viable for several years. Ideally these cultures are revived every two years and a fresh distilled water suspension is made from a typical sporulating colony.

Quality Control Cultures on Agar Slants

Stock cultures of molds are subcultured regularly to a fresh Sabouraud (Emmons modification) agar slant. *Cladosporium* (common species), *F. pedrosoi* and *M. gallinae* are subcultured at least once a month. When a culture mutates or dies, a fresh culture is obtained from the distilled water collection.

The following molds and actinomycetes are maintained for quality control tests:

A. fumigatus	*N. caviae*
B. dermatitidis	*S. schenckii*
Cladosporium (common species)	*Streptomyces* sp.
F. pedrosoi	*T. equinum*
H. capsulatum	*T. megnini*
M. canis	*T. mentagrophytes*
M. audouini	*T. rubrum*
M. gallinae	*T. tonsurans*
N. asteroides	*T. verrucosum*
N. brasiliensis	

BACTERIA

Stock cultures of *Staphylococcus* (coagulase positive) and *E. coli* or *Ps. aeruginosa* are subcultured to a brain-heart infusion agar slant every three months and at each time of use. Tubes are labeled with the name of organism, the date of inoculation, and identifying laboratory number.

CLINICAL FUNGAL ISOLATES

Yeast and mold clinical isolates are maintained in pure culture for at least one month after identification report has been made to physician. Significant isolates may be stored indefinitely in distilled water cultures in the manner described above.

MAINTENANCE OF TEACHING COLLECTION OF FUNGI

The maintenance of a large collection of fungi in working form with typical colony and microscopic morphologic characteristics, is a luxury that most laboratories cannot afford. Fungal strains "in captivity" will need to be coaxed by several means to produce characteristic morphologic features. Often they will simply mutate or die on repeated subcultures. A teaching laboratory will usually maintain many strains on distilled water and, in addition, will keep a working collection ready for demonstration. Haley and Callaway share with us their system for keeping good teaching cultures always ready for demonstration of typical gross and microscopic morphologic characteristics. Fungal subcultures are rotated on a battery of media tailored for each fungal strain. (See Haley and Callaway, p. 201, Table 1.)

The following system, in use at the University of Oregon Health Sciences Center, is suggested for laboratories with limited time available. Sabouraud agar (Emmons modification) is used. The teaching strains have been divided into three groups: (*1*) those subcultured every two weeks; (*2*) those subcultured every month; and (*3*) those subcultured at least every six months. Typical gross colonies are usually maintained in this way. For good sporulating strains, it is often necessary to revive a distilled water culture on potato dextrose agar.

The following list is given as a guide. Individual strains will vary, and this list should be revised as necessary.

Subcultures Made Every Two Weeks

Alternaria sp.
Aureobasidium pullulans
Neurospora sp.

Subcultures Made Every Four Weeks

Acremonium sp.
Aspergillus (*fumigatus* group)

Cladosporium sp. (common species)
Curvularia sp.

Drechslera sp.

Epicoccum sp.
Epidermophyton floccosum
Exophiala jeanselmei
Exophiala werneckii

Fonsecaea pedrosoi

Microsporum canis
Microsporum cookei
Microsporum distortum

Microsporum ferrugineum
Microsporum gallinae
Microsporum gypseum
Microsporum nanum
Mucor sp.

Nigrospora sp.

Phoma sp.
Phialophora verrucosa
Piedraia hortai

Rhizopus sp.

Sepedonium sp.
Stemphylium sp.
Syncephalastrum sp.

Subcultures Made Every Six Months

Absidia sp.
Actinomadura madurae
Aspergillus (*clavatus* group)
Aspergillus (*flavipes* group)
Aspergillus (*flavus* group)
Aspergillus (*glaucus* group)
Aspergillus (*nidulans* group)
Aspergillus (*niger* group)
Aspergillus (*terreus* group)
Aspergillus (*versicolor* group)

Basidiobolus haptosporus
Blastomyces dermatitidis[a]
Botrytis sp.

Candida albicans
Candida guillermondi
Candida krusei
Candida parapsilosis
Candida pseudotropicalis
Candida stellatoidea
Candida tropicalis
Chaetomium sp.

Chyrosporium keratinophilum
Chrysosporium pannorum
Chrysosporium parvum
Chrysosporium tropicum
Coccidioides immitis[a]
Cryptococcus albidus, var. *albidus*
Cryptococcus laurentii
Cryptococcus neoformans
Cunninghamella sp.

Fusarium sp.

Geotrichum sp.
Gliocladium sp.

Histoplasma capsulatum[a]

Madurella mycetomi
Microsporum audouini
Microsporum vanbreuseghemii

Nocardia asteroides
Nocardia brasiliensis
Nocardia caviae

[a]Major systemic pathogen, to be handled only by experienced workers.

Paracoccidioides brasiliensis[a]
Paecilomyces sp.
Penicillium sp.
Petriellidium boydii

Rhodotorula glutinis
Rhodotorula rubra

Saccharomyces cerevisiae
Scopulariopsis sp.
Sporothrix schenckii
Streptomyces sp.

Torulopsis glabrata
Trichoderma sp.
Trichophyton ajelloi
Trichophyton concentricum
Trichophyton equinum
Trichophyton fischeri

Trichophyton megninii
Trichophyton mentagrophytes
Trichophyton rubrum
Trichophyton schoenleinii
Trichophyton soudanense
Trichophyton terrestre
Trichophyton tonsurans
Trichophyton verrucosum
Trichophyton violaceum
Trichophyton yaoundei
Trichosporon cutaneum
Trichothecium roseum

Ustilago sp.

Verticillium sp.

Wangiella dermatitidis

REVIEW QUESTIONS

These are the kinds of questions that a mycology technologist will be asked. Answers will be found throughout the five chapters of this manual. Many of these are "think" questions. There is not necessarily only one correct answer.

Processing of Specimens

---

1. Describe the techniques for preparation and inoculation of expectorated sputum for fungal isolation.
2. Describe the techniques for processing tissue taken at biopsy for fungal isolation.
3. What is the best method for mailing a specimen taken at bronchoscopy for fungal isolation?
4. When a specimen is submitted with a request to rule out *Nocardia* and *Actinomyces* which media are inoculated?

Media

1. Name the antifungal antibiotic present in Mycosel or Mycobiotic agar.
2. Which significant fungi are inhibited by this antibiotic?
3. Which medium promotes optimal growth of *Histoplasma capsulatum*?
4. Which antibiotic is present in inhibitory mold agar (IMA)?
5. Why is Mycosel or Mycobiotic agar superior to IMA for the isolation of dermatophytes?

Microscopic Preparations

1. Describe some fungal elements that may be seen in a KOH preparation.
2. What is the advantage of a methenamine silver nitrate stain over a Gram stain or a KOH preparation?
3. Which kind of specimen for fungal isolation is routinely observed in India ink preparation?
4. What is the purpose of Mayer's mucicarmine stain in mycologic staining?
5. When is it appropriate to do a modified acid-fast stain?

Examination of Cultures

1. How long are cultures incubated for fungal isolation?
2. How often are blood cultures examined?
3. How often are other fungal cultures examined?
4. Why is the isolation of *Candida albicans* from expectorated sputum not usually considered significant?

Identification Procedures

1. What steps are taken when a moist colony grows on fungal media?
2. What are the steps in identifying molds isolated from skin, hair, or nails?

3. When a mold is isolated from any microbiology media, how is the possibility of *Coccidioides immitis* ruled out?
4. Why and when is *Coccidioides immitis* a hazard to laboratory personnel? What precautions are taken in a mycology laboratory to reduce this hazard?
5. Name the dimorphic fungi that are major pathogens and state the microscopic characteristics of each.

Microscopic Preparations

1. What is the purpose of a cover-slip culture?
2. What are the relative merits of KOH-DMSO and of 10% KOH?
3. What ingredients are present in lactophenol cotton blue and what is the purpose of each?

Differential Tests

1. Which tests are useful for yeast identification?
2. Which tests are used for dermatophyte identification?
3. How is dimorphism demonstrated?
4. What is the purpose of potato dextrose agar?
5. Name three uses of corn meal agar.
6. What is the use of Löeffler's serum slants in a mycology laboratory?

General Questions

1. What are the major taxonomic subdivisions?
2. What is meant by *perfect* and *imperfect* fungi?
3. Name a subcutaneous fungal disease and a fungus that causes it.
4. What does *tinea* mean?
5. Name a zoophilic fungus.

6. In what part of the world does blastomycosis occur? Coccidioidomycosis? Histoplasmosis? Cryptococcosis?

7. White mold growth is observed after three days of incubation from the sputum of a patient in Oregon with a history of lung disease. Which of the following is it most likely to be?

Coccidioides immitis

Aspergillus fumigatus

Cryptococcus neoformans

Histoplasma capsulatum

Blastomyces dermatitidis

Trichophyton rubrum

Which would it be if the patient lived in Mississippi? In California? Which of the above is it most unlikely to be?

8. Name at least three predisposing factors for opportunistic fungal disease.

9. What is the difference between a primary pathogenic fungus and an opportunistic fungus?

Yeast Identification

1. What are the distinguishing characteristics, if any, of the following yeasts on eosin–methylene blue agar (EMB) with tetracycline, incubated at 35° to 37°C in 5% to 10% CO_2? On corn meal agar?

Candida albicans

Candida tropicalis

Candida pseudotropicalis

Torulopsis glabrata

Cryptococcus neoformans

2. What is the purpose of seed agar?

3. When is it appropriate to include ascospore agar in a battery of yeast identification media?

4. When there is a mixed culture of two or more kinds of yeast, what is a way to separate the different strains?

5. Name three ways in which *C. albicans* can be identified in a clinical lab.

6. What are the minimal identifying criteria for *Cr. neoformans*?

7. Are assimilation tests aerobic or anaerobic?

Gross Morphologic Characteristics of Fungi

1. Name four black (dematiaceous) fungi.
2. Describe the gross appearance of most *Penicillium* species.
3. What is the characteristic gross morphology of *Histoplasma capsulatum*?
4. Name four fungi that are powdery and tan.
5. What is the distinguishing gross cultural characteristic of *M. canis*?
6. Which yeast is red or orange?
7. What are the colony characteristics of *Mucor* and *Rhizopus* species?
8. Name three waxy fungi.

Basic Structures

1. What is the difference between a hypha and a pseudohypha?
2. Draw a phialide.
3. Name three molds in which phialides are seen.
4. What is a conidiophore? Describe the conidophore of *Aspergillus;* of *Penicillium;* of *Blastomyces dermatitidis.*
5. Name two sexual forms seen in fungi in a medical laboratory.
6. When is a chlamydoconidium significant?
7. How do the conidia of the dermatophytes differ from those of *B. dermatitidis* and *H. capsulatum*?
8. What is an annellide?
9. What is meant by *conidiogenous cell*?

Common Molds

1. What is the difference between *Scopulariopsis* species and *Penicillium* species?
2. What are the identifying microscopic structures of *Cladosporium* species?
3. How are the pathogenic species of *Cladosporium* distinguished from the common species?
4. What are the differences between *Mucor* species and *Rhizopus* species?

5. To what subdivisions do *Mucor* and *Rhizopus* species belong? What class? What order?

6. Name a situation in which the isolation of *Aspergillus fumigatus* is significant?

Superfical Fungi

1. What is the difference between *Trichosporon cutaneum* and *Trichosporon beigelii*?

2. Why was the name *Cladosporium werneckii* changed to *Exophiala werneckii*?

3. What is the causative organism of tinea versicolor? How is it identified?

Dermatophytes

1. What are the identifying criteria of *Epidermophyton floccosum*? Gross colony? Microscopic structures?

2. How is *T. rubrum* identified? What special media may aid in the identification?

3. Describe a positive hair-penetration test.

4. Which media are useful in the identification of *T. verrucosum*? of *T. tonsurans*?

5. How are *Acremonium* species and *Chrysosporium* species distinguished from the dermatophytes?

6. Name a dermatophyte that causes tinea capitis. Is it zoophilic or anthropophilic?

7. Name a dermatophyte, a yeast, and a nondermatophyte that can cause onychomycosis.

8. Which fungi are most often isolated as causative agents of tinea cruris?

9. A slow growing white mold is isolated from a highly inflammatory lesion on the arm of a cattle farmer. What is it likely to be?

Subcutaneous Fungi

1. What are the microscopic characteristics of *Sporothrix schenckii*? Yeast phase? Mold phase?

2. Name the fungi that may cause chromomycosis. In what way are they alike?
3. Define the following:

Mycetoma

Maduromycetoma

Actinomycetoma

4. Name two organisms that may cause maduromycetoma. What is the tissue form of these?
5. Name an organism that may cause actinomycetoma.
6. How is a phaeomycotic cyst different from a lesion of chromomycosis?
7. What three kinds of conidium formation are seen in *Fonsecaea pedrosoi*?
8. Describe the gross colony characteristics of *Petriellidium boydii*.

Systemic Fungi

1. Name three major pathogenic dimorphic systemic fungi seen in the United States and describe the identifying criteria of each.
2. Which common molds are similar to each of these and how are they different from the pathogens that they resemble?
3. Describe the microscopic characteristics of *Coccidioides immitis* in tissue; in culture at 37°C on routine media; in culture at room temperature.
4. What antibiotic is used in the treatment of systemic fungal disease?

Aspergillus Review Questions

1. Which *Aspergillus* species is most commonly isolated as a pathogen?
2. How is *Aspergillus fumigatus* differentiated from *Aspergillus glaucus*?
3. Which group of *Aspergilli* are major toxin producers?
4. What are the identifying criteria of the *Aspergilli* in this group?
5. Which *Aspergillus* species are most often isolated from ear infections?
6. One group of *Aspergilli* that grows as tan to cream-colored colonies is the only group that produces secondary spores. What is the group?
7. Name two groups of *Aspergillus* that have biseriate phialides.

Nocardia and *Actinomyces* Species

1. How are *Streptomyces* species distinguished from *Nocardia* species?
2. Describe the procedure for setting up hydrolysis tests.
3. What distinguishes *N. asteroides* from *N. brasiliensis* on these tests?

Fungal Infections of the Eye

1. Name four opportunistic fungi that may invade the eye by trauma and describe the microscopic characteristics of each.
2. Name four fungi that may disseminate to the eye systemically.

Dematiaceous Fungi

1. Which dematiaceous fungi have budding forms and moist colonies in early culture?
2. How are *Drechslera* species different from *Alternaria* species?
3. Compare the microscopic forms of *Aureobasidium pullulans* with those of *Exophiala werneckii*.

BIBLIOGRAPHY

Ajello L, Georg L: *In vitro* cultures for differentiating between atypical isolates of *Trichophyton mentagrophytes* and *Trichophyton rubrum. Mycopathol Mycol Appl* 8:3, 1957.

American Type Culture Collection, Catalogue of Strains, Winter edition. Rockville, MD, 1970.

BBL Manual of Products and Laboratory Procedures, ed 5, Rohde, PA (ed), Cockeysville, MD: Baltimore Biological Laboratory, Division of Becton, Dickinson and Company, 1968.

Beneke ES, Rogers AL: *Medical Mycology Manual,* ed 3. Minneapolis: Burgess Publishing Co, 1970.

Castellani A: Miscellaneous mycological notes. *Ann NY Acad Sci* 83:147, 1962.

Conant NF, Smith DT, Baker RD, et al: *Manual of Clinical Mycology,* ed 3. Philadelphia: WB Saunders Co, 1971.

Converse JL: Effect of physico-chemical environment on Spherulation of *Coccidioides immitis* in a chemically defined medium. *J Bacteriol* 74:784, 1956.

Difco Manual of Dehydrated Culture Media and Reagents, ed 9. Detroit: Difco Laboratories, 1953.

Difco Supplementary Literature. Detroit: Difco Laboratories, 1972.

Dolan CT, Roberts GD: Mycology, Section III, in Washington JA (ed): *Laboratory Procedures in Clinical Microbiology.* Boston: Little Brown Co, 1974.

Emmons CW, Binford CH, Utz JP, et al: *Medical Mycology,* ed 3. Philadelphia: Lea and Febiger, 1977.

Fischer JB, Kane J: The laboratory diagnosis of dermatophytosis complicated with *Candida albicans. Can J Microbiol* 20:167, 1974.

Georg LK, Camp LB: Routine nutritional tests for the identification of dermatophytes. *J Bacteriol* 74:113, 1957.

Haley LD, Callaway CS: *Laboratory Methods in Medical Mycology.* ed 4. U.S. Department of Health Education and Welfare, HEW Publication No. (CDC) 78–8361, 1978.

Harold W, Snyder M: Scheme for cultural identification of *Candida* species of medical importance. *Difco Technical Information Bulletin* No. 0615, 1969.

Healey ME, Dillavou CL, Taylor GE: Diagnostic medium containing inositol, urea, and caffeic acid for selective growth of *Cryptococcus neoformans. J Clin Microbiol* 6:387, 1977.

Hopkins JM, Land GA: Rapid method for determining nitrate utilization by yeasts. *J Clin Pathol* 5:497, 1977.

Huppert M, Harper G, Sun HS, et al: Rapid methods for identification of yeasts. *J Clin Microbiol* 2(1):21, 1975.

Larsh HW, Goodman NL: Fungi of the systemic mycoses, in Lennette EH, Spaulding EH, Truant JP (eds): *Manual of Clinical Microbiology,* ed 2. Washington, DC: American Society for Microbiology, 1974, p 508.

Levine HB, Cobb JM, Smith CE: Immunity to coccicioidomycosis induced in mice by purified spherule, arthrospore and mycelial vaccines. *Trans NY Acad Sci* 22:436, 1960.

Mahan CT, Sale GE: Rapid methenamine silver stain for *Pneumocystis* and fungi. *Arch Pathol Lab Med* 102:351, 1978.

Oxoid Manual, ed 3. Southwark, London: Oxoid Ltd (reprint 1971).

Paik G, Suggs MT: Reagents, stains and miscellaneous procedures, in Lennette EH, Spaulding EH, Truant JP (eds): *Manual of Clinical Microbiology,* ed 2. Washington DC: American Society for Microbiology, 1974, p 430.

Philpot C: The differentiation of *Trichophyton mentagrophytes* from *Trichophyton rubrum* by a simple urease test. *Sabouraudia* 5(3):189, 1967.

Roberts GD, Washington JA: Detection of fungi in blood cultures. *J Clin Microbiol* 1:309, 1975.

Smith CD, Goodman NL: Improved culture methods for the isolation of *Histoplasma capsula-*

tum and *Blastomyces dermatitidis* from contaminated specimens. *Am J Clin Pathol* 63: 276, 1974.

Sun SH, Huppert M, Vukovich KR: Rapid in vitro conversion and identification of *Coccidioides immitis. J Clin Microbiol* 3(2):186, 1976.

Swartz JH, Medrek TF: Rapid contrast stain as a diagnostic aid in fungous infections. *Arch Derm* 99:494, 1969.

Taplin D, Zaias N, Rebell G, et al: Isolation and recognition of dermatophytes on a new medium (DTM). *Arch Dermatol* 99:203, 1969.

University of Oregon Health Sciences Center, Department of Clinical Pathology, Clinical Microbiology Procedure No 0330d-30, No 0330d-31, 1979.

University of Oregon Health Sciences Center, Department of Clinical Pathology, Clinical Microbiology Procedures: No 330a-46, 1974.

Vera HD, Dumoff M: Media, reagents, and stains, in Lennette EH, Spaulding EH, Truant JP (eds): *Manual of Clinical Microbiology* ed 2. Washington, DC: American Society for Microbiology, 1974, p 881.

Walker I, Huppert M: A rapid, reliable technique for the identification of *Candida albicans. Am J Clin Pathol* 31:551, 1959.

Weeks RJ: A rapid simplified medium for converting the mycelial phase of *Blastomyces dermatitidis* to the yeast phase. *Mycopathol Mycol Appl* 21:153, 1964.

Wolf PL, Russell B, Shimoda A: *Practical Clinical Microbiology and Mycology: Techniques and Interpretation.* New York: John Wiley & Sons, 1975.

Zaias N, Taplin D: Improved preparation for the diagnosis of mycologic diseases. *Arch Dermatol* 93:608, 1966.

Plates

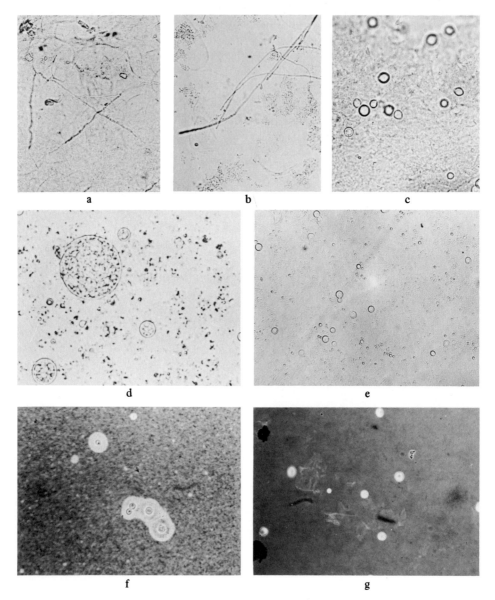

Plate 1. Wet-mount preparations of specimens

a. KOH (potassium hydroxide) preparation. Fungal hyphae in skin scales (high power).

b. KOH (potassium hydroxide) preparation. Hyphae and budding cells in sputum (high power).

c. KOH (potassium hydroxide) preparation. *Scopulariopsis* sp. conidia in nail (high power).

d. KOH (potassium hydroxide) preparation. *Coccidioides immitis*, spherules in sputum (high power).

e. KOH (potassium hydroxide) preparation. *Blastomyces dermatitidis*, budding cells in tissue (low power).

f. India ink preparation, positive. *Cryptococcus neoformans* (high power).

g. India ink preparation, negative. Red blood cells (high power).

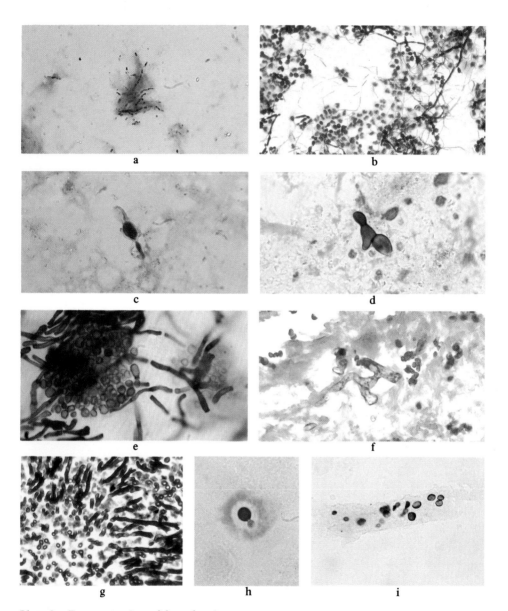

Plate 2. Demonstration of fungal stains

a. Modified acid-fast stain. *Nocardia asteroides* (oil immersion).

b. Gram's stain. Yeast and hyphae in urine (oil immersion).

c. Gram's stain. *Alternaria* sp. in skin scales (oil immersion).

d. Methenamine silver nitrate stain. *Alternaria* sp. in skin scales (oil immersion).

e. Periodic acid-Schiff stain. *Pityrosporum orbiculare* in skin scales (oil immersion).

f. Hematoxylin and eosin stain. *Rhizopus arrhizus* in necrotic tissue (high power).

g. Methenamine silver nitrate stain. *Aspergillus* hyphae in bronchial washings (high power).

h. Methenamine silver nitrate stain. *Cryptococcus neoformans* in mouse tissue (oil immersion).

i. Methenamine silver nitrate stain. *Pneumocystis carinii* in tissue (high power).

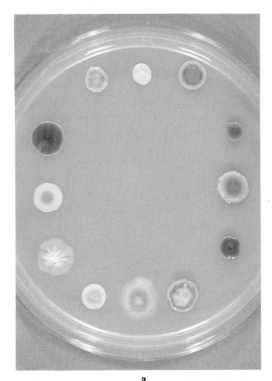

a

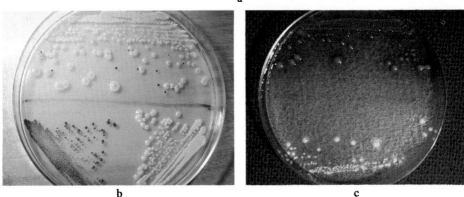

b   c

Plate 3. Media used for yeast differentiation

a. Colonies of yeasts on bromcresol green agar plate (one week at room temperature)
    (clockwise from 1 o'clock position): (1) *Cryptococcus neoformans*, (2) *Rhodotorula*
    sp., (3) *Saccharomyces cerevisiae*, (4) *Torulopsis glabrata*, (5) *Trichosporon cu-
    taneum*, (6) *Candida krusei*, (7) *Candida parapsilosis*, (8) *Candida tropicalis*, (9)
    Candida guillermondii, (10) *Candida pseudotropicalis*, (11) *Candida stellatoidea*,
    (12) *Candida albicans*. (Photo by Jim Phillips.)

b. Separation of yeast colonies on bromcresol green agar plate: *top:* mixed culture of
    Candida albicans and *Torulopsis glabrata*, *bottom left:* pure culture of *Torulopsis
    glabrata*, *bottom right:* pure culture of *Candida albicans*. (Photo by Phoebe Rich.)

c. Seed agar (Staib's medium) used for *Cryptococcus neoformans* identification: *top:*
    Cryptococcus neoformans (brown colonies), *bottom: Candida albicans* (white colo-
    nies). (Photo by Phoebe Rich.)

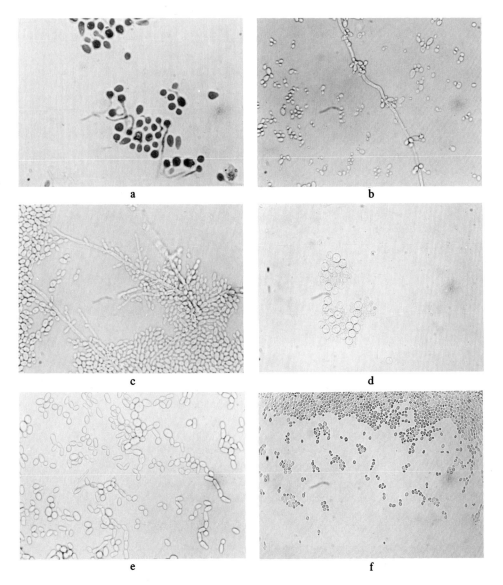

Plate 4. Yeast morphology on eosin methylene blue agar plate
(Plates are incubated in 10% CO_2 in a 37°C incubator.)

a. EMB: positive, 3 hours.
    Candida albicans; germ tubes (oil immersion).
b. EMB: positive, 24 hours.
    Candida albicans; hyphae and budding cells (high power).
c. EMB: negative, 24 hours.
    Candida tropicalis; pseudohyphae and budding cells (high power).
d. EMB: negative, 24 hours.
    Cryptococcus neoformans; budding cells only (high power).
e. EMB: negative, 24 hours.
    Trichosporon cutaneum; arthroconidia, budding cells and hyphae (high power).
f. EMB: negative, 24 hours.
    Torulopsis glabrata; budding cells only (high power).

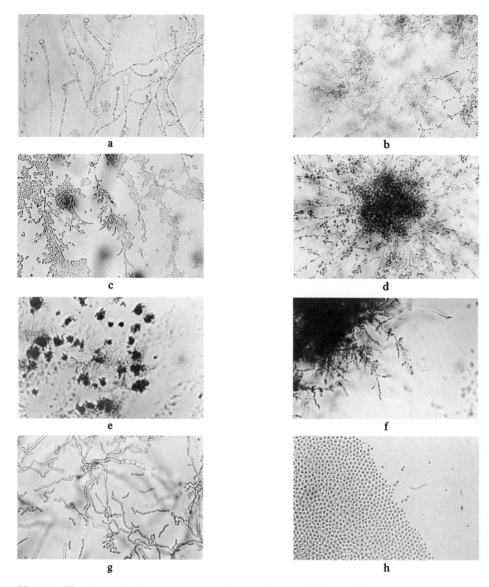

Plate 5. Yeast morphology on corn meal agar plate with Tween-80

a. *Candida albicans:* hyphae, chlamydospores, and groups of budding cells (low power).
b. *Candida parapsilosis:* hyphae and budding cells in small splattered colonies (low power).
c. *Candida pseudotropicalis:* hyphae and slender budding cells (low power).
d. *Candida tropicalis:* long hyphae and single budding cells in large stringy colonies (low power).
e. *Candida guillermondii:* hyphae and small budding cells compactly arranged (low power).
f. *Candida krusei:* hyphae and slender budding cells in parallel formation (low power).
g. *Trichosporon cutaneum:* hyphae, arthroconidia, and budding cells (low power).
h. *Cryptococcus neoformans:* budding cells only, showing "glass bead" effect (low power).

Index